Adult CCRN Certification Review

Ann J. Brorsen, RN, MSN, PHN, CCRN, CEN
Menifee, California

Keri R. Rogelet, RN, MSN, MBA/HCM, CCRN
Menifee, California

JONES AND BARTLETT PUBLISHERS
Sudbury, Massachusetts
BOSTON   TORONTO   LONDON   SINGAPORE

World Headquarters

Jones and Bartlett Publishers	Jones and Bartlett Publishers Canada	Jones and Bartlett Publishers International
40 Tall Pine Drive	6339 Ormindale Way	Barb House, Barb Mews
Sudbury, MA 01776	Mississauga, Ontario L5V 1J2	London W6 7PA
978-443-5000	Canada	United Kingdom
info@jbpub.com		
www.jbpub.com		

Jones and Bartlett's books and products are available through most bookstores and online booksellers. To contact Jones and Bartlett Publishers directly, call 800-832-0034, fax 978-443-8000, or visit our website www.jbpub.com.

Substantial discounts on bulk quantities of Jones and Bartlett's publications are available to corporations, professional associations, and other qualified organizations. For details and specific discount information, contact the special sales department at Jones and Bartlett via the above contact information or send an email to specialsales@jbpub.com.

The authors, editor, and publisher have made every effort to provide accurate information. However, they are not responsible for errors, omissions, or for any outcomes related to the use of the contents of this book and take no responsibility for the use of the products and procedures described. Treatments and side effects described in this book may not be applicable to all people; likewise, some people may require a dose or experience a side effect that is not described herein. Drugs and medical devices are discussed that may have limited availability controlled by the Food and Drug Administration (FDA) for use only in a research study or clinical trial. Research, clinical practice, and government regulations often change the accepted standard in this field. When consideration is being given to use of any drug in the clinical setting, the health care provider or reader is responsible for determining FDA status of the drug, reading the package insert, and reviewing prescribing information for the most up-to-date recommendations on dose, precautions, and contraindications, and determining the appropriate usage for the product. This is especially important in the case of drugs that are new or seldom used.

Production Credits

Publisher: Kevin Sullivan	Associate Marketing Manager: Ilana Goddess
Acquisitions Editor: Emily Ekle	Manufacturing and Inventory Control Supervisor: Amy Bacus
Acquisitions Editor: Amy Sibley	Composition: Arlene Apone
Associate Editor: Patricia Donnelly	Cover Design: Brian Moore
Editorial Assistant: Rachel Shuster	Printing and Binding: Courier Stoughton
Supervising Production Editor: Carolyn F. Rogers	Cover Printing: Courier Stoughton

Library of Congress Cataloging-in-Publication Data
Brorsen, Ann J.
  Adult CCRN certification review / Ann J. Brorsen, Keri R. Rogelet.
      p. ; cm.
  Includes bibliographical references and index.
  ISBN 978-0-7637-5934-6 (pbk.)
  1. Critical care medicine—Examinations—Study guides. I. Rogelet, Keri R. II. Title.
  [DNLM: 1. Critical Care—Examination Questions. 2. Critical Illness—nursing—Examination Questions. 3. Nursing Assessment—Examination Questions. WY 18.2 B873a 2009]
  RT120.I5B74 2009
  616.02'5076—dc22
                                        2008027308

6048

Printed in the United States of America
12 11 10 09 08   10 9 8 7 6 5 4 3 2 1

Dedication

This book is dedicated to all critical care nurses around the world. Thank you for your compassion, commitment, and love for your patients.

Contents

About the Authors

Ann J. Brorsen, RN, MSN, CCRN, CEN

Ann is a nationally known speaker and has presented certification review courses for the Adult and Pediatric CCRN, PCCN, and CEN. Ann has worked as a staff nurse, manager, nurse executive, consultant, and entrepreneur. Ann's clinical practice includes trauma ED and ICU. Ann holds memberships in Sigma Theta Tau, the American Association of Critical-Care Nurses, the Emergency Nurses' Association, the Society of Critical Care Medicine, and the National Nurses in Business Association. Ann is co-author of the *PCCN Certification Review*, also published by Jones and Bartlett. She is also the Chief Operating Officer and Director of Clinical Applications for Pro Ed in Menifee, California.

Keri R. Rogelet, RN, MSN, MBA/HCM, CCRN

Keri has presented national programs on adult health issues, the Neonatal CCRN, the Pediatric CCRN, and neonatal developmental care. Keri has worked in an adult cardio-thoracic ICU and currently works as a team leader in a Level III NICU. Keri holds memberships in Sigma Theta Tau, the American Association of Critical-Care Nurses, the National Association of Neonatal Nurses, and the Academy of Neonatal Nursing. In addition, she works as a consultant for adult, pediatric, and neonatal product applications. Keri recently co-authored the *PCCN Certification Review*, also published by Jones and Bartlett. She is currently the Chief Financial Officer and Director of Clinical Development for Pro Ed in Menifee, California.

Contact Information

Web: www.forproed.com
Email: proedcertify@yahoo.com

Contributor

Melissa R. Christiansen, RN, MSN, NP-C, CCRN, CNRN

Melissa has more than 23 years of experience as a critical care nurse in neurological, cardiac, and trauma ICUs. She is currently working as a family nurse practitioner in Southern California. Melissa has presented programs on neurological-neuroscience topics, adult critical care certification reviews, and courses on postanesthesia nursing. Melissa is a member of Sigma Theta Tau, the American Association of Critical-Care Nurses, the American Association of Neuroscience Nurses, and the American Academy of Nurse Practitioners. Melissa served as the regional Vice President of the California Association for Nurse Practitioners. Melissa is also on the faculty for the BSN and MSN programs at the University of Phoenix.

Acknowledgments

Mary Margaret Forsythe, RN, and Nancy O. Roberts, RN

Two instructors who were ultimate professionals and passed before their time.

Karen S. Ehrat, RN, PhD

For seeing potential in a new grad and making education a joy and a privilege. You will be missed.

Laura Gasparis-Vonfrolio, RN, PhD

The consummate nursing leader, educator, and innovator. This book is proof that success is possible.

Keri and Melissa

Thanks for all the hard work, late hours, your professionalism, and hanging in there.

A.J.B.

To Ann

To the best friend and mentor a nurse could ever have. Thank you for encouraging and motivating me to be a better nurse, professional, leader, and person.

To Melissa

For your assistance, patience and late nights, thank you.

K.R.R.

Preface

Congratulations! You are one step closer to achieving certification as a CCRN. Even if you plan to use this book only as a study guide for critical care nursing, it will be an invaluable resource. This book will present an introduction to the CCRN credential, guide you through the process of registering for the CCRN exam, and offer some helpful test-taking strategies. We will even provide you with the resources and paperwork you need to complete the process. All you have to do is send us an e-mail.

This book contains test questions and their answers, along with the rationale for each answer. The questions cover a broad range of topics and are representative of the type of questions you will find on the actual CCRN examination. In addition, a written 150-question exam with answers and rationales appears at the end of the book. This exam is also available on the enclosed CD. If you use the CD to take a practice test, the questions will be randomly selected and will enable you to time yourself and practice as if you were taking the actual examination.

We are dedicated to helping you successfully pass this exam and achieve certification as a CCRN. Please feel free to contact us if you have any questions or would like to schedule a CCRN Review for your facility or group.

The CCRN Credential

Traditionally, nurses have worked in a variety of roles and environments. For most of the twentieth century, when nurses graduated from their programs, they had spent many hours in clinical situations and were prepared to practice in any area. Nursing eventually had to adjust from the general practitioner to a nurse who would concentrate practice in one area. Nurses worked in emergency rooms, operating rooms, recovery rooms, obstetrics, and medical surgical units. Those nurses who worked in operating rooms or who administered anesthesia were considered specialized. With the advent of emerging technology, the post–World War II population boom, and a trend toward increasingly more acute patients, nursing and hospitals adjusted by placing patients in more subspecialized areas.

One critical issue that arose in the twentieth century related to patients with poliomyelitis, who were increasing both in number and special needs. The "iron lung" had been around for years. In the 1930s, the machine cost $1,500, which was also the median cost for a home at that time. Patients who could afford such treatment began to recover, only to develop sequelae that required specialized care. Tilt beds and hot pack treatments were initiated. At one time, even curare was used to combat the severe muscle spasms suffered by polio victims. All of these treatments required time and resources, including larger numbers of nurses.

In 1931, the American Association of Nurse Anesthetist (no "s" on the end) formed. On June 4, 1945, the organization held the first-ever certification examination for a nursing specialty. In 1952, the first accredited program for nurse anesthetists was started.

In 1955, Jonas Salk announced the discovery of a vaccine for polio. The vaccine would help prevent spread of the disease, but thousands of victims still required care. Technology in general was improving and becoming more broadly available. Although the first EKG machines were available in the United States as early as 1909, they were not widely used until the late 1950s.

In the 1960s, many patients required around-the-clock specialized care that required resources and practitioners who were experts or who had a great deal of experience with the particular condition or disease process. Veterans of previous wars and the escalating Vietnam War required increasingly more medical resources. Hospitals began placing cardiac, trauma, burn, and acute medical patients in areas of the hospital designated as providing more "intensive" care. Patient survival rates improved so the numbers of specialized areas increased.

In 1967, nurses from Nashville Baptist Hospital were frustrated at the lack of educational opportunities for continuing education for intensive care nurses, so they sent inquiries to other nurses to see if interest existed to form an association or some type of national association to provide education to other intensive care nurses. At that time, most of the ICUs served cardiac patients. A year later, more than 400 nurses attended a symposium and affirmed the need for an organization. In 1969, the American Association of Cardiovascular Nurses was formed. In 1971, the name was changed to the

American Association of Critical-Care Nurses (AACN) in recognition of the broad area covered by critical care.

AACN is now the largest specialty nursing organization in the world. In 1975, the AACN Certification Corporation was established and began offering the CCRN examination. We invite you to visit the AACN Web site at www.aacn.org to learn more about the CCRN credential. Thousands of nurses have successfully completed the Adult CCRN exam and we are here to help you become successful. The next section will explain the registration procedure for the examination. You can do it!

REFERENCES

http://www.aacn.org
(accessed February 19, 2008).

http://www.aacn.org/AACN/mrkt.nsf/vwdoc/HistoryofAACN?opendocument
(accessed February 19, 2008).

http://americanhistory.si.edu/polio/howpolio/index.htm
(accessed February 20, 2008).

http://www.anesthesia-nursing.com/wina.html
(accessed February 20, 2008).

The Synergy Model

The Synergy Model was originally developed to match clinical competency with patient needs and outcomes. The nurse and the care provided are driven by the needs of the patients and their families. Nurses begin practice as novices and, as they gain experience, may reach the expert level. The expert nurse is able to synthesize information, integrate that information, and then formulate a plan of care based on the patient's unique needs. A given patient may have either simple needs or very complex needs. Each patient also has characteristics that reflect his or her physical, emotional, cultural, family, financial, and social resources. The nurse must take all of the patient's characteristics into consideration

The patient must be the focus of the care, and the patient's needs must come first. When the needs and characteristics of the patient are matched with the competencies of the nurse, synergy is the result. For example, it would not be in the best interest of a critically ill patient who requires multiple medications and hemodynamic monitoring to assign that patient to a new graduate who lacks experience and knowledge to care for a patient with complex needs.

Synergy is applicable to education, the corporate world, small business, and anywhere the characteristics of the individual must be matched by the competencies of another entity. In nursing, the goal of synergy is to provide optimal outcomes for both the patient and the nurse.

Until 1999, the Adult CCRN examination was entirely based on clinical judgment. If you could memorize a lot of facts, you would probably be successful on the exam. Today, 80% of the exam is based on clinical judgment, but the other 20% focuses on professional caring and ethical practice.

There is no question that the Synergy Model can be confusing and intimidating. However, excellent resources are available to help you understand the model and its underlying concepts. At the end of this section is a list of those resources—we hope you will take the time to investigate each of them. AACN has posted on their Web site the information about nurse and patient characteristics that appear on the next 2 pages. We also recommend 2 excellent books about the Synergy Model: *Critical Care Nursing: Synergy for Optimal Outcomes,* by Roberta Kaplow, RN, PhD, CCRN, CCNS, CCNS and Sonya R. Hardin, RN, PhD, CCRN and *Synergy for Clinical Excellence: The AACN Synergy Model for Patient Care,* by Sonya R. Hardin, RN, PhD, CCRN and Roberta Kaplow, RN, PhD, CCRN, CCNS, CCNS.

Recently, AACN expanded available information about the Synergy Model patient and nurse characteristics. We thank AACN for the information that appears below.

Remember, the CCRN exam does not test terminology specific to the Synergy Model, but rather your ability to integrate these concepts into the care of patients.

PATIENT CHARACTERISTICS

Resiliency

The capacity to return to a restorative level of functioning using compensatory/coping mechanisms; the ability to bounce back quickly after an insult.

Level 1—Minimally resilient

Unable to mount a response; failure of compensatory/ coping mechanisms; minimal reserves; brittle

Level 3—Moderately resilient

Able to mount a moderate response; able to initiate some degree of compensation; moderate reserves

Level 5—Highly resilient

Able to mount and maintain a response; intact compensatory/coping mechanisms; strong reserves; endurance

Vulnerability

Susceptibility to actual or potential stressors that may adversely affect patient outcomes.

Level 1—Highly vulnerable

Susceptible; unprotected, fragile

Level 3—Moderately vulnerable

Somewhat susceptible; somewhat protected

Level 5—Minimally vulnerable

Safe; out of the woods; protected, not fragile

Stability

The ability to maintain steady-state equilibrium.

Level 1—Minimally stable

Labile; unstable; unresponsive to therapies; high risk of death

Level 3—Moderately stable

Able to maintain steady state for limited period of time; some responsiveness to therapies

Level 5—Highly stable

Constant; responsive to therapies; low risk of death

Complexity

The intricate entanglement of two or more systems (e.g., body, family, therapies).

Level 1—Highly complex

Intricate; complex patient/family dynamics; ambiguous/ vague; atypical presentation

Level 3—Moderately complex

Moderately involved patient/family dynamics

Level 5—Minimally complex

Straightforward; routine patient/family dynamics; simple/clear cut; typical presentation

Resource availability

Extent of resources (e.g., technical, fiscal, personal, psychological, and social) the patient/family/ community bring to the situation.

Level 1—Few resources

Necessary knowledge and skills not available; necessary financial support not available; minimal personal/psychological supportive resources; few social systems resources

Level 3—Moderate resources

Limited knowledge and skills available; limited financial support available; limited personal/psychological supportive resources; limited social systems resources

Level 5—Many resources

Extensive knowledge and skills available and accessible; financial resources readily available; strong personal/psychological supportive resources; strong social systems resources

PATIENT CHARACTERISTICS (CONTINUED)

Participation in care | **Extent to which patient/family engages in aspects of care.**

Level 1—No participation | Patient and family unable or unwilling to participate in care

Level 3—Moderate level of participation | Patient and family need assistance in care

Level 5—Full participation | Patient and family fully able to participate in care

Participation in decision-making | **Extent to which patient/family engages in decision-making.**

Level 1—No participation | Patient and family have no capacity for decision-making; requires surrogacy

Level 3—Moderate level of participation | Patient and family have limited capacity; seeks input/advice from others in decision-making

Level 5—Full participation | Patient and family have capacity, and makes decision for self

Predictability | **A characteristic that allows one to expect a certain course of events or course of illness.**

Level 1—Not predictable | Uncertain; uncommon patient population/illness; unusual or unexpected course; does not follow critical pathway, or no critical pathway developed

Level 3—Moderately predictable | Wavering; occasionally-noted patient population/illness

Level 5—Highly predictable | Certain; common patient population/illness; usual and expected course; follows critical pathway

Source: American Association of Critical-Care Nurses. (n.d.) *The AACN Synergy Model for patient care.* Available at: http://www.aacn.org/WD/Certifications/content/synmodel.content. Used with permission.

NURSE COMPETENCIES

Clinical judgment | **Clinical reasoning, which includes clinical decision-making, critical thinking, and a global grasp of the situation, coupled with nursing skills acquired through a process of integrating formal and informal experiential knowledge and evidence-based guidelines.**

Level 1 | Collects basic-level data; follows algorithms, decision trees, and protocols with all populations and is uncomfortable deviating from them; matches formal knowledge with clinical events to make decisions; questions the limits of one's ability to make clinical decisions and delegates the decision-making to other clinicians; includes extraneous detail

(continues)

NURSE COMPETENCIES (CONTINUED)

Level 3	Collects and interprets complex patient data; makes clinical judgments based on an immediate grasp of the whole picture for common or routine patient populations; recognizes patterns and trends that may predict the direction of illness; recognizes limits and seeks appropriate help; focuses on key elements of case, while shorting out extraneous details
Level 5	Synthesizes and interprets multiple, sometimes conflicting, sources of data; makes judgment based on an immediate grasp of the whole picture, unless working with new patient populations; uses past experiences to anticipate problems; helps patient and family see the "big picture"; recognizes the limits of clinical judgment and seeks multidisciplinary collaboration and consultation with comfort; recognizes and responds to the dynamic situation
Advocacy and moral agency	**Working on another's behalf and representing the concerns of the patient/family and nursing staff; serving as a moral agent in identifying and helping to resolve ethical and clinical concerns within and outside the clinical setting.**
Level 1	Works on behalf of patient; self assesses personal values; aware of ethical conflicts/issues that may surface in clinical setting; makes ethical/moral decisions based on rules; represents patient when patient cannot represent self; aware of patients' rights
Level 3	Works on behalf of patient and family; considers patient values and incorporates in care, even when differing from personal values; supports colleagues in ethical and clinical issues; moral decision-making can deviate from rules; demonstrates give and take with patient's family, allowing them to speak/represent themselves when possible; aware of patient and family rights
Level 5	Works on behalf of patient, family, and community; advocates from patient/family perspective, whether similar to or different from personal values; advocates ethical conflict and issues from patient/family perspective; suspends rules—patient and family drive moral decision-making; empowers the patient and family to speak for/represent themselves; achieves mutuality within patient/professional relationships
Caring practices	**Nursing activities that create a compassionate, supportive, and therapeutic environment for patients and staff, with the aim of promoting comfort and healing and preventing unnecessary suffering. Includes, but is not limited to, vigilance, engagement, and responsiveness of caregivers, including family and healthcare personnel.**

NURSE COMPETENCIES (CONTINUED)

Level 1   Focuses on the usual and customary needs of the patient; no anticipation of future needs; bases care on standards and protocols; maintains a safe physical environment; acknowledges death as a potential outcome

Level 3   Responds to subtle patient and family changes; engages with the patient as a unique patient in a compassionate manner; recognizes and tailors caring practices to the individuality of patient and family; domesticates the patient's and family's environment; recognizes that death may be an acceptable outcome

Level 5   Has astute awareness and anticipates patient and family changes and needs; fully engaged with and sensing how to stand alongside the patient, family, and community; caring practices follow the patient and family lead; anticipates hazards and avoids them, and promotes safety throughout patient's and family's transitions along the healthcare continuum; orchestrates the process that ensures patient's/family's comfort and concerns surrounding issues of death and dying are met

Collaboration   **Working with others (e.g., patients, families, healthcare providers) in a way that promotes/encourages each person's contributions toward achieving optimal/realistic patient/family goals. Involves intra- and interdisciplinary work with colleagues and community.**

Level 1   Willing to be taught, coached and/or mentored; participates in team meetings and discussions regarding patient care and/or practice issues; open to various team members' contributions

Level 3   Seeks opportunities to be taught, coached, and/or mentored; elicits others' advice and perspectives; initiates and participates in team meetings and discussions regarding patient care and/or practice issues; recognizes and suggests various team members' participation

Level 5   Seeks opportunities to teach, coach, and mentor and to be taught, coached, and mentored; facilitates active involvement and complementary contributions of others in team meetings and discussions regarding patient care and/or practice issues; involves/recruits diverse resources when appropriate to optimize patient outcomes

Systems thinking   **Body of knowledge and tools that allow the nurse to manage whatever environmental and system resources exist for the patient/family and staff, within or across healthcare and non-healthcare systems.**

Level 1   Uses a limited array of strategies; limited outlook—sees the pieces or components; does not recognize negotiation as an alternative; sees patient and family within the isolated environment of the unit; sees self as key resource

(continues)

NURSE COMPETENCIES (CONTINUED)

Level 3	Develops strategies based on needs and strengths of patient/family; able to make connections within components; sees opportunity to negotiate but may not have strategies; developing a view of the patient/family transition process; recognizes how to obtain resources beyond self
Level 5	Develops, integrates, and applies a variety of strategies that are driven by the needs and strengths of the patient/family; global or holistic outlook—sees the whole rather than the pieces; knows when and how to negotiate and navigate through the system on behalf of patients and families; anticipates needs of patients and families as they move through the healthcare system; utilizes untapped and alternative resources as necessary
Response to diversity	**The sensitivity to recognize, appreciate, and incorporate differences into the provision of care. Differences may include, but are not limited to, cultural differences, spiritual beliefs, gender, race, ethnicity, lifestyle, socioeconomic status, age, and values.**
Level 1	Assesses cultural diversity; provides care based on own belief system; learns the culture of the healthcare environment
Level 3	Inquires about cultural differences and considers their impact on care; accommodates personal and professional differences in the plan of care; helps patient/family understand the culture of the healthcare system
Level 5	Responds to, anticipates, and integrates cultural differences into patient/family care; appreciates and incorporates differences, including alternative therapies, into care; tailors healthcare culture, to the extent possible, to meet the diverse needs and strengths of the patient/family
Facilitation of learning	**The ability to facilitate learning for patients/families, nursing staff, other members of the healthcare team, and community. Includes both formal and informal facilitation of learning.**
Level 1	Follows planned educational programs; sees patient/family education as a separate task from delivery of care; provides data without seeking to assess patient's readiness or understanding; has limited knowledge of the totality of the educational needs; focuses on a nurse's perspective; sees the patient as a passive recipient
Level 3	Adapts planned educational programs; begins to recognize and integrate different ways of teaching into delivery of care; incorporates patient's understanding into practice; sees the overlapping of educational plans from different healthcare providers' perspectives; begins to see the patient as having input into goals; begins to see individualism

NURSE COMPETENCIES (CONTINUED)

Level 5	Creatively modifies or develops patient/family education programs; integrates patient/family education through-out delivery of care; evaluates patient's understanding by observing behavior changes related to learning; is able to collaborate and incorporate all healthcare providers' and educational plans into the patient/family educational program; sets patient-driven goals for education; sees patient/family as having choices and consequences that are negotiated in relation to education
Clinical inquiry (innovator/evaluator)	**The ongoing process of questioning and evaluating practice and providing informed practice. Creating practice changes through research utilization and experiential learning.**
Level 1	Follows standards and guidelines; implements clinical changes and research-based practices developed by others; recognizes the need for further learning to improve patient care; recognizes obvious changing patient situation (e.g., deterioration, crisis); needs and seeks help to identify patient problem
Level 3	Questions appropriateness of policies and guidelines; questions current practice; seeks advice, resources, or information to improve patient care; begins to compare and contrast possible alternatives
Level 5	Improves, deviates from, or individualizes standards and guidelines for particular patient situations or populations; questions and/or evaluates current practice based on patients' responses, review of the literature, research and education/learning; acquires knowledge and skills needed to address questions arising in practice and improve patient care; (The domains of clinical judgment and clinical inquiry converge at the expert level; they cannot be separated)

Source: American Association of Critical-Care Nurses. (n.d.) *The AACN Synergy Model for patient care.* Available at: http://www.aacn.org/WD/Certifications/content/synmodel.content. Used with permission.

RESOURCES

AACN certification information. Retrieved on March 15, 2008, from http://web.aacn.org/WD/Certifications/Content

Becker, D., Kaplow, R., Muenzen, P. M., & Hartigan, C. (2006). Activities performed by acute and critical care advanced practice nurses: American Association of Critical-Care Nurses study of practice. *American Journal of Critical Care, 15*(2), 130–148.

Brewer, B. B., Wojner-Alexandrov, A. W., Triola, N., & et al. (2007). AACN synergy model's characteristics of patients: Psychometric analyses in a tertiary care health system. *American Journal of Critical Care, 16*(2), 158–167.

Burns, S. M. (Ed.). (2007). *American Association of Critical-Care Nurses (AACN): AACN protocols for practice: Healing environments* (2nd ed.). Sudbury, MA: Jones and Bartlett.

Cline, M., Nottingham, M., & Lockhart, J. S. (2006). Synergy for clinical excellence: The AACN Synergy Model for Patient Care. *Critical Care Nurse, 26*(2), 139–140.

Copstead, L., & Banasik, J. L. (2000). *Pathophysiology: Biological and behavioral perspectives* (2nd ed.). Philadelphia: W. B. Saunders/Elsevier.

Curley, M. A. Q. (1998). Patient nurse synergy: Optimizing patients' outcomes. *American Journal of Critical Care, 7,* 64–72.

Dossey, B. M., Keegan, L., & Guzzetta, C. (2003). *Holistic nursing: A handbook for practice* (3rd ed.). Sudbury, MA: Jones and Bartlett.

Edwards, D. F. (1999). The Synergy Model: Linking patient needs to nurse competencies. *Critical Care Nurse, 19*(1), 88–98.

Hardin, S. R., & Kaplow, R. (2005). *Synergy for clinical excellence: The AACN Synergy Model for Patient Care.* Sudbury, MA: Jones and Bartlett.

Hardin, S. R., & Kaplow, R. (Eds.). (2004). *Synergy for clinical excellence: The AACN Synergy Model for Patient Care.* Sudbury, MA: Jones and Bartlett.

Kaplow, R. (2004). Applying the Synergy Model to nursing education. *Critical Care Nurse: AACN Critical Care Careers, 20*(22), 24–26.

Kelleher, S. (2006). Providing patient-centered care in an intensive care unit. *Nursing Standard, 21*(13), 35–40.

Lipson, J. G., Dibble, S. L., & Minarik, P. A. (Eds.). (1996). *Culture and nursing care: A pocket guide.* San Francisco, CA: UCSF Nursing Press.

McQuillan, K. A., Von Rueden, K. T., Hartsock, R. L., Flynn, M. B., & Whalen, E. (Eds.). (2002). *Trauma nursing: From resuscitation through rehabilitation* (3rd ed.). Philadelphia: W. B. Saunders/Elsevier.

Smith, A.R. (2006). Using the Synergy Model to provide spiritual nursing care in critical care settings. *Critical Care Nurse, 26*(4), 41–47.

Registering for the CCRN Examination

The first thing you must do is determine if you are eligible for the exam. To be able to take the CCRN exam, you must not have any encumbrances on your current registered nurse license in any state—in other words, no restrictions, disciplinary actions, attached conditions, or provisions of any kind that would affect your ability to practice as a nurse. You need to have completed 1,750 hours of direct bedside care for a critically ill patient population during the past 2 years. There are 3 CCRN exams: Adult, Pediatric, and Neonatal. For you to qualify for the Adult CCRN exam, all of your practice hours must involve care of adult patients. You may not split the hours between, say, a pediatric ICU and an adult ICU.

Of the 1,750 hours of direct care, 875 hours must have been completed in the past year. If you are an educator, a CNS, or a manager, you can still qualify. If you directly supervise students or nurses at the bedside, you will qualify. You must, however, participate in the care of the patient. For example, if you demonstrate a procedure or supervise a nurse or student performing the procedure, that activity would be acceptable.

Nurses must have a certain level of experience to qualify for the CCRN exam. Many questions require integration of knowledge and critical thinking, and the test covers advanced concepts such as hemodynamics and ventilator management. It would be difficult, though not impossible, to pass the test if you have not had experience with either of these clinical situations.

Other questions test your familiarity with technology such as arterial lines, pulmonary artery catheters, intra-aortic balloon pumps, and intracranial pressure monitoring. Passing the test would certainly be easier if you have experience with this technology, but not every critical care area utilizes these therapies. For example, some nurses do not have direct experience with patients undergoing open heart surgery or neurosurgery. In such cases, the relevant concepts can be learned from reading appropriate critical care texts or by consulting another nurse with experience in the particular area. Nursing is a mobile profession, and quite often a person you work with may have experiences and qualifications unknown to you. Some nurses have the opportunity to work via registries or as travelers and have a wide base of experience. Other nurses will seek out new experiences within their own facility or work part-time in other facilities. We are not trying to scare you. Thousands of nurses have passed this exam and it is certainly feasible to do so even without experience in certain areas.

Candidates for the CCRN come from a variety of critical care settings: ICU, CCU, telemetry, catheterization lab, PACU, step-down units, emergency room, and progressive care. Critical care patients are found in all these areas. To see what the CCRN exam covers, you can download a copy of the Adult CCRN Test Plan from AACN at www.aacn.org. The Test Plan is an outline, or blueprint, of the major areas to be tested. The Test Plan also indicates the percentage of questions tested in that particular section or system. Specific conditions and pathophysiologies are listed on the Test Plan, allowing you to better focus your study time and resources. If you would like us to send you an application and current Adult CCRN Test Plan, please email us your name and address (please do not forget your ZIP code!).

When you sign up for the CCRN exam, you can sign up as either a member or a nonmember of AACN. The cost is lower if you are a member. You can join AACN at the time you register to receive the member discount. Just email us if you have any questions. After your documents are received by AACN, you must allow several weeks for processing. You will then be sent a postcard stating that, from that date, you will have 90 days to complete the exam.

Once you sign up, you will be provided with a list of examination locations near you, based on your ZIP code. The test is administered at Applied Measurement Professional (AMP) sites around the United States and you may take the exam at any AMP testing center.

Your next step is to call the AMP testing center you select and make an appointment for the exam. The testing center will authorize the time and day when you will take the test. Visit the AACN Web site or the AMP Web site for updated information. Please note: You will be sent a specific authorization code to access the AMP Web site to register for the exam. Specific rules apply when you want to change an appointment, so make sure you have the most current information on this process.

The CCRN exam is now computer based and given year round. You may take the CCRN exam the old-fashioned way, by pencil and paper. These written exams are given only a couple times a year and require special registrations and arrangements. Please contact AACN directly if you wish to test in this manner.

Remember, thousands of nurses have passed this examination and you can, too!

Test-Taking Strategies

When preparing for the CCRN exam, the first thing to do is be absolutely honest with yourself about how you study. If you have good study habits and plenty of time, you are very fortunate. If you are a procrastinator, studying a little bit at a time might help. Nurses have to juggle so many roles that take up their time: parent, child, employee, student, teacher, and on and on. One of the biggest struggles is simply finding time and a place to study. Discovering your learning style will help you find a better way to absorb information.

Three types of learners are commonly identified: visual, auditory, and kinesthetic. There is no perfect strategy for learning because every person is unique. Not everyone has a single style of learning; you may use a mix of styles depending on your situation.

Visual learners learn better from reading and writing than from hearing and talking about information. Background noise, such as music or television, is distracting to these types of learners. Finding a quiet space is a problem for some people. You may have to stay awake after family members have gone to bed. Flashcards often work and some people use colored markers to highlight important information.

Auditory learners learn information effectively by listening and talking. Playing music, listening to audiotapes, or being part of a study group often works.

Kinesthetic learners prefer to learn via a "hands-on" approach. Nurses often learn this way because we have to listen to lectures and then demonstrate skills. This approach focuses on the use of models, manikins, or patients and works well for many healthcare providers. Kinesthetic people are often "antsy" and cannot sit still for long periods of time, so lectures may be difficult for them without frequent breaks. If you are a kinesthetic learner, some of the things that might help while studying include taking frequent breaks, walking around, or riding a stationary cycle.

No matter what your personal learning style, your test-taking skills can be improved. How? Practice! That is why we wrote this book in a question-and-answer format. Keep practicing the questions until you can answer at least 80% correctly. Research has shown that two-thirds of study time should be spent taking sample tests, and only one-third of study time should be spent reviewing content.

Studying, like regular exercise, is good for the brain. As nurses, we must always keep abreast of the professional literature and spend time studying to keep our knowledge and skills up-to-date. In addition, many states require continuing education to renew a professional license. The CCRN requires 100 hours of continuing education to be obtained within a 3 year period. Anything worthwhile studying takes time, effort, and sacrifice. There is no way around studying for this certification. There are no shortcuts!

If you have been out of school for a while, don't despair! It may be slow going at first, so take things a little at a time. Just like going to the gym, you should make a plan to study in one particular place and at the same time if possible. This is your space and your time—claim it. Have all your books, tapes, and other study materials handy. If you need snack food, make sure it is not all sugar and include some salty food. Caffeine tends to make people jittery, but if you need it, it may be right for you.

The Adult CCRN Test Plan is a blueprint of the exam's content. The major sections are broken down into subheadings and topics. If you study only a little at a time, you will be fine. One day you may feel like studying cardiomyopathy; the next day, you may focus on chest tubes. You may download the current Adult CCRN Test Plan from AACN at www.aacn.org. We did not include a Test Plan in this book because the exam changes frequently and you should have a copy of the current plan.

If you study with a group, you can save a lot of time and effort by breaking up the topics for that study period and having each person present his or her topic(s) and provide handouts and practice questions for the rest of the group. When you can make up a test question about a subject, you really will be prepared. Study for short periods of time, say 30 to 45 minutes, and then take a break. Set small goals and, after you have accomplished each one, reward yourself!

EXAM CONTENT

The Adult CCRN certification exam consists of 150 multiple-choice test questions. Twenty-five of those questions do not count; they are there to be validated. In other words, every question is tried first to see if it is written well and if a certain percentage of people answer it correctly. At this point in the process, a question can still be "tweaked" for use on future exams.

Your results are determined by how many answers you get correct. Some answers are a bit harder than others. The final score usually indicates a pass if you get at least 70% correct. If you do not know an answer, take your best guess, because you have at least a 25% chance of guessing correctly. You get points only for questions answered correctly.

The Test Plan shows the breakdown of questions by topic and section. AACN uses the Synergy Model as a basis for practice. We will give you a brief overview of the Synergy Model in another section of this book. Here is the good news: There are no questions on the test that deal specifically with the terminology of the Synergy Model. Instead, the answers to questions are based on best practice that utilizes and synthesizes the Synergy Model.

STUDY TIPS

A multiple-choice test question consists of three parts: an introductory statement, a stem (question), and options, from which you must select the correct answer. The introductory statement provides information about a clinical issue, pathophysiology, or a nursing action or duty.

Stems are worded in different ways. Some stems are in the form of a question; others are in the form of an incomplete statement. Additionally, a stem will usually request 1 of 2 types of responses: a positive response or a negative response. More good news: The test was recently changed so that it does not include negative stem questions! This means stems such as "all of the following except" are no longer part of the exam. (The questions you will practice from in this book may have an occasional negative stem to facilitate learning.) More good news: There are no longer any multiple-multiple-choice questions on the exam!

Key words are important words or phrases that help focus your attention on what the question is asking. Examples of key words include *always, most, first response, earliest, priority, first, on admission, common, best, least, not, immediately,* and *initial.*

You should always be looking for a *therapeutic response.* The nurse is *always* therapeutic. In other words, your *initial response* as a nurse is *always* the therapeutic response—you must acknowledge and validate the patient's feelings. Communication skills learned in Nursing 101 are important components of successful test-taking strategies. More than one option may contain a therapeutic response. When in doubt, validate, validate, validate. Always validate the feelings before you present information. A medical emergency would, of course, take precedence.

Who is actually the focus of the question? You need to be able to identify this person. Sometimes questions are asked about a friend, a relative, or a significant other instead of a patient. A lot of information in the question may be deliberately distracting. Also, you must, when applicable, validate that person's feelings first.

WHEN IN DOUBT

When answering questions, remember Maslow's hierarchy of needs and the ABCs (airway, breathing, circulation). When these goals are met, then safety is the priority. After safety, the psychological needs are a priority. Assessment always comes before diagnosis and treatment (intervention). Learning takes place only if the patient is motivated.

Eliminate incorrect options. This gives you a 50% chance of guessing the correct answer. Here are some hints:

- Select the most general, all-encompassing option.
- Eliminate similar options or those that contain words such as "always" or "never." If two options say essentially the same thing, then neither is correct. If three of the four options sound similar, choose the one that sounds different.
- Eliminate any options that contain the words "always" or "never."
- Look for the longest option. It is usually the correct answer.
- Watch for grammatical inconsistencies between the stem and options.

IT'S TIME FOR THE CCRN EXAM!

Well, you are finally ready! The night before the exam, get a good night's sleep. Do not cram the night before, although that is easier said than done. Do something relaxing and enjoyable, like going to a movie or out to dinner. Try to avoid caffeine or any other stimulant.

Take the exam and pass it!

REFERENCES

Kobel Lamonte, M. (2007). Test-taking strategies for CNOR certification. *Association of Operating Room Nurses. AORN Journal, 85*(2), 315–332.

Ludwig, C. (2004). Preparing for certification: Test-taking strategies. *Medsurg Nursing, 13*(2), 127–128.

Cardiovascular

QUESTIONS

1. Calculate the cardiac output for a patient with a heart rate of 60 and a stroke volume of 70 mL.
   A. 0.85%
   B. 4.2 L/min
   C. 1.16 mL/min
   D. 3,800 cc/min

2. What percentage of the cardiac cycle is provided by the atrial kick?
   A. 15%
   B. 20%
   C. 30%
   D. 35%

3. A normal value for an ejection fraction (EF) would be:
   A. 65%
   B. 40%
   C. 30%
   D. 25%

4. The ejection fraction (EF) most closely represents:
   A. RVEDP
   B. PAOP
   C. RVP
   D. LVEDP

5. Stroke volume is comprised of which of the following factors?
   A. Blood volume, viscosity, impedance
   B. Cardiac output, heart rate, compliance
   C. Contractility, preload, afterload
   D. Compliance, impedance, heart rate

6. A reflex tachycardia caused by stretch of right atrial receptors is known as the
   A. Herring–Sines law.
   B. Renin–angiotensin system.
   C. Starling's law.
   D. Bainbridge reflex.

7. Diastole comprises what percentage of the cardiac cycle?
   A. One-half
   B. Two-thirds
   C. One-fourth
   D. One-third

8. What is the mean arterial pressure (MAP) for a patient with a blood pressure of 120/50 and a heart rate of 70?
   A. 73
   B. 2.4
   C. 50
   D. 85

9. Your patient has the following parameters:
   HR 80
   BP 110/70
   SV 60
   BSA 2.0 m^2

   Calculate the cardiac index (CI) for this patient.
   A. 4.8 L/min
   B. 55 L/min/m^2
   C. 2.4 L/min/m^2
   D. 30 mL/m^2

10. The resistance against which the right ventricle must use to eject its volume is known as:
    A. PAOP
    B. SVR
    C. PAP
    D. PVR

11. Pressures in the left side of the heart and pulmonary filling pressures are represented by the
    A. CI.
    B. PAD.
    C. PAOP.
    D. SVR.

12. Normal values for pulmonary artery pressures should be:
    A. PAS 30–40 mm Hg, PAD 20–25 mm Hg, PAM 25–30 mm Hg
    B. PAS 20–30 mm Hg, PAD 4–10 mm Hg, PAM 10–15 mm Hg
    C. PAS 10–20 mm Hg, PAD 6–12 mm Hg, PAM 8–10 mm Hg
    D. PAS 5–10 mm Hg, PAD 4–8 mm Hg, PAM 6–9 mm Hg

13. The mean pressure difference in the systemic vascular bed divided by blood flow is known as:
    A. SVR
    B. LAP
    C. PVRI
    D. PCW

14. Which heart murmur is associated with acute valvular regurgitation?
    A. S_3
    B. S_2
    C. S_1
    D. S_4

15. Which of the following leads is best for monitoring for a RBBB?
    A. Lead II
    B. Lead I
    C. Lead V_1
    D. Lead V_6

16. Tall, peaked T waves on an EKG may be indicative of
    A. Hypocalcemia.
    B. Non-STEMI.
    C. Hyperkalemia.
    D. LBBB.

17. Ethyl suffered a cardiac arrest at home. The family did not perform CPR and the paramedics arrived 6 minutes after the arrest. The patient was found in pulseless V-tach. Defibrillation was performed and CPR was continuous during transport to the ED. The patient was transferred to the ICU because of a bed shortage in the ED. The physician initiated hypothermic measures and administered vecuronium. This medication was used to:
    A. Control ventricular dysrhythmias
    B. Prevent shivering
    C. Act as a sedative
    D. Relieve pain

18. Your patient was admitted for malaise, severe dyspnea, and he had a syncopal episode at work. The patient states he has a midline burning sensation in his chest that worsens when he is supine. You suspect
    A. A pleural effusion.
    B. Pericardial tamponade.
    C. GERD.
    D. Myocarditis.

19. A definitive diagnosis of myocarditis can be made via
    A. An endomyocardial biopsy.
    B. Transesophageal ultrasound.
    C. Transmural catheterization.
    D. Chest X ray.

20. What volume of fluid is required to cause pericardial tamponade?
    A. 25–50 mL
    B. 50–75 mL
    C. 100–150 mL
    D. 200–300 mL

21. Beck's triad is a combination of symptoms useful in diagnosing tamponade. The symptoms include
    A. Pericardial friction rub, hypertension, and RV failure.
    B. Increased pulse pressure, increased JVD, and tachycardia.
    C. Tachycardia, hypertension, and LV failure.
    D. Distended neck veins, muffled heart sounds, and hypotension.

22. Which of the following hemodynamic changes will occur with a cardiac tamponade?
    A. Increased cardiac output
    B. Decreased stroke volume
    C. Increased contractility
    D. Decreased heart rate

23. If your patient had a cardiac tamponade, which of the following findings would you expect on a chest X ray?
    A. A dilated superior vena cava
    B. Increased JVD
    C. Narrowed mediastinum
    D. Delineation of the pericardium and epicardium

24. Your patient was admitted for severe dyspnea, dysphagia, palpitations, and an intractable cough. On auscultation, you hear a loud S_1 and a right-sided S_3 and S_4. A pulmonary artery catheter is placed and large A waves are seen in the PAOP tracing. The patient probably has:
    A. Mitral insufficiency
    B. Myocarditis
    C. Atrial stenosis
    D. Mitral stenosis

25. Quincke's sign is usually seen in
    A. Mitral stenosis.
    B. Endocarditis.
    C. Aortic insufficiency.
    D. Pericarditis.

26. In patients with aortic insufficiency, the popliteal blood pressure is often higher than the brachial blood pressure by at least 40 mm Hg. This is known as
    A. DeMusset's sign.
    B. Hill's sign.
    C. Holmes' sign.
    D. Rochelle's sign.

27. In stable angina, which of the following statements is true?
    A. A positive treadmill test will indicate CAD.
    B. A thallium test will not diagnose LV dysfunction.
    C. The treadmill test will miss up to 20% of single-vessel diseases.
    D. CK-MB isoenzymes and troponins will not increase.

28. **Actions of beta blockers include**
    A. Increased myocardial oxygen demand.
    B. Increased heart rate.
    C. Increased diastolic filling time.
    D. Increased afterload.

29. **If the inferior wall of the heart is infarcted, the leads that will most directly reflect the injury are:**
    A. II, II, aVF
    B. I, aVL
    C. V_1–V_2
    D. V_5–V_6

30. **An anterior wall infarction may be seen in leads**
    A. V_4, R.
    B. V_5–V_6.
    C. V_7–V_9.
    D. V_2–V_4.

31. **Pulsus alternans is most often noted with**
    A. Mitral stenosis.
    B. Constrictive pericarditis.
    C. Aortic stenosis.
    D. LV failure.

32. **Which of the heart valves is most commonly affected by infective endocarditis?**
    A. Aortic
    B. Pulmonic
    C. Mitral
    D. Tricuspid

33. **Alpha-adrenergic effects of norepinephrine include**
    A. Increased force of myocardial contraction.
    B. Increased SA node firing.
    C. Increased AV conduction time.
    D. Peripheral arteriolar vasoconstriction.

34. **Stimulation of the vasomotor center in the medulla occurs when the partial pressure of oxygen changes. This is initiated by:**
    A. Baroreceptors
    B. Chemoreceptors
    C. The Purkinge system
    D. Bainbridge reflex

35. **When attempting to auscultate the aortic area, where should the stethoscope be placed?**
    A. At the second intercostal space, left sternal border
    B. Over the apical area
    C. At the second intercostal space, right sternal border
    D. At the fifth intercostal space, left sternal border

36. When preparing to teach your 30-year-old female patient about goals for weight control, the BMI should be assessed. What is the recommended range for the BMI?
    A. 12.6–15.0
    B. 11.2–15.8
    C. 18.0–24.9
    D. 28.6–24.7

37. Symptoms of right-sided heart failure include
    A. Pulmonary edema.
    B. Elevated PAD and PAOP.
    C. Hepatomegaly.
    D. Orthopnea.

38. NSAIDs are contraindicated in the treatment of patients with heart failure because they
    A. Decrease myocardial contractility.
    B. Cause atrial fibrillation in patients with heart failure.
    C. Promote fluid retention.
    D. May cause hypocalcemia.

39. Contraindications for use of an intra-aortic balloon pump (IABP) would include
    A. Cardiogenic shock.
    B. Aortic valve regurgitation.
    C. Left ventricular failure.
    D. Unstable angina.

40. Complications with use of the intra-aortic balloon pump (IABP) may include
    A. Decreased cardiac output.
    B. Gangrene of lower extremities.
    C. Ruptured papillary muscle.
    D. Preoperative use prior to CABG.

41. An absolute contraindication for use of a fibrinolytic would be:
    A. Traumatic CPR
    B. Cerebrovascular disease
    C. Subacute bacterial endocarditis
    D. Oral anticoagulants

42. Which of the following statements is true about lidocaine?
    A. Lidocaine causes hypotension.
    B. Lidocaine is associated with moderate gastrointestinal intolerance.
    C. Lidocaine does not impair normal contractility.
    D. Lidocaine can cause nystagmus.

43. Which drug listed below has a high iodine content?
    A. Flecanide
    B. Lidocaine
    C. Mexilitene
    D. Amiodarone

44. **The drug of choice to treat AV nodal and atrioventricular re-entrant arrhythmias is:**
    A. Amiodarone
    B. Clonidine
    C. Quinidine
    D. Adenosine

45. **Sometimes certain medications prolong the QT interval, potentially causing polymorphic ventricular tachycardia. The drug of choice to treat this rhythm is:**
    A. Magnesium
    B. Calcium
    C. Digoxin
    D. Lidocaine

46. **Calcium channel blockers act primarily on**
    A. Cardiac output (decreases).
    B. Arteries to arterioles.
    C. Lung receptors only.
    D. Venules to veins.

47. **The fourth heart sound (S_4) is**
    A. Heard as the mitral valve opens.
    B. A low-pitched murmur.
    C. Heard during atrial contraction.
    D. Produced in congestive heart failure.

48. **Which of the following is an example of a systolic murmur?**
    A. Tricuspid stenosis
    B. Tricuspid insufficiency
    C. Mitral stenosis
    D. Pulmonic insufficiency

49. **Which of the following is an example of a pansystolic murmur?**
    A. Pulmonic insufficiency
    B. Tricuspid insufficiency
    C. Atrial stenosis
    D. Mitral stenosis

50. **Gloria Y. was admitted for increased exercise intolerance, severe edema, and dyspnea at rest. A pulmonary artery catheter was placed and the following pressures were obtained: RAP = 18, PA = 65/30, RV = 68/26, PAOP = 14. You would suspect which of the following conditions?**
    A. Cardiac tamponade
    B. Congestive heart failure
    C. Pulmonary embolus
    D. Pulmonary hypertension

51. Norman is a 45-year-old steel worker admitted for acute dyspnea and chest pain. A pulmonary artery catheter was placed and the following readings were obtained: RAP = 16, RV = 70/26, PA = 68/34, PAOP = 24. What is the probable diagnosis?
    A. Congestive heart failure
    B. Restrictive pericarditis
    C. Pulmonary embolus
    D. Pulmonary hypertension

52. If the international normalized ratio (INR) is above 5.0, the patient is at significant risk of bleeding. A drug that can cause a significant rise in the INR is:
    A. Ethacrinic acid
    B. Penicillin
    C. Amiodarone
    D. A statin

53. A drug that will significantly decrease the INR is:
    A. Naficillin
    B. Vitamin K
    C. High-dose vitamin C
    D. Cyclosporine

54. Your patient has a temporary pacemaker and has been requiring adjustments to raise the energy output (milliamps). This is probably due to
    A. Hyperkalemia.
    B. Necrotic tissue.
    C. Lidocaine toxicity.
    D. An atrioventricular block.

55. Kenneth is a 54-year-old who was admitted with a non-STEMI inferior wall MI. He is complaining of dyspnea, weakness, bilateral crackles, and demonstrates orthopnea. He also has an S_3 heart sound. You suspect he has developed:
    A. A pulmonary embolus
    B. Pulmonary hypertension
    C. A fat embolism
    D. Cardiogenic shock

56. Your patient suddenly complains of chest pain and has increased pulmonary artery and wedge pressures. You auscultate a new holosystolic murmur at the lower-left sternal border. Your patient has probably experienced a
    A. Dissecting thoracic aneurysm.
    B. Pulmonary embolus.
    C. Ventricular septal rupture.
    D. Lateral wall MI.

57. Darlene was admitted 3 days ago for management of a deep vein thrombosis. During your initial assessment this morning, you found her sitting on the side of the bed leaning forward. She states that this position relieved her newly developed chest pain. She also states that the pain is worse on inspiration. You notify the

physician, and she orders a chest X ray and lab work. The results show that Darlene's sedimentation rate and WBCs are elevated. Darlene most likely has:

A. Pericarditis

B. A thoracic aneurysm

C. A pulmonary embolus

D. Pulmonary edema

58. **A probable candidate for a coronary artery bypass graft might have**

A. An ejection fraction of 55% and diabetes.

B. Right main artery disease.

C. An ejection fraction of 35% and coronary artery disease.

D. A previous history of cardiac surgery.

59. **You are performing cardiopulmonary resuscitation on a patient with an endotracheal tube in place. The placement of the tube has been confirmed. The patient should be ventilated every:**

A. 6–8 seconds

B. 5 compressions

C. 15 compressions

D. Every 3–5 seconds

60. **If you are using a biphasic defibrillator on an adult, the energy setting should be set at:**

A. 360 joules

B. 50–100 joules

C. 300 joules

D. 200 joules

61. **You have administered 40 mg of furosemide to your patient to help treat pulmonary edema. What change would you expect to see first with regard to the pulmonary artery catheter parameters?**

A. Increased RV

B. Decreased PAOP

C. Decreased RAP

D. Increased LAP

62. **Wellen's syndrome**

A. Is the same as Prinzmetal's angina.

B. Occurs with proximal stenosis of the LAD.

C. Is called crescendo angina.

D. Is variant angina.

63. **A vasodilator used in the treatment of anginal pain is:**

A. Morphine

B. Ticlid

C. Aspirin

D. NTG

64. A patient is at high risk for ventricular septal defect or rupture or even a ventricular aneurysm if an infarct occurs in the
    A. Left anterior descending artery.
    B. Left main coronary artery.
    C. Left circumflex artery.
    D. Right coronary artery.

65. If a chronic fluid accumulation occurs, the pericardial sac may hold as much as _____ before the signs of a cardiac tamponade will appear.
    A. 200 mL
    B. 400 mL
    C. 1,000 mL
    D. 2,000 mL

66. Which of the following statements is true about pericardial effusion?
    A. This is a painless, hard-to-diagnose condition.
    B. On chest X ray, a "water bottle" silhouette is noted.
    C. Diastolic filling is increased.
    D. The voltage of the QRS complex is increased.

67. Increased afterload would be seen with:
    A. Polycythemia
    B. Aortic insufficiency
    C. Hypovolemia
    D. Sepsis

68. Auto-regulatory control of cardiac vessels becomes impaired if the coronary perfusion pressure drops below
    A. 35 mm Hg.
    B. 40 mm Hg.
    C. 50 mm Hg.
    D. 60 mm Hg.

69. Renin is secreted by the
    A. Pancreas.
    B. Lungs.
    C. Liver.
    D. Kidneys.

70. If blood pressure is lower by at least 10–11 mm Hg on inspiration than on expiration, this is known as:
    A. Pulsus alternans
    B. Pulse pressure
    C. Pulsus paradoxus
    D. Pulsus parvus

71. Your patient, Robert, has suffered an MI and is in critical but stable condition. Seven family members arrive at the ICU, demanding to see the patient. Your best response would be to:

A. Notify social services

B. Identify a responsible family spokesperson and contact

C. Refuse to admit more than 1 person

D. Call security to remove the visitors

72. Continuing with the scenario from Question 71, after you have identified Robert's significant other, his estranged wife arrives at the ICU. Robert is intubated, but writes a note stating he wants no information given to the estranged wife. She becomes belligerent when told of Robert's wishes and threatens the hospital staff with a lawsuit. The most appropriate nursing action would be to:

A. Request an ethics/multidisciplinary care conference to discuss communication and dissemination of the patient's medical status and review the visitation policy

B. Immediately call the hospital attorney to speak with the wife

C. Give the wife any information she wants, but do not inform the patient

D. Request the patient's physician to write a non-visitation order for the wife

73. Rebecca is a Jehovah's Witness who has just undergone a cardiac surgical procedure. Her Hgb and Hct are falling and are now 6.5 and 24. Her chest tubes have drained 1750 mL in the last 4 hours. The anticipated treatment would be to:

A. Administer 1 unit of type-specific whole blood

B. Administer 500 mL of albumin

C. Administer 250 mL of fresh frozen plasma

D. Administer continuous-circuit autotransfusion

74. The major advantage to using an internal mammary artery for cardiac bypass is:

A. Ease of harvesting

B. Postsurgical patency

C. Lowered infection rate

D. Lower rate of reperfusion rhythms

75. Your patient just underwent a percutaneous intervention for stent placement, then was returned to the ICU. You note a rash over the patient's trunk and arms. This is probably due to

A. An allergic reaction to contrast dye.

B. Petechiae from a fat emboli.

C. A reaction to the indwelling stent.

D. A rash secondary to a *Candida* infection.

76. A sign of necrosis on an EKG would include

A. Acute ST elevation.

B. A right BBB.

C. A left BBB.

D. A Q wave in Lead III.

77. Karen received 4 mg of morphine IV and now is unresponsive and her respiratory rate and depth are diminished. The antidote for morphine is:

A. Regitine

B. Bicarbonate

C. Naloxone

D. Atropine

78. **Complications associated with ventricular assist devices (VADs) include**
    A. Thromboembolism.
    B. Thrombocytopenia.
    C. Dissection of the aorta.
    D. Septicemia.

79. **Indications for use of a ventricular assist device (VAD) are:**
    A. Dysrhythmias
    B. As destination therapy
    C. Prolonged cardiac arrest
    D. Extensive organ damage

80. **The most common infection in patients with a ventricular assist device (VAD) is:**
    A. Septicemia
    B. Pericarditis
    C. Pneumonia
    D. Pericardial effusion

81. **The most commonly used type of ventricular assist device (VAD) is the:**
    A. RVAD
    B. VAD
    C. BIVAD
    D. LVAD

82. **The most common major impediment to family education regarding placement of a ventricular assist device (VAD) is:**
    A. Language
    B. Technology
    C. Time
    D. Physician availability

83. **The physician has just informed your patient that she needs an LVAD. The patient is crying and says, "I just know I am going to die. What's the point? It must be my time." The patient is obviously quite stressed. The priority for the nurse at this time is:**
    A. Tell the patient she will not die
    B. Explore possible suicidal ideation
    C. Immediately place the patient in a single room
    D. Notify the hospital's spiritual advisor

84. **Your patient has just returned from an abdominal aortic aneurysm repair. He is intubated and is somewhat restless. Vital signs are stable. The patient keeps pointing at the lumbar area of his back. This may indicate**
    A. A blister from the surgical ground pad.
    B. Need for repositioning.
    C. Irritation from the dressing.
    D. Retroperitoneal bleeding.

85. **The definitive invasive diagnostic procedure to diagnose an aortic dissection is:**
    A. A left lateral recumbent chest X ray
    B. Computerized tomography (CT) scan
    C. Transesophageal ultrasound
    D. Aortogram

86. **Which of the following statements about aortic aneurysms is true?**
    A. The mortality increases when the patient is between 25 and 35 years old.
    B. Aortic aneurysm is more common in men than in women.
    C. There are no warning signs.
    D. Aortic aneurysms are the result of aortic stenosis.

87. **An aneurysm that is dissecting upward (ascending) produces pain**
    A. In the chest and midscapular area.
    B. In the back of the neck and left shoulder.
    C. From the umbilical area to the shoulder.
    D. In the left shoulder and midsternal area.

88. **An aortic aneurysm that extends more than _____ will require surgical repair.**
    A. 3 cm
    B. 5 cm
    C. 7 cm
    D. 9 cm

89. **When an arterial aortic dissection occurs, it is usually due to weakness in which area of the artery?**
    A. Tunica intima
    B. Tunica adventicia
    C. Tunica media
    D. Tunica externa

90. **The most common area affected by aortic aneurysms is:**
    A. Aortic arch
    B. Abdominal
    C. Thoracic
    D. Lumbar

91. **Your patient has just returned from a three-vessel CABG. The mediastinal tubes are draining frank blood. The anesthesiologist orders protamine to be administered to the patient. This drug is given to counteract the effects of:**
    A. Beta blockers
    B. Catecholamines
    C. Heparin
    D. Cardiopulmonary bypass

92. **A possible complication of cardiopulmonary bypass is**
    A. Bleeding.
    B. Dysrhythmias.
    C. Hypertension.
    D. A systemic inflammatory response.

93. Your patient was admitted for pneumonia. He is 2 years post heart transplant. When you place the EKG monitoring leads, you note sinus tachycardia with PVCs and a 2-mm ST elevation. The patient denies pain. This finding is
    A. Impossible.
    B. Normal.
    C. Indicative of a RBBB.
    D. Indicative of an inferior MI.

94. The primary cause of acquired valvular heart disease is:
    A. Heredity
    B. Smoking
    C. Drug abuse
    D. Rheumatic fever

95. The patient who is status post heart transplant may have significant bradycardia. The drug of choice is:
    A. Atropine
    B. Isuproterenol
    C. Apresoline
    D. Adenosine

96. The most common precipitating cause of dissecting aneurysms is:
    A. Weakness of the vessel wall
    B. Heart failure
    C. Hypertension
    D. Atheroembolism

97. Your patient is 36 hours status post right femoral bypass graft. The patient complains of pain with even slight movement of the limb. You suspect
    A. An arterial obstruction.
    B. A DVT.
    C. A venous obstruction.
    D. A leg cramp from prolonged bed rest.

98. Terrance had a pulmonary artery catheter placed. When a wedge pressure was initially obtained, large V waves were noted and the PAOP was 27. The probable cause of this reading is:
    A. A ventricular septal defect
    B. Left heart failure
    C. Papillary muscle rupture
    D. Right heart failure

99. Your patient received streptokinase about 30 minutes ago for a lateral wall STEMI. You would expect which of the following events to occur?
    A. Lowered CPK isoenzymes
    B. Reperfusion rhythms
    C. Transient increased chest pain
    D. Mild CHF

100. A quadriplegic patient has undergone a CABG and has had no complications. You are about to teach his wife how to change the chest dressings and the graft site dressings on the patient's legs. Principles of teaching include
    A. Teaching all the information at once.
    B. Teaching the information as fast as possible.
    C. Explaining the rationale for the procedure, and then demonstrating it.
    D. Speaking slowly so the patient can hear.

101. Your patient had a cardiac arrest. You are doing CPR near his implanted ICD generator. If the ICD defibrillates, you would feel
    A. A powerful shock.
    B. Nothing.
    C. Mild tingling.
    D. A mild shock.

102. Newer ICDs use the most efficient shock waveforms for defibrillation and cardioversion. The most efficient waveform would be:
    A. Square wave technology
    B. Monophasic
    C. Fixed curve
    D. Biphasic

103. Your patient requires emergent programming of her ICD. How high should the defibrillation output level be set?
    A. 10 joules
    B. 20 joules
    C. 30 joules
    D. 40 joules

104. When you receive report on your patient, you are told his ICD was reset. You notice a large magnet on the table outside the room. What is the purpose of this magnet?
    A. It inhibits all output from the ICD.
    B. It inhibits the shocking portion only.
    C. It inhibits the pacemaker function.
    D. It allows timing of the ICD to be set.

105. Tachyarrhythmias that are refractive to conventional therapies may have to be treated with radio-frequency ablation. This treatment is usually successful on reentry tachyarrhythmias. The radio-frequency destroys myocardial tissue via:
    A. Radiation
    B. Heat
    C. Cold
    D. Over riding signal to ablate the pacemaker

106. Your patient has atrial fibrillation and needs to be cardioverted. The patient was medicated for pain and anxiety with morphine and Versed. Which additional medication will help the process of cardioversion from atrial fibrillation to a normal sinus rhythm?
    A. Digitalis
    B. Amiodarone
    C. Pronestyl
    D. Ibutilide

107. Which of the following pulmonary artery pressures would be considered normal?
    A. PAP = 38/22, PAOP = 17
    B. PAP = 16/8, PAOP = 3
    C. PAP = 24/12, PAOP = 9
    D. PAP = 36/28, PAOP = 24

108. If the PAWP shows a dampened waveform, this may be due to
    A. Overwedging.
    B. Balloon over-inflation.
    C. Balloon under-inflation.
    D. A clot.

109. A sudden change in a pulmonary artery waveform or pressure reading may be caused by
    A. A displaced catheter.
    B. Incorrect calibration.
    C. Blood on the transducer.
    D. Balloon rupture.

110. During insertion of the pulmonary catheter, your patient has a short run of V-tach and shows unifocal PVCs. Your immediate response should be to:
    A. Administer lidocaine 1 mg/kg
    B. Hang an amiodarone drip
    C. Notify the physician
    D. Have the physician completely withdraw the catheter

111. Your patient has a PAOP (PCWP) of 3. The patient is restless and mildly tachycardic. You anticipate which of the following interventions?
    A. Administer nitroprusside to decrease preload
    B. Administer volume replacement
    C. Increase afterload with a vasoconstrictor
    D. Administer an inotrope

112. Which of the following conditions would manifest with elevated pulmonary artery pressures and a normal wedge pressure?
    A. Pericarditis
    B. Pulmonary hypertension
    C. Right ventricular failure
    D. Pulmonary emboli

113. A way to assess the afterload of the left ventricle is to:
    A. Calculate the PVR and add it to the RAP
    B. Calculate the systemic vascular resistance
    C. Calculate the MAP
    D. Calculate the cardiac index

114. Gina was admitted to the CCU with cough, fever, chills, anorexia, malaise, and headache. She has a pericardial friction rub and a history of rheumatic fever. While examining Gina, you note fine, dark lines in her nail beds and some flat lesions on her palms. These flat lesions are known as:
    A. Janeway lesions
    B. Roth spots
    C. Osler's nodes
    D. Pella's sign

115. If you utilize the Fontaine classification for peripheral vascular disease, intermittent claudication occurs at
    A. Stage I.
    B. Stage II.
    C. Stage III.
    D. Stage IV.

116. Which of the following nursing actions would be important in the care of a patient with occlusive disease of the terminal aorta and a nonhealing wound on the left foot?
    A. Elevate the legs
    B. Place the patient in high Fowler's position
    C. Maintain normothermia
    D. Restrict fluids

117. In a patient with cardiogenic shock, an undesirable outcome would produce
    A. Increased cardiac output.
    B. Increased systemic vascular resistance.
    C. Decreased ventricular preload.
    D. Decreased pulmonary artery pressures.

118. Your patient required a pulmonary artery catheter placement to help monitor fluid and oxygenation. While the catheter was being inserted, blood gas samples were obtained from the right atrium (O_2 saturation 75%), from the right ventricle (92%), and from the pulmonary artery (92%). These results probably indicate
    A. Pericarditis.
    B. A ventral septal defect.
    C. A monitor or catheter malfunction.
    D. Pneumonia.

119. If your patient's temporary pacemaker is not sensing, your first action should be to
    A. Place the patient on their right side.
    B. Increase mA output.
    C. Check the sensitivity control for the proper setting.
    D. Immediately turn off the pacemaker and notify the physician.

120. **A diastolic murmur will occur as a result of regurgitant blood flow over which of the following valves?**
   A. Mitral, aortic
   B. Mitral, tricuspid
   C. Pulmonic, aortic
   D. Tricuspid, pulmonic

121. **Blood flow that moves forward through stentotic valves can also cause a diastolic murmur. The valves involved are the:**
   A. Mitral, aortic
   B. Mitral, tricuspid
   C. Pulmonic, aortic
   D. Tricuspid, pulmonic

122. **Sid is a 30-year-old motorcyclist who lost control of his motorcycle in the rain. Although Sid was wearing a helmet and protective gear, he suffered a fractured left femur, left flail chest, a cervical sprain, and road rash on his face and neck. Sid was admitted with a blood pressure of 84/44, HR 100, RR 26 and shallow, T 98.4°F. His 12-lead EKG shows ST elevation in the anterior leads. His chest X ray shows a normal cardiac silhouette and no infiltrates. His Hgb is 9.0, Hct is 32, and MB is 18%. Sid is restless and complains of pain in his chest and left leg. What condition would you anticipate?**
   A. Systolic dysfunction
   B. Hypovolemic shock
   C. Pulmonary hypertension
   D. Pulmonary edema

Use the following scenario for Questions 123 and 124.

Four days ago, Sue, age 70, was admitted to your unit status post laparotomy for an unknown abdominal mass. During the surgery, she had minimal blood loss and an uneventful course. Her history includes smoking since she was 15 (unknown number of packs per day), Type II diabetes, a permanent pacemaker, an anterior MI, and a right-sided stroke 20 years ago with no deficits.

Three days ago, Sue had a hypotensive episode. Her BP dropped to 82/48 and her heart rate was 70. The hospitalist ordered dobutamine, and Sue's blood pressure increased until the MAP was 72.

Today, Sue remains on dobutamine at 4 μg/kg/min, the BP is 108/60, MAP is 76, and the heart rate is 70. Attempts at weaning dobutamine have failed: Sue's blood pressure drops precipitously if the dobutamine dose is lowered.

123. **What do you think is the cause of Sue's initial hypotensive episode?**
   A. Hypovolemic shock
   B. Previous MI
   C. Rapid rewarming postoperatively
   D. Cell-mediated response

124. **What additional action could be taken to improve Sue's cardiac output and help wean her from the dobutamine?**
    A. Initiate a fluid challenge
    B. Start dopamine
    C. Place a pulmonary artery catheter
    D. Increase the rate on the pacemaker

125. **What does the acronym AICD stand for?**
    A. Automated internal cardiac defibrillator
    B. Autocardiac internal converting defibrillator
    C. Automated implantable cardioverter/defibrillator
    D. Automatic implanted coronary defibrillator

126. **Fred has had an AICD for 6 months. He has been admitted to the ICU for syncope. You notice his pulse is very irregular and he is complaining of getting "zapped" often. On his monitor, the rhythm is sinus bradycardia with numerous pacemaker spikes. What could be wrong?**
    A. Fred's AICD has a faulty lead.
    B. Fred has had a myocardial infarction.
    C. The battery in Fred's AICD is losing power.
    D. Fred has a generator failure of his AICD.

127. **Which physical finding is significant for carotid stenosis?**
    A. Heberden's nodules
    B. Systolic murmur, Grade IV/VI
    C. Carotid bruit
    D. Broussard's nodules

128. **Barry has Wolf-Parkinson-White Syndrome. He is having increasing bouts of tachycardia. It has been decided to utilize overdrive pacing to correct this problem. How do you explain this type of pacemaker to a new orientee?**
    A. The pacemaker or AICD is set at a constant rate of 70 bpm and is synchronized.
    B. The pacemaker or AICD is set on demand mode and is asynchronous.
    C. The pacemaker or AICD is set on demand mode and is synchronous.
    D. The pacemaker or AICD is set on inhibit mode and is synchronous.

129. **Which pacemaker/AICD program code would you expect for a patient with complete heart block?**
    A. VVI
    B. DDD
    C. VVT
    D. DDI

130. **Gene had a DDD pacemaker inserted 3 years ago. He has been admitted for pacemaker syndrome. What symptoms do you expect to see?**
    A. Fatigue, agitation, dyspnea
    B. Fatigue, dizziness, confusion
    C. Fatigue, agitation, forgetfulness
    D. Fatigue, dizziness, syncope

131. **Tina, a 44-year-old with an acute myocardial infarction, suddenly develops complete heart block. Her blood pressure drops, her heart rate falls to 27, and her color ashen. What should you do?**
    A. Apply an external pacemaker, medicate the patient, and notify the physician.
    B. Wait for the physician to return your call and give atropine 4 mg intravenously.
    C. Apply a transvenous pacemaker, medicate the patient, then notify the physician.
    D. Call a Code Blue and prepare to start CPR.

132. **Your acute myocardial infarction patient waited for 16 hours before coming to the hospital. He has a right bundle branch block and a left anterior fascicular block. What is the significance of this?**
    A. He has extensive myocardial damage.
    B. He needs a pacemaker as soon as possible.
    C. He needs to be transferred to a facility that can perform a heart transplant.
    D. This problem will resolve itself over the next few weeks.

133. **Ted has had an anterolateral myocardial infarction. Where do you expect to see changes on the 12-lead EKG?**
    A. V_1, V_2, I, AVL
    B. V_2, V_3, V_4, I, AVL
    C. V_2, V_3, V_4, II, III, AVF
    D. V_1, V_2, II, III, AVF

134. **What do abnormal Q waves signify on a 12-lead EKG?**
    A. They are of no significance.
    B. Repolarization of the myocardium
    C. Complete-thickness infarction of myocardium
    D. Partial-thickness death of myocardium

135. **Marge has had an inferior wall MI. Where do you expect to see the changes on her 12-lead EKG?**
    A. II, III, AVF
    B. I, II, AVL
    C. I, III, AVF
    D. V_1, V_2

136. **Your patient has had an anteroseptal MI. Where do you expect to see changes on the 12-lead EKG?**
    A. V_1, V_2, V_3, V_4
    B. V_2, V_3, V_4, V_5, V_6
    C. V_1, V_2, II, III, AVF
    D. V_1, V_2, I, AVL

137. **What is measured by the vertical lines on the EKG paper?**
    A. Velocity
    B. Time
    C. Voltage
    D. Intensity

138. **What is measured by the horizontal lines on the EKG paper?**
    A. Velocity
    B. Time
    C. Voltage
    D. Intensity

139. **V_1 and V_2 leads show which type of bundle branch block?**
    A. Right bundle branch block
    B. Left bundle branch block
    C. Dual bundle branch block
    D. V_1 and V_2 leads do not show bundle branch blocks.

140. **What are the most valuable pieces of information evaluated with a 12-lead EKG?**
    A. Rate, arrhythmias, infarction
    B. Rate, rhythm, axis, hypertrophy, infarction
    C. Rate, bundle branch block, hypertrophy
    D. Rate, rhythm, arrhythmias

141. **Which of the following conditions are associated with ST-T wave abnormalities?**
    A. Ventricular hypertrophy, pericarditis, COPD
    B. COPD, axis deviation
    C. Atrial hypertrophy, axis deviation
    D. Pericarditis, axis deviation

142. **12-lead EKG changes that would you expect in a patient with COPD would include**
    A. Low-voltage P waves and tachycardia.
    B. Tall P waves and left ventricular hypertrophy.
    C. Tall, peaked P waves, right ventricular hypertrophy, and low-voltage QRS.
    D. Low-voltage QRS and left atrial hypertrophy.

143. **What are some common reasons for pacemaker insertion?**
    A. Tachycardia, Wenkebach, bradycardia
    B. Symptomatic bradycardia, overdrive pacing, acute MI with sinus dysfunction
    C. Complete heart block, Wenkebach, tachycardia
    D. Bundle branch block, Wenkebach, tachycardia

144. **Quinidine and hypomagnesemia can both lead to**
    A. Torsades de pointe.
    B. Ventricular tachycardia.
    C. Ventricular fibrillation.
    D. Atrial tachycardia.

145. **What is required for a diagnosis of hospital-acquired pneumonia (HAP)?**
    A. Recent common cold prior to admission
    B. Cigarette smoking
    C. Acute myocardial infarction
    D. Hospitalization for more than 2 days

146. **What is the most common causative organism in hospital-acquired pneumonia (HAP)?**
    A. Methicillin-Resistant *Staphylococcus aureus* (MRSA)
    B. *Pseudomonas aeruginosa*
    C. *Streptococcus pneumoniae*
    D. *Acinetobacter* species

147. **What are some risk factors for developing hospital-acquired pneumonia (HAP)?**
    A. Altered level of consciousness, urinary catheter, sedation
    B. COPD, ill hospital staff, beta blockers
    C. H_2 blockers, age, history of smoking
    D. H_2 blockers, postpartum patient, age

148. **Millie is a 78-year-old patient admitted to ICU postoperatively 2 days ago after a colon resection for cancer. She has a nasogastric tube through which she is receiving routine doses of antacids. Her morning labs are: WBCs 14.8, neutrophils 9,600. Her chest X ray is inconclusive. What is Millie's problem?**
    A. Pulmonary embolism
    B. Hospital-acquired pneumonia
    C. Congestive heart failure
    D. Atelectasis

149. **How does hospital-acquired pneumonia (HAP) differ from ventilator-acquired pneumonia (VAP)?**
    A. There is no difference.
    B. HAP and VAP result from infection with different causative organisms.
    C. The main difference is that the VAP patient is intubated.
    D. Therapies differ.

150. **What does SVO_2 measure?**
    A. Oxygen saturation of the blood in the brachial vein
    B. Oxygen saturation of the blood returning to the lungs
    C. Oxygen saturation of the blood in the coronary sinus
    D. Oxygen saturation in the capillary bed

151. **Ben, a victim of a gunshot wound to his left chest, has a pneumo-hemothorax. His saturations are decreasing. The physician orders mixed venous gases, and the results show an SVO_2. What does this information tell you about the patient's condition?**
    A. How much shunting is occurring
    B. CO_2 levels
    C. HCO_3 levels
    D. PO_2 level

152. **Continuing the scenario from Question 151, later that day Ben's SVO_2 is 22%. What does this indicate about his condition?**
    A. It is a normal reading.
    B. His shunt is improving.
    C. His shunt is worsening.
    D. His shunt is stable.

153. **Promethazine is contraindicated with fluoroquinolone antibiotics because**
     A. It produces increased sedation.
     B. This combination leads to QT prolongation and arrhythmias.
     C. Promethazine is inactivated.
     D. Fluoroquinolone is inactivated.

154. **What is the infusion rate for Lasix (furosemide)?**
     A. It may be given intravenous push at any dose.
     B. 4 mg/minute
     C. 1 mg/minute
     D. It should always be given as a piggyback.

155. **Why is Lasix given slowly?**
     A. Rapid infusion can cause nausea.
     B. Rapid infusion can cause rash.
     C. Rapid infusion can cause hyperkalemia.
     D. Rapid infusion can lead to hearing loss.

156. **Your patient has had an angiogram today with stent placement. He is to start Plavix. You are teaching him about this medication when you learn he takes numerous herbal remedies daily. Which ones should he avoid while he is taking Plavix?**
     A. Dong quai, gingko biloba, saw palmetto
     B. Aloe extract, bilberry
     C. Calendula, clove
     D. Fenugreek, licorice

157. **What history should you know before starting an infusion of Reo Pro (abciximab)?**
     A. Chest pain
     B. Any bleeding history
     C. Previous myocardial infarction
     D. Family history

158. **Warfarin is indicated for which of the following conditions?**
     A. DVT, CHF, atrial fibrillation
     B. DVT, atrial fibrillation, heart valve replacement
     C. Pulmonary embolism, DVT, COPD
     D. Pulmonary embolism, atrial fibrillation, CHF

159. **You are teaching Anne about her Coumadin (warfarin) therapy. Part of your teaching must include foods to avoid. Which of the following foods should be avoided?**
     A. Broccoli, soybean oil, spinach
     B. Olive oil, peanut butter, kale
     C. Avocado, broccoli, peas
     D. Broccoli, green beans, spinach

160. **Integrilin (eptifbatide) is indicated for which of the following conditions?**
     A. A patient with a DVT
     B. A patient with a pulmonary embolism
     C. A patient with acute coronary syndrome (ACS)
     D. A patient with an occlusive cerebrovascular accident

161. Javier is a 30-year-old patient with a history of Type II diabetes. He was admitted for multiple syncopal episodes, dyspnea, and tachycardia. A pulmonary artery catheter was placed and the following pressures obtained: wedge pressure (PAOP) of 20 mm Hg, pulmonary artery pressure of 52/22 mm Hg, and a right atrial pressure (RAP) of 4 mm Hg. Likely diagnostic possibilities include all the following *except*
    A. Pulmonary embolism.
    B. Aortic stenosis.
    C. Mitral regurgitation.
    D. Aortic insufficiency.

162. Pete had a pulmonary artery catheter placed because he was being evaluated for lung function. His initial readings show a wedge pressure of 7 mm Hg, pulmonary artery pressure of 40/12 mm Hg, and right atrial pressure of 19 mm Hg. The cardiac index is 2.0 L/min/m². These results would indicate all of the following possibilities *except*
    A. Right ventricular infarct.
    B. LAD obstruction.
    C. Pulmonary stenosis.
    D. Right ventricular dysfunction.

163. Edward had a four-vessel coronary bypass and was admitted to the CVICU about an hour ago. On admission, he was borderline ST with PVCs, for which he is receiving potassium replacement, arterial line BP 116/70 mm Hg, cuff correlated, PAD 12 mm Hg, RAP 6 mm Hg. Now, Edward's mediastinal tubes have ceased draining, the PAOP has increased to 20 mm Hg, and the RAP is now 14 mm Hg. His heat rate is 92 with isolated PVCs, and the arterial line BP is 124/72. The changes in his cardiac index are negligible. The most likely cause of these changes is:
    A. An increase in auto PEEP
    B. Pericardial tamponade
    C. Transducer change in position/level
    D. A tension pneumothorax

164. Pulmonary artery wedge pressure should be measured at which point in the respiratory cycle?
    A. At the end of inspiration
    B. At the midpoint between inspiration and expiration
    C. At the end of expiration
    D. There are no criteria for this measurement.

165. You are attempting to use a pulmonary artery wedge pressure (PCWP) to estimate the LVEDP. Which of the following conditions might make this measurement more difficult?
    A. Heart rate of 150
    B. Aortic stenosis
    C. Mitral regurgitation
    D. Tricuspid regurgitation

166. Roger was initially admitted to your MICU with a diagnosis of congestive heart failure. After further study, it was determined that he has restrictive cardiomyopathy. A common cause of restrictive cardiomyopathy is:
    A. Unknown
    B. Glycogen storage disease
    C. History of diabetes
    D. Viral infection

167. The type of cardiomyopathy that is characterized by replacement of normal cells by fatty tissue is known as:
    A. Hypertrophic
    B. Dilated
    C. Arrhythmogenic
    D. Restrictive

168. Which of the following hemodynamic effects would be seen in a patient with hypertrophic cardiomyopathy?
    A. Decreased CO, decreased ejection fraction
    B. Normal CO, increased ejection fraction
    C. Increased CO, increased ejection fraction
    D. Decreased CO, increased ejection fraction

169. Dilated cardiomyopathy is characterized by dilation of the ventricles and impaired systolic function. Common causes are valvular heart disease and ischemic heart disease; other causes are idiopathic. The most common cause of idiopathic dilated cardiomyopathy is:
    A. Alcohol
    B. Familial
    C. Genetic
    D. Autoimmune

170. Peripartum cardiomyopathy is a form of
    A. Restrictive cardiomyopathy.
    B. Hypertrophic cardiomyopathy.
    C. Viral cardiomyopathy.
    D. Dilated cardiomyopathy.

171. Your patient was admitted for ascites, orthopnea, paroxysmal nocturnal dyspnea, and excessive fatigue. On physical examination, you note S_3 and S_4 gallops, and basilar crackles. The EKG shows sinus tachycardia. These symptoms are usually indicative of which of the following types of cardiomyopathy?
    A. Dilated
    B. Restrictive
    C. Alcohol induced
    D. Hypertrophic

172. The most common new-onset dysrhythmias seen in a patient with pulmonary edema is:
    A. Supraventricular tachycardia
    B. RBBB
    C. Ventricular tachycardia
    D. Atrial fibrillation

173. Your patient will be having an LVAD placed this evening and will be cared for in your unit. Family members are quite anxious to learn more about the device and to participate in the patient's care. An important point when teaching caregivers is to make certain they understand what changes in the patient's condition should be reported immediately to the staff. A complication that should be reported immediately would be:
    A. Irritation or redness at the incision
    B. A temperature of 99.6°F
    C. Any change in the mentation of the patient
    D. A rise in blood pressure greater than 10 mm Hg

174. A 46-year-old construction worker was seen in the ED after falling into a trench. He sustained a left fractured tibia and fibula and a fractured left scapula. He required a splenectomy and was just admitted to your care. Your initial assessment results are as follows:
    EKG: ST at 126 with isolated PVC
    Arterial line BP: 84/50 mm Hg; cuff BP: 88/50 mm Hg
    Skin pale, cool, clammy
    RR 26, breath sounds clear, slightly diminished RLL
    O_2 2 L/min via NC
    Mentation: responds to questions slowly, oriented to self and time
    Pulmonary artery catheter readings: PAP 22/8, PAOP 6, RAP 4
    Cardiac Output: 3.2
    Cardiac Index: 1.4

    Which of the following conditions do you believe this patient is developing?
    A. Cardiogenic shock
    B. Hypovolemic shock
    C. Septic shock
    D. Left ventricular failure

175. James is a 60-year-old night watchman. When he returned home from work this morning, he was short of breath and overly fatigued. His wife mentioned that his ankles were quite swollen. James went to bed and, when his wife could not arouse him, she called paramedics. James arrived in your MICU about 30 minutes ago. He is being mechanically ventilated at TV 700, FiO_2 0.80, AMV 14. He remains unresponsive. A pulmonary artery catheter was placed. His assessment findings are as follows:
    EKG: ST at 108
    Arterial line BP: 68/42 mm Hg; cuff BP: 64/46 mm Hg
    Skin pale, cool, clammy

Doppler-only dorsalis pedis

RR 15, breath sounds = crackles LLL, RLL

Marked pretibial edema

Mentation: unresponsive to painful stimuli

Pulmonary artery catheter readings: PAP 46/28, PAOP 26, RAP 18

Cardiac Output: 3.2

Cardiac Index: 1.2

James is probably developing?
   A. Right heart failure
   B. Pulmonary hypertension
   C. Cardiogenic shock
   D. Pulmonary effusion

176. **Continuing with the scenario from Question 175, which of the following medications would you anticipate using to improve James' current condition?**
   A. Dobutamine
   B. Epinephrine
   C. Diltiazem
   D. Isoproterenol

177. **Yesterday, Frank was shoveling snow when he became short of breath and felt diffuse chest discomfort. He went inside for lunch and the pain disappeared. Frank resumed shoveling snow and felt more fatigued than ever. Today, Frank was admitted to your unit with orthopnea and profound dyspnea. He is constantly saying, "I'm 56 years old and have been outside all my life. I'm not sick enough to be in here." His girlfriend reports that over the past 3 weeks Frank has been more tired than usual, even when performing small tasks around the house. Frank agreed to placement of a pulmonary artery catheter, and the following information was obtained:**

EKG: Borderline ST at 100 with rare PACs

Cuff BP: 142/74 mm Hg

Skin warm, pale; capillary refill 4 seconds; 2+ pitting edema (pretibial)

RR 20; breath sounds: crackles in posterior lobes

O_2 2 L/min via NC

ABGs: drawn, but results are unavailable

Mentation: alert, oriented $\times$ 4

Pulmonary artery catheter readings: PAP 40/20, PAOP 20, RAP 5

Cardiac Output: 3.6

Cardiac Index: 2.0

Frank probably has developed?
   A. A mild pericarditis
   B. Pulmonary edema (noncardiac)
   C. Chylothorax
   D. Left ventricular failure

178. Erin is 63 years old and has a history of COPD. Today, she was admitted with an inferior wall MI. About 30 minutes ago, she complained of increasing shortness of breath. When she changed her position, the dyspnea abated. Now she is again complaining of dyspnea. You perform a 12-lead EKG because your unit monitor allows monitoring of only leads II and MCL_1. The EKG shows lead V_1–V_4 ST-segment depression. Other physical and laboratory findings are as follows:

EKG: Sinus arrhythmia at 97

Cuff BP: 104/70 mm Hg

Skin pale, cool, clammy; sacral edema, pedal and pretibial edema

RR 20; breath sounds: bilateral crackles

O_2 2 L/min via NC

ABGs: pH 7.38, pCO_2 48, paO_2 66, HCO_3 34

Mentation: alert, oriented $\times$ 4

Pulmonary artery catheter readings: PAP 46/26, PAOP 24, RAP 13

Cardiac Output: 3.2

Cardiac Index: 2.1

What is the interpretation of the ABGs?
   A. Uncompensated metabolic acidosis
   B. Compensated respiratory acidosis
   C. Uncompensated metabolic alkalosis
   D. Compensated respiratory alkalosis

179. Continuing with the scenario from Question 178, Erin is probably developing
   A. Pulmonary effusion.
   B. Left ventricular failure.
   C. Pericarditis.
   D. Congestive heart failure.

180. What is the normal value for the right ventricular end diastolic pressure?
   A. 2–8 mm Hg
   B. 6–12 mm Hg
   C. 12–20 mm Hg
   D. 18–24 mm Hg

181. Changes in which of the following leads will identify a lateral MI?
   A. II, III, aVF
   B. V_1–V_4
   C. V_2–V_6
   D. I, aVL, V_5, V_6

182. Aaron was admitted to your unit about 6 hours ago with an inferior MI. He has been medicated for pain and is resting comfortably at this time. His wife is visiting. She approaches you and says Aaron is dizzy and cannot catch his breath. His EKG now shows a sinus bradycardia with multifocal PVCs at 4 per minute. Other findings are as follows:

EKG: sinus bradycardia at 52 with rare multifocal PVCs

Cuff BP: 86/48 mm Hg

Skin pale, cool, clammy

Previous BP: 108/72 mm Hg

RR 28, O_2 2 L/min via NC

Mentation: anxious, oriented $\times$ 4

Aaron's current arrhythmia will probably be

    A. Permanent and asymptomatic.

    B. Transient and possibly symptomatic.

    C. Permanent and symptomatic.

    D. Transient and asymptomatic.

183. **Joanne had a VVI pacemaker inserted. What does the first "V" in this acronym stand for?**

    A. Paced, ventricular

    B. Paced, inhibited

    C. Ventricular inhibited

    D. Ventricular

184. **Continuing with the scenario from Question 183, what does the second "V" in the acronym for Joanne's pacemaker stand for?**

    A. Ventricular paced

    B. Ventricular inhibited

    C. Ventricular sensed

    D. Ventricular programmed

185. **Josephine is 71 years old. She was alert and active last evening, but was found this morning sitting in her kitchen, hardly able to move. At first, it was thought she had suffered a stroke, but she was admitted because her EKG showed large R waves in leads V_1 and V_2. A pulmonary artery catheter was placed without incident. Physical parameters are as follows:**

EKG: SR at 92, no ectopy

Cuff BP: 94/62 mm Hg

Skin pale, cool, clammy

RR 18; breath sounds: clear, slightly diminished LLL

O_2 2 L/min via NC

Moderate jugular venous distention, no bruits

Mentation: lethargic

Pulmonary artery catheter readings: PAP 26/12, PAOP 10, RAP 18

Cardiac Output: 4.8

Cardiac Index: 2.5

An expected diagnosis for Josephine would be:

    A. Aortic insufficiency

    B. LV hypertrophy

    C. RV infarction

    D. Pericarditis

186. **Nitroprusside has which of the following sets of hemodynamic effects?**

	HR	MAP	CVP	SVR	CO
A.	↑	↓	↓	↓	↑
B.	↑	↑	↓	↓	↑
C.	↓	↑	↓	↓	↓
D.	↓	↑	↑	↓	↑

187. **Epinephrine has which of the following sets of hemodynamic effects?**

	HR	MAP	CVP	SVR	CO
A.	↑	↓	↑	↓	↑
B.	↑/↓	↓	↑	↓	↑
C.	↑	↑	↑	↑/↓	↑
D.	↑/↓	↑	↓	↑	↑

188. **Phenylephrine has which of the following sets of hemodynamic effects?**

	HR	MAP	CVP	SVR	CO
A.	↓	↓	↓	↑	↑/↓
B.	0/↓	↑	↑	↑	↑/↓
C.	↑/↓	↓	↓	↑	↓
D.	↑	↑	↓	↓	↓

189. Digoxin has which of the following sets of hemodynamic effects?

	HR	MAP	CVP	SVR	CO
A.	↑/↓	↑	↓	↓	↑
B.	↓	0	0/↓	↑	↑
C.	↑/↓	↓	↑	↑	↑
D.	↓	↓	↓	↓	↓

190. Lidocaine has which of the following sets of hemodynamic effects?

	HR	MAP	CVP	SVR	CO
A.	↑	↓	↓	↑/↓	0
B.	↑	↑	↑	↓	↓
C.	↓	↓	↓	↓	↑/↓
D.	0	0/↓	0	0/↓	0/↑

191. Dobutamine has which of the following sets of hemodynamic effects?

	HR	MAP	CVP	SVR	CO
A.	0/↑	0/↑	0/↓	0/↓	↑
B.	↑	↑	↑	↑	↑
C.	↓	↑	↓	↑	↑
D.	↑	0/↓	↓	0/↓	↑

192. Dopamine has which of the following sets of hemodynamic effects?

	HR	MAP	CVP	SVR	CO
A.	↑	↓	↓	0/↑	↓
B.	0/↑	0/↑	0/↑	0/↑	↑
C.	↑	↑/↓	↑	0/↓	↑
D.	↑/↓	↑	↑	↑/↓	↓

193. Milrinone has which of the following sets of hemodynamic effects?

	HR	MAP	CVP	SVR	CO
A.	↑	↑	↓	↑	↑
B.	↑/↓	↑	↓	↑	↓
C.	0/↑	↓	0/↓	↓	↑
D.	↑	↓	↑/↓	↓	↓

194. Roy was working on his roof yesterday when he slipped and fell, impaling himself on a wooden fencepost. The post was removed, and Roy is now in your SICU.
Today, you note the following parameters and symptoms:
EKG: ST at 120 without ectopy
Arterial line BP: 92/60 mm Hg; cuff BP 90/64 mm Hg
Skin warm, dry; capillary refill 2 seconds
RR 22; breath sounds: clear
O_2 3 L/min via NC
Temperature: 100.8°F
Mentation: Alert, oriented × 4
Pulmonary artery catheter readings: PAP 20/8, PAOP 6, RAP 3, SVR 820
Cardiac Output: 7.6
Cardiac Index: 4.0

Roy is probably developing?
   A. A pericardial tamponade
   B. Left heart failure
   C. Distributive shock
   D. Septic shock

195. Susan was flying cross country and ate the snack the airline provided. After about 5 minutes, she began to wheeze and her respirations became labored. A physician on board administered epinephrine, and the symptoms abated. The physician did not explain the reason for the reaction to Susan. Two days later, Susan was sharing some of her snack mix with her nephew and again began wheezing. She became severely tachypneic and was transported to the ED. She required treatment with epinephrine and steroids. She was intubated and sent to your unit. Susan is 8 months pregnant. She is currently exhibiting the following signs and symptoms:

    EKG: ST at 128 without ectopy

    Cuff BP: 88/58 mm Hg

    Skin cool, pale; capillary refill 4 seconds

    Ventilator settings: AMV 14, TV 650, FiO_2 100%

    RR 30

    Temperature: 99.4°F (rectal)

    Mentation: awake, restless

    Pulmonary artery catheter readings: PAP 34/18, PAOP 16, RAP 8, SVR 816

    Cardiac Output: 3.2

    Cardiac Index: 2.0

    Susan is probably developing?
     A. Anaphylactic shock
     B. Cardiogenic shock
     C. Hypovolemic shock
     D. Distributive shock

196. Luigi is a 70-year-old who was admitted following a two-vessel coronary artery bypass graft and mitral valve replacement. He now complains of upper left anterior chest pain and is becoming dyspneic. During the past hour, his mediastinal tubes have drained 30 cc. Luigi has the following vital signs and parameters:

    EKG: ST at 126 without ectopy

    Heart sounds somewhat muffled, no shift in PMI

    Arterial line BP: 82/50 mm Hg; cuff BP: 84/50 mm Hg

    Skin pale, cool, clammy

    RR 26, breath sounds: diminished

    O_2 2 L/min via NC

    BSA: 1.9

    Mentation: alert, oriented × 4

    Pulmonary artery catheter readings: PAP 30/22, PAOP 20, RAP 20

    Cardiac Output: 3.2

    Cardiac Index: not calculated

    Which of the following conditions does Luigi probably have?
     A. Left ventricular failure
     B. Pericardial tamponade
     C. Right ventricular failure
     D. Pericarditis

197. Continuing with the scenario from Question 196, calculate the mean arterial pressure for Luigi.
    A. 60
    B. 66
    C. 132
    D. 40

198. Continuing with the scenario from Question 196, calculate the cardiac index for Luigi.
    A. 2.5
    B. 1.7
    C. 2.9
    D. 1.9

199. Your patient is a 45-year-old ironworker. He was admitted for cardiomyopathy. His initial ejection fraction was 21%, and the patient has been confused most of the time since his admission yesterday. On admission, his EKG showed ST depression in leads V_1–V_4. He has since become more dyspneic and is getting restless. Current vital signs and parameters are as follows:

    EKG: ST at 116

    Arterial line BP: 110/64 mm Hg; cuff BP: 102/70 mm Hg

    Skin pale, cool; bilateral pretibial and pedal edema, sacral edema

    Temperature: 99°F

    RR 30; breath sounds: clear, slightly diminished RLL

    O_2 4 L/min via mask

    Mentation: oriented to self, confused at times

    Pulmonary artery catheter readings: PAP 50/22, PAOP 20, RAP 16

    Cardiac Output: 3.4

    Cardiac Index: 2.2

    What condition does this patient appear to be suffering from at this time?
    A. An anterior MI
    B. Inferior wall MI
    C. Biventricular failure
    D. Right ventricular failure

200. Sandra is a 54-year-old who has a long time history of primary pulmonary hypertension and has been getting more exercise intolerant the past 2 months. Her vital signs and other parameters are as follows:

    EKG: ST at 116; 4-mm R wave in V_1, V_2; 4-mm S wave in V_1

    Cuff BP: 140/80 mm Hg

    Skin pale, cool; bilateral pretibial and pedal edema, sacral edema

    Temperature: 98.3°F

    RR 26; breath sounds: diminished crackles throughout

    O_2 4 L/min via mask

    Mentation: oriented × 4

    Pulmonary artery catheter readings: PAP 68/40, PAOP 16, RAP 24

    Cardiac Output: 3.4

    Cardiac Index: 2.7

Which of the following conditions is Sandra probably developing?
   A. Pulmonary edema
   B. Atrial septal defect
   C. Right ventricular hypertrophy
   D. Dilated cardiomyopathy

201. Yolanda is 53 years old and was admitted to your unit directly from the cardiac catheterization lab. She required an emergency angioplasty of the right coronary artery. She now has an intra-aortic balloon pump in place, with the augmentation currently set at 1:2. The balloon inflation point is appropriate, the dressing is dry with old bloody drainage, and a small hematoma is noted at the balloon insertion site. Yolanda has an uneventful night and was medicated once for a headache. She was easily weaned from the IABP this morning. Her BP is 138/76 mm Hg, and her cardiac output is 4.8. She was medicated again about an hour ago with Tylenol #3 (acetaminophen + codeine 30 mg). Yolanda's headache is probably due to?
   A. The contrast dye used for the procedure
   B. The augmented blood pressure
   C. Pain from the procedure
   D. An intracerebral bleed

202. Daniel was involved in a gang fight last week, during which he was stabbed several times in the anterior chest and twice in the abdomen. He has undergone 2 surgeries and is now recovering from a splenectomy, small bowel repair, and repair of a small laceration to the left subclavian artery. Daniel has received multiple units of blood and blood products. He was extubated this morning, but now complains of increasing shortness of breath. He is easily fatigued and his pulse oximeter is reading 0.94, down from 0.97. His morning chest X ray shows "bilateral widespread infiltrates." Other lab results and parameters are as follows:

EKG: ST at 114, isolated PACs

Arterial line BP: 118/76 mm Hg; cuff BP: 114/76 mm Hg

Skin warm

Temperature: 101°F

RR 30; breath sounds: clear, slightly diminished RLL

O_2 4 L/min via mask

ABGs: pH 7.32, $PaCO_2$ 29, paO_2 70, HCO_3 19

Mentation: oriented × 4 most of time, two episodes of confusion, easily reoriented

Pulmonary artery catheter readings: PAP 19/8, PAOP 6, RAP 5

Cardiac Output: 7.2

Cardiac Index: 3.8

Which condition do you believe Daniel is developing?
   A. ARDS
   B. Pneumonia
   C. Pulmonary emboli
   D. Sepsis

203. Continuing the scenario from Question 202 and based on your findings, which treatment do you anticipate for Daniel?
    A. Placement on a ventilator with PEEP
    B. Anticoagulant therapy
    C. Antibiotics with goal-directed therapy
    D. An immediate V/Q scan

204. Some patients require the use of nitroprusside and dobutamine at the same time. What is the desired effect of this combination?
    A. Decreased preload and afterload
    B. Increased preload and afterload
    C. Decreased SVR, increased contractility
    D. Increased SVR, decreased contractility

This concludes the Cardiovascular questions.

ANSWERS

1. **Correct Answer: B**

   Normal cardiac output should be 4 to 8 L/min. The formula for calculating this value is CO = HR × SV.

2. **Correct Answer: B**

   Atrial kick is a term that represents the amount of the total cardiac output that is supplied via atrial contraction. If the patient has a condition or dysrhythmia that impairs or eliminates the atrial contraction, the patient may be compromised.

3. **Correct Answer: A**

   The ejection fraction should be over 50%. This is the amount of blood ejected from the left ventricle compared to the total amount available. This amount is expressed as a percentage. For example, if the ventricle contains 90 mL of blood and 50 mL is ejected, the amount would be represented as a percentage—in this case, 55%. An ejection fraction of 35% or less indicates a problem with contractility, outflow, or filling.

4. **Correct Answer: D**

   EF and LVEDP (left ventricular end diastolic pressure) are closely related. The LVEDP is the volume of blood left at the end of the contraction.

5. **Correct Answer: C**

   Answer A are the components of afterload. Answers B and D are mixed components of cardiac output.

6. **Correct Answer: D**

   It is believed that the Bainbridge reflex exists to speed up the heart rate if the right side becomes overloaded and helps to equalize pressures in both sides.

7. **Correct Answer: B**

   Some people believe that the heart is virtually static during diastole. During this period, the cardiac vessels and chambers fill with blood.

8. **Correct Answer: A**

   The MAP (mean arterial pressure) takes into account that the diastolic phase of the cardiac cycle comprises two-thirds of the cycle. The calculation for the MAP is MAP = 2(DBP) + (SBP)/3. If you took the average of the two pressures, it would not account for the importance of the diastolic phase. The heart rate is not entered into this calculation. Patients should maintain a MAP of at least 60 mm Hg to ensure adequate perfusion of the brain and kidneys.

9. **Correct Answer: C**

   The CI is a more specific indicator of hemodynamic status. The CO has a broad range of 4–8 L/min. To make the numbers specific to an individual, body surface area is entered in the equation. Then the normal range becomes 2.5–4.5 L/min/m^2. To determine the cardiac index, you must first calculate the cardiac output (CO). Then, use the following equation: CI = CO/BSA.

10. **Correct Answer: D**
This pressure represents a mean pressure in the pulmonary vasculature that is divided by the blood flow. Normal range is 100–200 dynes/sec/cm^{-5}.

11. **Correct Answer: C**
When the balloon of a pulmonary artery catheter is inflated, it eventually "wedges" in the pulmonary artery. The turbulence behind it is blocked, and it senses what is in front of it: the pulmonary vascular bed and left side of the heart. This pressure was formerly known as PAWP (pulmonary artery wedge pressure); it is now known as PAOP (pulmonary artery occlusive pressure) or sometimes PCWP (pulmonary capillary wedge pressure). The normal value should be 5–12 mm Hg.

12. **Correct Answer: B**
Answer B represents the normal range of values.

13. **Correct Answer: A**
This is the resistance the left ventricle must pump against. The normal value is 900–1400 dynes/sec/cm^{-5}.

14. **Correct Answer: D**
S_1 and S_2 are normal sounds. S_3 is associated with fluid status. S_4 is associated with compliance.

15. **Correct Answer: C**
This is the best lead to monitor for RBBB and should definitely be used when inserting a pulmonary artery catheter.

16. **Correct Answer: C**
The PR interval may become prolonged. If the potassium level is above 8, a wide-complex tachycardia may result. Keep in mind that low levels of calcium or sodium may potentiate the cardiac effects. A low pH may also potentiate the cardiac effects.

17. **Correct Answer: B**
Vecuronium is a paralytic and will prevent shivering. If the patient shivers, his or her temperature will rise.

18. **Correct Answer: D**
Myocarditis can also present with inspiratory pain. Pain when supine is a cardinal sign of myocarditis. Other findings can include symptoms that are consistent with a respiratory infection, S_3, S_4, and a possible pericardial friction rub.

19. **Correct Answer: A**
This is the only definitive way to diagnose myocarditis.

20. **Correct Answer: B**
Although this amount may be small, the pressure in the intrapericardial space may equal or exceed atrial and ventricular diastolic pressures, causing an acute tamponade.

21. **Correct Answer: D**
Tachycardia is an early sign of tamponade. A narrowed pulse pressure occurs and fluid cannot be ejected from the heart. The muffled heart sounds occur because the fluid in the sac minimizes the transmission of sound waves.

22. **Correct Answer: B**
Because the heart cannot adequately fill or eject its contents adequately, stroke volume decreases and causes a decreased cardiac output. Contractility decreases because the muscle cannot adequately stretch and, therefore, will not be able to contract effectively.

23. **Correct Answer: A**
The vena cava is dilated because blood cannot empty into the right atrium. JVD would not be visible on a chest X ray. The mediastinum would be widened. The chest X ray will not show delineation of the pericardium or epicardium.

24. **Correct Answer: D**
The large A waves will been seen with increased pressure during atrial contraction. This wave form could be caused by mitral stenosis, an ischemic left ventricle, or failure of a left ventricle.

25. **Correct Answer: C**
Quincke's sign is elicited by pressing down on the fingertip and observing a visible pulsation in the nail bed. This effect results from a rapid initial hard pulsation followed by a sudden collapse as blood flows back through an incompetent valve.

26. **Correct Answer: B**
Hill's sign reflects a rapid rise in pulsation. DeMusset's sign is also found in aortic insufficiency and is demonstrated by the bobbing of the head in time with the forceful pulse. Answers C and D are not diagnostic signs.

27. **Correct Answer: D**
Treadmill stress testing may miss as much as 40% of single-vessel disease. LV dysfunction may be diagnosed via a thallium test (myocardial scintigraphy). A positive treadmill test may not be positive for CAD.

28. **Correct Answer: C**
The parameters in answers A, B, and D are all increased.

29. **Correct Answer: A**
Leads I and aVL will show damage to the higher areas of the lateral wall. Leads V_1 and V_2 show septal wall damage. Leads V_5 and V_6 show damage to the apical area.

30. **Correct Answer: D**
Leads V_4 and R indicate right ventricular damage. Leads V_5 and V_6 indicate apical injury. Leads V_7–V_9 are specific to the posterior wall.

31. **Correct Answer: D**
Pulsus alternans occurs when a weakened myocardium cannot maintain an even pressure with each contraction. The pulses alternate between strong and weak. This finding is also seen in CHF.

32. **Correct Answer: C**
The mitral valve is the most common site; the aortic valve is the next most common valve affected. The valve least affected is the pulmonic valve. The tricuspid valve is often involved secondarily as a result of IV drug abuse.

33. **Correct Answer: D**
Answers A, B, and C are the effects of beta-adrenergic sympathetic stimulation.

34. **Correct Answer: B**
Minute changes in the partial pressure of oxygen, pH, and the partial pressure of carbon dioxide result in changes in the heart and respiratory rate. These changes are initiated by the chemoreceptors located in the carotid and aortic bodies.

35. **Correct Answer: C**
Answer A is the pulmonic area, answer B is the location of the mitral valve, and answer C is the tricuspid area.

36. **Correct Answer: C**
A body mass index over 30 indicates obesity. A BMI between 25–30 means the patient is overweight. In addition, a waist circumference of less than 36 inches is considered normal for females. A waist circumstance of less than 41 inches is considered normal for males. To calculate the BMI, use this formula: BMI = (weight in pounds) (height in inches)^2 × 703.

37. **Correct Answer: C**
Answers A, B, and D are symptoms of left-sided heart failure. When the right side of the heart fails, it is often due to left-sided heart failure. The right ventricle cannot adequately pump blood out, so filling pressures rise and the blood backs up, resulting in hepatomegaly. Thus the CVP and RV pressures are elevated. Additional symptoms may include splenomegaly, ascites, abdominal pain, S_3, S_4, and weight gain.

38. **Correct Answer: C**
NSAIDs cause fluid retention and can contribute to renal insufficiency.

39. **Correct Answer: B**
Other contraindications include coagulopathy, aortic aneurysm, aortic dissection, and irreversible brain damage. Absolute contraindications include history of hemorrhagic stroke, acute pericarditis, pregnancy, bleeding disorders, and current abdominal bleeding.

40. **Correct Answer: B**
The size of the femoral sheath may occlude or diminish circulation to the lower extremities. A thrombus could form. Rarely, tearing or rupture of the aorta will occur. Other complications include infection, emboli, equipment malfunction, balloon leaks, and aortic dissection.

41. **Correct Answer: A**
Answers B, C, and D are relative contraindications. Additional absolute contraindications include hypertension and bleeding disorders.

42. **Correct Answer: C**
Answers A, B, and D are effects of phenytoin, another class 1B drug. Lidocaine may shorten the QT interval, and its side effects usually involve the CNS: slurred speech, drowsiness, confusion, paresthesias, seizures, and convulsions.

43. **Correct Answer: D**
The high iodine content can actually exert an effect on the thyroid and thus produce an antiarrhythmic action.

44. **Correct Answer: D**
Amiodarone and quinidine are antiarrhythmics; clonidine is an antihypertensive. Adenosine occurs naturally in the body and has a very short half-life (only a few seconds). Adenosine slows AV nodal conduction or can interrupt it altogether, potentially causing a transient AV block (seen as asystole). The patient may experience mild to moderate chest discomfort, slight hypotension, bradycardia, and possibly flushing.

45. **Correct Answer: A**
The QT interval may be prolonged by tricyclic antidepressants, erythromycin, quinidine, or terfenidine. Magnesium acts on the calcium transfer across the cell membrane and within the cell itself. If high doses of magnesium are given, AV conduction may slow.

46. **Correct Answer: B**
Large-lumen vessels in the arterial system are affected. The advantage of this action is that both systolic and diastolic pressures are reduced and the patient will not have a drop in blood pressure. The blood pressure may be lowered slightly and initiates a reflex baroreceptor response to speed up the heart rate to maintain cardiac output.

47. **Correct Answer: C**
The S_4 heart sound is also known as an atrial gallop. When the atria contract and blood fills the ventricle, there is naturally some resistance to that pressure because the ventricle is already about 80% full. If the patient has a problem such as hypertension, an MI, an anginal episode, or aortic stenosis, the S_4 may become quite pronounced.

48. **Correct Answer: B**
A heart murmur is a sound produced by turbulent blood flow. By definition, a systolic murmur would be heard during systole when the ventricles are contracting. The mitral and tricuspid valves should be closed. If these valves are incompetent (insufficiency), blood will flow back through the valve (regurgitation). Thus, pulmonic and aortic stenosis, and mitral and tricuspid insufficiency, are systolic murmurs.

49. **Correct Answer: B**
By definition, pansystolic means the murmur is heard throughout systole. The only systolic murmur listed is tricuspid insufficiency. Answers A, C, and D are diastolic murmurs.

50. **Correct Answer: D**
The elevated right ventricular pressure and the elevated right atrial pressure indicate pulmonary hypertension. The wedge pressure is normal. The wedge pressure reflects the status of the left side of the heart. Fluid cannot clear the lungs, so pressure builds and the right-side pressures rise due to the increased workload. Edema results from the fluid backup. The dyspnea and exercise intolerance are caused by the presence of excess fluid in the lungs.

51. **Correct Answer: B**
All of the pressures are higher than normal. In restrictive pericarditis, the entire heart is affected and compressed, leading to abnormally high pressures.

52. **Correct Answer: C**
Answers A, B, and D cause only a moderate rise in INR. Other drugs that significantly raise INR include aspirin, sulfonamides, cimetidine, fluoroquinolones, and macrolide antibiotics.

53. **Correct Answer: B**
Answers A, C, and D decrease the INR only moderately. Other drugs that significantly decrease the INR include rifampin, phenobarbital, and glutethimide. Vitamin K is widely used as an antidote for warfarin and can actually decrease the INR too far and may result in increased warfarin resistance. Careful monitoring of the patient is required if the INR reaches a critical level. Warfarin breakdown is also accelerated by barbiturates.

54. **Correct Answer: B**
Necrotic tissue cannot conduct an impulse. Ischemic tissue may impair conduction. If the patient were hypokalemic, the mA would have to be raised because a low potassium level depresses the myocardium.

55. **Correct Answer: D**
The MI has impaired the heart's ability to pump effectively. The cardiac output falls and the body reacts by vasoconstricting peripheral circulation and increasing the heart rate. Tachycardia is also the result of catecholamine release, and myocardial oxygen consumption is increased. The left ventricle works harder, but has been compromised by the MI. Preload increases because fluid cannot be pumped out of the chambers effectively. The S_3 heart sound is a signal of increased preload. Pulmonary congestion occurs due to increased left heart pressures.

56. **Correct Answer: C**
A new holosystolic murmur at the lower-left sternal border means that turbulent blood flow is occurring there. This turbulence is caused by a hole that allows blood to flow through a previously closed area. The SvO_2 will increase due to the mixing of blood. This condition must be corrected surgically.

57. **Correct Answer: A**
The chest X ray will probably show a pericardial effusion. The elevated sedimentation rate and WBC indicate infection. In pericarditis, leaning forward often relieves chest pain and lying supine makes the pain worse. If the pain worsens on inspiration, it is because the lungs expand and come in contact with the pericardium. The patient will probably also have a fever. Monitor for any signs of a cardiac tamponade and be diligent with the use of anticoagulants.

58. **Correct Answer: C**
New evidence indicates that an ejection fraction of 35% or less may predispose an individual to sudden cardiac death. When that condition is combined with existing CAD, the likelihood of a cardiac event is increased. Generally, if an individual has disease in the left main artery, three vessels, proximal LAD with one additional vessel, then the patient is a candidate for a CABG. Emergent conditions for a CABG include MI with shock, or refractory pain, or unstable angina. Patients who dissect during a stent placement require immediate surgery.

59. **Correct Answer: A**
The new AHA guidelines specify that ventilation should occur every 6 to 8 seconds. The compressions should continue at a rate of 100. The ventilation rate approximates a normal adult rate and allows for cardiac fill. Ventilating too fast raises intrathoracic pressure and interferes with cardiac fill.

60. **Correct Answer: D**

    The delivery of 200 joules on a biphasic defibrillator is as effective as delivery of 360 joules on a monophasic defibrillator. The purpose of defibrillation is to deliver enough electricity to cause a large-enough mass of myocardium to depolarize simultaneously. If that occurs, it is then possible for a normal rhythm to reemerge or become the primary rhythm. It is important to identify the initial cause of the dysrhythmia and treat it if possible to prevent recurrence.

61. **Correct Answer: B**

    In addition to its diuretic properties, furosemide is a mild vasodilator. The fluid in the lungs will decrease due to venous pooling, thereby decreasing the PAOP.

62. **Correct Answer: B**

    Wellen's syndrome is a type of angina that occurs when the LAD is stenosed proximally. The ST segment is not elevated more than 1 mm in V_1–V_3, there is mild T-wave inversion in V_2–V_3, and Q waves are not pathologic (greater than 25% of the total length). Because of the location of the stenosis, surgery is required emergently. Variant angina is the same as Prinzmetal's angina. The pain occurs at rest and is associated with vasospasm. Crescendo angina means that, over time, it takes less to initiate the pain and the pain lasts longer.

63. **Correct Answer: D**

    Nitroglycerin is a vasodilator for both arterial and venous systems. Sometimes the diseased coronary vessels are stiff and calcified. If the patient has good collateral circulation, oxygen and blood can reach the ischemic areas. Nitroglycerin is now available in metered-dose oral spray, pressed tablet, paste, and intravenously (nitroprusside).

64. **Correct Answer: B**

    An infarct in the left main coronary artery is ominous. Sudden death may occur, along with heart blocks and atrial and ventricular dysrhythmias.

65. **Correct Answer: D**

    In a chronic condition, as much as 2,000 mL of fluid may collect in the pericardial sac before symptoms appear. This buildup is usually due to a chronic pleural effusion or uremia. An acute tamponade may occur with as little as 50 mL.

66. **Correct Answer: B**

    The classic description of the chest X ray is the "water bottle" silhouette. QRS amplitude is decreased. Diastolic filling is decreased as well.

67. **Correct Answer: A**

    Both hypovolemia and sepsis decrease afterload, as does aortic insufficiency. Aortic stenosis increases afterload, as do peripheral vasoconstriction and hypertension.

68. **Correct Answer: C**

    A pressure of at least 50 mm Hg is required to maintain auto-regulatory control.

69. **Correct Answer: D**

    Renin is a protease and will be secreted if the sodium concentration falls, or there is an increase in sympathetic output, or a decrease in blood pressure. Blood pressure may be lowered by diuretics, hemorrhage, dehydration, or sodium depletion. Something as simple as NG tube drainage can decrease blood pressure, so in the ICU setting it is critical to monitor and maintain accurate intake and output.

70. **Correct Answer: C**
Pulsus paradoxus may be present in people with asthma, emphysema, cardiac tamponade, restrictive pericarditis, or hemorrhagic shock. Pulse pressure is the difference between systolic and diastolic blood pressure. Pulsus parvus means a small or weak pulse. Pulsus alternans means the upstroke is more powerful than the downstroke.

71. **Correct Answer: B**
Visitation policies vary by institution. However, it is best to identify 1 person as the point of contact. HIPAA regulations require limitations on the dissemination of any medical information. The patient must specify whom is to receive the information if the patient is able to communicate his or her wishes. If the patient is not able to communicate his or her wishes, the next of kin may be designated as a contact person.

72. **Correct Answer: A**
The best response would be to respond collaboratively and interact with other professionals.

73. **Correct Answer: D**
The religious preference of the patient must be respected. The only acceptable form of transfusion in this case is via autotransfusion.

74. **Correct Answer: B**
Utilizing the internal mammary artery means grafts do not have to come from the saphenous veins in the leg, thereby minimizing risk for infection from another site. The internal mammary artery is also separated only at one end and reanastomosed to the affected coronary artery distal to the affected area. Patency is quite good. After 10 years, approximately 90% of mammary artery grafts are still patent.

75. **Correct Answer: A**
Iodine dye is used and will cause a rash, itching, swelling, and may lead to laryngospasm and anaphylaxis. It is imperative to determine whether the patient is allergic to iodine, shellfish, or horses prior to performing the procedure.

76. **Correct Answer: A**
Along with the acute ST elevation, another indicator of necrosis would be an abnormal Q wave. If the Q wave appears within about 6 hours of a transmural MI, it is an ominous sign. If the Q wave is more than 0.04 seconds long, it is a sign of necrosis. In an inferior MI, the Q wave should not exceed 0.03 seconds or it is indicative of necrosis.

77. **Correct Answer: C**
The antagonist for morphine or other opioids is Narcan (naloxone). Generally, the naloxone dose is 0.4 mg IV. This dose can be repeated about every 3 to 4 minutes three times. When you give Narcan, you must always be alert for the patient to relapse once the dose wears off. Administering multiple follow-up doses is not uncommon.

78. **Correct Answer: A**
Answers B, C, and D are complications of an intra-aortic balloon pump (IABP). Other common complications from VADs include infection and bleeding.

79. **Correct Answer: B**
    Prolonged cardiac arrest, especially with neurological damage, is a contraindication to use of a VAD. Extensive organ damage is another contraindication. VADs are not indicated for dysrhythmias. Other indications for a VAD include use as a bridge to transplant, cardiogenic shock, and inability to wean from cardiopulmonary bypass. Always be aware of the possibility of device failure.

80. **Correct Answer: C**
    Pneumonia secondary to immobility is the primary reason for infection with VADs. Many patients with VADs also need some type of ventilatory support, and the placement of tubes into the body is always a potential source of infection. This risk is usually minimized by good handwashing and aseptic technique.

81. **Correct Answer: D**
    The left ventricular assist device is the most commonly used because left heart failure is more prevalent and usually precedes right ventricular failure.

82. **Correct Answer: C**
    Quite often the patient develops cardiogenic shock and requires emergent placement of a VAD. If the nurse is able to at least explain the function of the device, it can be a great relief to family.

83. **Correct Answer: B**
    The patient is approaching crisis and may feel hopeless. The nurse should take the time to fully explore and validate the patient's feelings, and then decide on the appropriate course of action.

84. **Correct Answer: D**
    If the patient is bleeding, the blood may settle into the lumbar area. Blood is heavy and will flow into the retroperitoneal area because of gravity. It may be over an hour and loss of several hundred milliliters of blood before vital signs are affected.

85. **Correct Answer: D**
    The aortogram is the established standard for a definitive diagnosis and is the only invasive procedure listed. This test is sometimes called an aortic angiogram with (radiopaque) contrast dye.

86. **Correct Answer: B**
    Men (70+%) definitely have more aneurysms than women (30+%). Aortic regurgitation is often a cause for an aneurysm, rather than stenosis. Advanced age contributes to mortality; younger patients have a better chance of survival.

87. **Correct Answer: A**
    Quite often the patient will describe a ripping or tearing sensation and severe pain. Hypotension may be present as the dissection progresses. Warning signs include hypertension, a new murmur (aortic insufficiency), weak peripheral pulses, and possible deterioration of level of consciousness. Aneurysms that dissect downward radiate pain to the lower abdomen, lower back, and legs.

88. **Correct Answer: B**
    Any aortic aneurysm that extends over 4 cm will generally need surgical repair. Other criteria for immediate repair include impending rupture, limb ischemia, uncontrolled pain, cardiac tamponade, and increasing size.

89. **Correct Answer: A**

The inner layer of the vessel becomes separated, and blood enters the area under pressure.

90. **Correct Answer: B**

The abdominal area is most commonly affected and usually offers good surgical access. Aneurysms in the aortic arch are sometimes not accessible surgically and may pose a high risk during the procedure.

91. **Correct Answer: C**

Protamine is used as an antagonist of heparin. Although cardiopulmonary bypass procedures use heparin, the more precise answer is C. Sometimes protamine may cause a severe adverse reaction, resulting in vasodilation that leads to profound hypotension.

92. **Correct Answer: D**

CAB (coronary artery bypass) is often associated with damage to the cells. Sometimes fibrin, platelet aggregates, catecholamines, and bubbles circulate. Venous tone can increase due to catecholamines within the system.

93. **Correct Answer: B**

Patients with heart transplants do not feel cardiac pain because the heart has been denervated.

94. **Correct Answer: D**

Rheumatic fever remains the most common cause of acquired valvular disease. The valves are a perfect place for bacteria to colonize, and blood is a perfect medium for bacterial growth. The causative organism is beta-hemolytic *Streptococcus*.

95. **Correct Answer: B**

When the heart is denervated, it has no connection to the autonomic nervous system, so reflexive response does not occur. A sympathetic stimulant must be used. If no other complications occur, the ventricle will eventually adjust to not receiving autonomic input.

96. **Correct Answer: C**

The conditions listed in answers A, B, and D may contribute to an aneurysm, but hypertension remains the primary cause. Constant pressure on the vessel walls will weaken the vessel.

97. **Correct Answer: A**

Pain is a cardinal sign of an arterial obstruction. The nurse should check for pallor, sensation, and the quality of pulses. If the obstruction is venous, the limb may exhibit cyanosis.

98. **Correct Answer: C**

The large V wave may be mistaken for the right ventricular tracing or even a pulmonary artery tracing. Large V waves usually occur with a papillary muscle rupture (sometimes ischemia) secondary to mitral regurgitation or an acute lateral wall MI.

99. **Correct Answer: B**

Reperfusion rhythms such as ventricular tachycardia, sinus bradycardia, accelerated idioventricular rhythm, and underlying sinus rhythms with ventricular ectopy may occur. The patient should experience less chest pain. The CPK isoenzymes may actually become elevated temporarily as blood flows freely through newly opened arteries. CHF is not a result of this therapy.

100. **Correct Answer: C**

Family members are probably quite familiar with the process of providing care for this patient. Do not ignore the patient. There is no point in speaking slowly unless either the caregiver or the patient has difficulty understanding instructions. Teaching quickly is counterproductive and may be considered rude and unprofessional. Allow time for a return demonstration of skills and encourage questions.

101. **Correct Answer: C**

You should feel only a mild tingling. You should not fear this device to the point of not performing CPR, and CPR should not be delayed. If the ICD fires, anyone touching the patient at that moment may feel the tingling sensation.

102. **Correct Answer: D**

Biphasic defibrillation works by sending electricity from the cathode to the anode and then reversing the current. It takes less energy to cause mass depolarization of the myocardium. Cardioversion is much more successful as well. Both defibrillation and cardioversion take less energy to convert patients. Be certain to follow the latest American Heart Association guidelines when using these devices.

103. **Correct Answer: A**

The ICD should be set 10 joules above the defibrillation threshold on at least 2 successive attempts. The threshold varies from patient to patient and depends on existing catecholamine levels. Some physicians just set the ICD 10 joules below the maximum output; although this measure saves time, it does not really fine-tune the ICD to the patient.

104. **Correct Answer: B**

The magnet is used to inhibit the shocking (tachy) feature of the ICD and can shut down a malfunctioning ICD. Patient teaching includes educating the patient about the dangers of being in close proximity to large magnets. Most ICDs have a warning tone built in. If the patient comes too close to a magnet, the device emits the tone. The type of tone varies with the manufacturer.

105. **Correct Answer: B**

These waves heat the tissue around the active sites and prevent reentry loop. Once the temperature reaches 50°C, cell damage and death occur. The continuing heat creates a lesion that is approximately 2–5 mm in diameter. This "burned" area causes necrosis and will not conduct electricity.

106. **Correct Answer: D**

Ibutilide is a relatively new class III/IV medication. It must be used at the time of the cardioversion and will be ineffective if used prior to the cardioversion.

107. **Correct Answer: C**

Normal pulmonary artery pressures are as follows:

PAS = 29–30 mm Hg
PAD = 5–6 mm Hg
PAM = 10–20 mm Hg
PAOP (PCWP) = 4–12 mm Hg

108. **Correct Answer: D**

The presence of a clot, an air bubble, or the catheter tip up against the vessel can all dampen the waveform.

109. **Correct Answer: B**

Most often, the transducer has not been calibrated correctly or has not been leveled appropriately. Air or blood in the system will also dampen the waveform. If the balloon ruptures, no wedge pressure will be obtainable.

110. **Correct Answer: C**

If the catheter is in the right ventricle and touches the myocardium, PVCs can result. When the catheter floats past the RV and into the pulmonary artery, the PVCs will disappear. Occasionally, the physician will withdraw the catheter a centimeter or two, and then allow it to "refloat" into the correct position.

111. **Correct Answer: B**

The low wedge pressure indicates hypovolemia and will require volume replacement.

112. **Correct Answer: B**

In pulmonary hypertension, the wedge pressure remains normal. It reflects pressures in the left side of the heart. The pulmonary artery pressures reflect pressures in the pulmonary vasculature.

113. **Correct Answer: B**

The systemic vascular resistance is the definition of left ventricular afterload. PVR is the afterload of the right ventricle.

114. **Correct Answer: A**

Gina has endocarditis. Janeway lesions are flat, painless, erythematous areas that predominately appear on the palms of the hands and the soles of the feet. Osler's nodes are small, painful nodules also associated with endocarditis and found on fingers and toes. Roth spots are seen when examining the retina. They are rounded, white spots and associated with endocarditis. Pella's sign is not a medical term. It is thought that microvascular clots form in the heart and pass through the microcirculation and impede peripheral circulation, sometimes causing necrosis.

115. **Correct Answer: B**

With Stage I, there is disease (pathological arterial changes) but no symptoms. Stage II is representative of a 75% occlusion and the patient will have intermittent claudication. Stage III represents a 90–95% occlusion and the patient will have pain at rest. Stage IV is a 99–100% occlusion and necrosis will result if not treated.

116. **Correct Answer: C**

Patients with peripheral vascular disease are often hypothermic because of poor circulation. Healing is slowed because of the decrease in circulation. The nurse should provide proper alignment without impeding circulation and monitor peripheral pulses for presence and quality. The color and temperature of the extremity should be monitored and results charted.

117. **Correct Answer: B**

A primary goal in cardiogenic shock is to improve the pumping action of the heart (improve myocardial contractility), reduce the workload, reduce oxygen demand, and improve cardiac output. If possible, systemic vascular resistance should be decreased and the left ventricle augmented with an inotrope. Nitroprusside will reduce preload and afterload. Both the cardiac workload and the myocardial oxygen demand will be reduced.

118. **Correct Answer: B**
Deoxygenated blood returns from the body with an O_2 saturation rate of approximately 75%. The right atrial value is normal. The values for the right ventricle and pulmonary artery should also reach this level. The high level means that some of the oxygenated blood from the left side of the heart has mixed with the deoxygenated blood through a ventricular septal defect. This would be called a left-to-right shunt, because the blood flows from an area of high pressure to an area of low pressure.

119. **Correct Answer: C**
The first thing to do is check the sensitivity control. Even though most of these pacemakers have a cover, the dial may have been moved and indicate that a fixed rate is set. If the pacer continues to fire, it may cause an R-on-T phenomenon and cause ventricular tachycardia or fibrillation. If the patient has an adequate rhythm, you can turn off the pacemaker and notify the physician. If the patient has a nonsustaining rhythm, try positioning the patient on his or her left side to see if the wire will come in contact with the myocardium. You can also try turning up the mA level. Either way, the physician must be notified and vital signs carefully monitored until the physician can reposition the electrodes.

120. **Correct Answer: C**
During ventricular diastole, both the aortic and pulmonic valves close. If a valve is incompetent, the blood will flow backward through the valve, causing turbulent blood flow—that is, a murmur.

121. **Correct Answer: B**
During diastole, the tricuspid and mitral valves close just prior to systole. If the valve is stentotic, it will not close completely. When the atria contract, a murmur is heard as blood passes through the narrow opening.

122. **Correct Answer: A**
The injuries to the chest may have caused a pulmonary artery laceration or a cardiac contusion (the latter condition is more likely). The patient's blood pressure is low, and the EKG shows ST-segment elevation in the anterior leads. If the myocardium is contused, it will react the same way as if an MI had occurred. The ST elevation may be the result of a physiologic insult to a coronary artery, and an area of the myocardium is ischemic. The pumping function of the myocardium is compromised and may need additional support with inotropes and possibly an intra-aortic balloon pump (IABP). As a consequence, the patient may undergo angiography and/or surgery. Volume replacement may be necessary. This patient is in the first stage of cardiogenic shock.

123. **Correct Answer: D**
Approximately 24 hours after a surgical procedure, inflammatory cell mediators can lead to vasodilation. Sue has a permanent pacemaker, and apparently her heart rate cannot compensate for the drop in blood pressure. The cardiac output was not increased as a result of the reduced systemic resistance. The patient's pacemaker did not allow the heart rate to climb above 70. The dobutamine acted on the pump and increased the contractility. This patient also has a history of a previous MI.

124. **Correct Answer: D**

Turning up the rate should allow for weaning off the dobutamine. This patient is also in the beginning stage of cardiogenic shock, but can easily be helped by simply changing the rate on the pacemaker.

125. **Correct Answer: C**

Automated implantable cardioverter/defibrillators (AICD) can be implanted for patients with recurrent ventricular tachycardia. They can also be programmed to act as pacemakers.

126. **Correct Answer: A**

Fred has probably dislodged a lead, or the lead may have been damaged on insertion. Either way, Fred needs a new AICD or new leads.

127. **Correct Answer: C**

Carotid bruit is the significant physical finding associated with carotid stenosis. Heberden's nodules and Broussard's nodules are seen with arthritis. The systolic murmur is an indication of a valvular problem.

128. **Correct Answer: B**

This patient needs a pacemaker or AICD that can deliver a more powerful impulse. The asynchronous mode will override Barry's internal pacemaker.

129. **Correct Answer: B**

A dual-lead pacemaker/AICD is necessary to maintain the atrial kick. Single-chamber pacing can lead to pacemaker syndrome. The letters on pacemaker modes are interpreted as follows:

Chamber Paced	Chamber Sensed	Mode of Response	Programmability, Rate Modulation	Antiatachyarrhythmia Function
V = Ventricle	V = Ventricle	I = Inhibit	P = Simple programmable	P = Pacing
A = Atrium	A = Atrium	T = Triggered	M = Multi-programmable	S = Shock
D = Dual chamber	D = Dual chamber	D = Dual (T & I)	R = Rate modulation	Dual = Dual (P & S)

130. **Correct Answer: C**

Pacemaker Syndrome results from the loss of atrial kick or regurgitation against a closed A-V valve. Gene's atrial lead may have been damaged or failed.

131. **Correct Answer: A**

The most important action is to improve the cardiovascular status of this patient. The transcutaneous-paced patient must be sedated for comfort. The physician must be notified that a transvenous or permanent pacemaker insertion may be necessary. It would be acceptable to give atropine for this condition, but not at the dose listed in the question.

132. **Correct Answer: B**

Because your patient has lost 2 of the 3 main fascicles that innervate the heart, he is at great risk for sudden death. He needs a pacemaker as soon as possible.

133. **Correct Answer: B**

The V_2, V_3, V_4, I, and AVL leads are indicative of an anterolateral MI. The MI could also include V_5 and V_6, which are also lateral leads.

134. **Correct Answer: C**

When the tissue dies due to myocardial infarction, it becomes electrically dead causing the opposing energy to become the dominant feature. Partial-thickness myocardial death would be classified as a non-Q-wave MI.

135. **Correct Answer: A**

You would identify an inferior wall MI in leads II, III, and AVF.

136. **Correct Answer: A**

The anteroseptal MI is seen in leads V_1, V_2, V_3, and V_4. The septal leads are V_1 and V_2, and the anterior leads (which overlap) are V_2, V_3, and V_4.

137. **Correct Answer: B**

Time is measured by the vertical lines on the EKG graph paper. When conduction defects occur, the tracings are wider because it takes more time to travel the same distance.

138. **Correct Answer: C**

Voltage is measured by the horizontal lines on the EKG graph paper. If a ventricle is enlarged, there will be a larger voltage on the 12-lead EKG.

139. **Correct Answer: A**

Leads V_1 and V_2 show right bundle branch blocks. A simple way to remember which type of bundle branch block has occurred with a QRS wider than 0.12 seconds is to think of the turn signals on your car. For a right turn, you must push the lever up; for a left turn, the lever must go down. Looking at leads V_1 and V_2, if the QRS is upright, then there is a right bundle branch block. If V_1 and V_2 are downward in force, then it is a left bundle branch block.

140. **Correct Answer: B**

Rate, rhythm, axis, hypertrophy, and infarction are the most valuable areas examined in a 12-lead EKG.

141. **Correct Answer: A**

Ventricular hypertrophy, pericarditis, and COPD all create ST-T wave abnormalities on the 12-lead EKG.

142. **Correct Answer: C**

COPD causes changes in the 12-lead EKG due to the increased workload on the right side of the heart. Common changes seen in patients with COPD are tall, peaked P waves; right axis deviation; right ventricular hypertrophy; and low-voltage QRS.

143. **Correct Answer: B**

Pacemakers are inserted for many reasons, including symptomatic bradycardia, bradycardia with escape beats, overdrive pacing, bradycardia/arrest, acute MI with sinus dysfunction, Mobtiz type II, complete heart block, and development of a new bundle branch block.

144. **Correct Answer: A**
Quinidine and hypomagnesemia can lead to torsades de pointe, a recurrent ventricular tachycardia that turns on its axis every 6–8 beats, giving the EKG a twisting or "turning on point" look. Hypomagnesemia can occur when the patient receives total parenteral nutrition.

145. **Correct Answer: D**
Hospitalization for more than 2 days is required for a diagnosis of hospital-acquired pneumonia (HAP). If pneumonia occurs before the patient has been hospitalized for 2 days, it is classified as community-acquired pneumonia.

146. **Correct Answer: B**
Pseudomonas aeruginosa is the organism that most commonly causes HAP. Methicillin-Resistant *Staphylococcus aureus* is the second most common cause of HAP.

147. **Correct Answer: C**
Factors increasing the risk for HAP include altered level of consciousness, nasogastric tube, elderly, COPD, postoperative patients, H_2 blockers, antacids, periodontal work, and acute illness or injury.

148. **Correct Answer: B**
Millie's age, her time in the hospital, her nasogastric tube, and her use of antacids are all risk factors for HAP. That her chest X ray is inconclusive is not unusual with elderly patients, as these individuals often have other underlying disease that makes it difficult to identify pneumonia.

149. **Correct Answer: C**
The major difference between HAP and VAP is that the VAP patient is intubated. Both types of pneumonia are caused by the same organism, *Pseudomonas aeruginosa*.

150. **Correct Answer: B**
SVO_2 measures the oxygen saturation of venous blood as it returns to the lungs for oxygenation. Normal SVO_2 is 60–80%. This percentage decreases as lung function worsens, meaning the blood leaving the left ventricle has less oxygen to deliver in the first place.

151. **Correct Answer: A**
SVO_2 shows shunting. There is a normal 5% physiologic shunt due to the presence of blood in the bronchial, pleural, and thebesian veins. When an individual has an infection, trauma, or ARDS, blood is shunted at a higher rate, which is observed as a lowered SVO_2.

152. **Correct Answer: C**
The patient's shunt is worsening. PEEP must be added to decrease the shunt and raise the SVO_2. A chest X ray should also be done to assess his pneumo-hemothorax for possible worsening. In addition, the patient's chest tube drainage system should be examined for the possibility of clots blocking drainage.

153. **Correct Answer: B**

Concomitant use of promethazine and fluoroquinolones is contraindicated because this combination can cause prolongation of QT interval and increase the risk of arrhythmias.

154. **Correct Answer: B**

The rate should not exceed 4 mg/min. An administration rate faster than 4 mg/min can cause the patient to develop tinnitus or hearing loss.

155. **Correct Answer: D**

Rapid infusion of Lasix can cause tinnitus and hearing loss.

156. **Correct Answer: A**

Dong quai, gingko biloba, and ginseng can increase bleeding times. Saw palmetto decreases the effectiveness of Plavix.

157. **Correct Answer: B**

Use of Reo Pro, like any other platelet inhibitor, requires that the patient be carefully questioned about any bleeding history.

158. **Correct Answer: B**

DVT, atrial fibrillation, heart valve replacement, and myocardial infarction are all conditions that require the use of warfarin. DVT, atrial fibrillation, and heart valve replacement patients take warfarin on a ongoing basis. MI patients may be weaned off warfarin in 3 to 4 months.

159. **Correct Answer: A**

There are numerous foods to be avoided when a patient is taking warfarin. The foods highest in vitamin K are broccoli, Brussels sprouts, cabbage, spinach, turnip greens, endive, scallions, parsley, red leaf lettuce, watercress, and soybean, canola, and salad oils. All of these foods decrease the effectiveness of warfarin.

160. **Correct Answer: C**

Integrilin (eptifbatide) is used primarily for patients with acute coronary syndrome to inhibit platelet aggregation.

161. **Correct Answer: A**

Pulmonary embolism is probably not the cause of Javier's condition. The high wedge pressure in association with a low CVP indicates a problem on the left side of the heart. A pulmonary embolism would have resulted in a high right atrial pressure and equal right atrial and wedge pressures. A clue to his condition is the increase in the pulmonary capillary wedge pressure along with increase in the pulmonary artery pressure. The pulmonary diastolic pressure roughly equals the wedge pressure, indicating no increase in pulmonary venous resistance. Thus the problem most likely involves the left heart. Possibilities include coronary artery disease, cardiomyopathy, aortic stenosis, mitral regurgitation or stenosis, and aortic insufficiency.

162. **Correct Answer: B**

The least likely diagnosis is obstruction of the left anterior descending coronary artery. Pete is not exhibiting chest pain or EKG changes. He also has a normal PAOP, indicating normal left-sided cardiac function, but the pressures in the right heart are elevated

(RAP and PAP). Therefore, the problem is in the right heart. Conditions that would produce these findings include RV dysfunction, pulmonary embolism, pulmonary stenosis, and RV hypertrophy.

163. **Correct Answer: C**

This question can be quite tricky. The first thing to notice is that the pressures all rose by 8 mm Hg. Unless there was some major coincidence, this would not happen. The patient had no change in his BP or cardiac index. The mediastinal tubes may stop draining or dramatically slow down soon after surgery. The patient is currently not showing any signs of a tamponade, nor do the hemodynamics support that diagnosis. A change in the position or level of the transducers would produce this change. Most units keep the transducer for the arterial pressure and central hemodynamics on the same manifold. Changes in the bed position or transducers are very common in a CVICU.

164. **Correct Answer: C**

The pulmonary arterial wedge pressure should always be measured at the end of expiration. Pleural pressure will be closest to zero at this time, and an accurate estimate of transmural pressure can be obtained. If the pleural pressure is measured at the end of inspiration, then it will be negative if the patient is breathing spontaneously. The pleural pressure will be positive if the patient is being ventilated with positive-pressure ventilation. If the patient is being treated with positive end-expiratory pressure (PEEP), then pleural pressure may remain somewhat positive at the end of expiration.

165. **Correct Answer: A**

A heart rate of 150 may make it nearly impossible to obtain a stable wedge pressure reading. Tricuspid regurgitation should have no effect on a wedge pressure measurement because the wedge reflects pressure to the left atrium. Aortic stenosis also is not a problem because obstruction of the aortic valve would produce an increase in left atrial pressure if the patient has heart failure. Measurement of wedge pressure can be a problem in patients with severe mitral regurgitation because they may have a superimposed V wave on the wedge tracing.

166. **Correct Answer: B**

Amyloidosis and mochromatosis are additional causes of restrictive cardiomyopathy. The myocardium (especially the left ventricle) becomes rigid from fibrosis, which results in inadequate left ventricular filling and increased atrial dilatation. Left ventricular diastolic dysfunction occurs and the LVEDP is markedly increased. Systolic function remains normal in this type of cardiomyopathy. Fluid backs up into the lungs and the patient appears to have congestive heart failure. There is no cure for this condition, and symptoms are treated as they occur.

167. **Correct Answer: C**

"Arrhythmogenic" is a relatively new classification for cardiomyopathy. In this condition, the normal myocardial cells are replaced by fatty tissue and fibrous tissue. The right ventricle is primarily affected. Conduction cannot occur normally, and the patient will have multiple ventricular arrhythmias and right ventricular failure. Young people with arrhythmogenic cardiomyopathy are at risk for sudden death. The cause of this condition is unknown, but some research has shown a possible link to an autosomal dominant gene.

168. **Correct Answer: B**
In hypertrophic cardiomyopathy, the myocardium thickens, but not symmetrically: There is more thickening of the ventricular septum than of the ventricle. If you were to look at a heart with this condition, it could appear normal externally. When the septum is thicker, it creates a hyperdynamic state by increasing contractility, so the ejection fraction is increased. In rare conditions where the septum is asymmetrically thickened, left ventricular outflow will be impaired, so cardiac output would be decreased.

169. **Correct Answer: A**
Although the exact causes of this condition are unknown, a large number of alcoholics develop dilated cardiomyopathy. Three reasons postulated as causes have been identified:
  - The alcohol or its metabolites have a toxic effect.
  - Alcohol sometimes contains additives, such as cobalt.
  - The cause may be nutritional in origin, such as a thiamine deficiency.
New research suggests that there may also be a viral link to chronic alcoholism. Interestingly, this type of cardiomyopathy might reverse itself if the drinking is stopped. Other types of cardiomyopathy are not reversible.

170. **Correct Answer: D**
Peripartum cardiomyopathy develops during the first 3 to 4 months after completion of pregnancy. Sometimes the cause is myocarditis.

171. **Correct Answer: A**
Dilated cardiomyopathy causes systolic dysfunction. You will hear S_3 and S_4 gallops, and the EKG may show atrial fibrillation, ventricular dysrhythmias, or a sinus tachycardia most of the time. The patient may have a systolic murmur of the AV valves. The patient will probably also have peripheral edema or ascites, hepatomegaly, and pale, cool extremities. It is possible to have changes in mentation. Hypertrophic and restrictive cardiomyopathies are diastolic dysfunctions.

172. **Correct Answer: D**
Atrial fibrillation is the result of the constant stretching and disruption of normal pathways in the atrium due to increased preload from the pulmonary congestion.

173. **Correct Answer: C**
The nurse would monitor the patient's vital signs. This family is so eager to help and they would probably have someone at the bedside for many hours during the day. Any change in mentation is very significant, and the family can help monitor the patient when the nurse is away from the room. The family will be ready to embrace learning and assume more tasks as time passes if they are positively reinforced for their efforts.

174. **Correct Answer: B**
The blood pressure, PAS/PAD pressures, and RAP are low. The cardiac output and cardiac index are low, as are the heart rate and respiratory rate. The patient's mentation is also diminished. The values indicate that the patient is in hypovolemic shock.

175. **Correct Answer: C**
James is developing cardiogenic shock. When the left ventricle fails, fluid backs up into the pulmonary vasculature. Since the wedge pressure is high, it means the fluid is already

backed up in the left heart. The PAP and RAP are also high, indicating pulmonary congestion. Cardiac output and cardiac index are low, and BP is not being maintained.

176. **Correct Answer: A**
Dobutamine is an inotrope that improves the pumping action of the heart. This alpha-, $beta_1$-, and $beta_2$-agonist increases contractility and cardiac output with little or no increase in myocardial oxygen consumption. It has a very mild vasodilatory effect, though high doses can cause ischemia.

177. **Correct Answer: D**
Frank has increased exercise intolerance, edema, dyspnea, and increased PAP and wedge pressures. The RAP is normal. These findings are all signs of left ventricular failure.

178. **Correct Answer: B**
The pH is normal (compensated), the CO_2 level is high (respiratory acidosis), and the HCO_3 level is normal.

179. **Correct Answer: D**
Erin's left heart pressures are elevated, as is her RAP. This indicates inability of the heart to eject fluid. The preload is high. Crackles indicate pulmonary congestion. Edema indicates third spacing.

180. **Correct Answer: A**
The RAP (CVP) is equal to the RVEDP. During diastole, the tricuspid valve opens and the right ventricle and right atrium fill with blood. The pressures are equal.

181. **Correct Answer: D**
A lateral MI is identified by changes in leads I, aVL, V_5, and V_6.

182. **Correct Answer: B**
Because the RCA perfuses the SA node in just over half the population, and because it supplies the proximal bundle if His and the AV node in more than 90% of individuals, conduction defects may occur.

183. **Correct Answer: A**
Using ICHD nomenclature, the first "V" is the chamber paced.

184. **Correct Answer: C**
Using ICHD nomenclature, the second "V" is the chamber sensed.

185. **Correct Answer: C**
Of the choices given here, the problem is in the right ventricle. The PAP and wedge pressures are normal. The RAP is high and there is some jugular distention. These findings would indicate a problem with the right ventricle: It cannot pump effectively. The lungs do not seem to be the problem because the pulmonary artery pressures are normal. The lethargy may be unrelated and needs to be evaluated because it is a significant change for this patient.

Questions 186–193 are exercises to match up hemodynamic effects of frequently used medications.

186. **Correct Answer: A**

187. **Correct Answer: C**

188. **Correct Answer: B**

189. **Correct Answer: B**

190. **Correct Answer: D**

191. **Correct Answer: A**

192. **Correct Answer: B**

193. **Correct Answer: C**

194. **Correct Answer: D**
Roy is in the hyperdynamic ("warm") stage of septic shock. The endotoxins are causing an increase in metabolism and act as vasodilators. The temperature is elevated because of the increased metabolism and infection. The RAP, PAP, SVR, and PAOP are decreased because of vasodilation. The cardiac output and cardiac index are high because they are compensating. Hypotension occurs because of vasodilation. Urine output should be quite high. Roy needs immediate treatment with large quantities of fluids, vasopressors, antibiotics, and anti-endotoxins.

195. **Correct Answer: D**
Susan was admitted for anaphylactic shock. She is 8 months pregnant, and the baby is probably pressing on her aorta and vena cava. A simple change of position might fix the problem. In anaphylactic shock, the PAP would be low in the initial stages because of vasodilation. In obstructive shock, the PAP and PAOP can be either normal or high. Symptoms usually resolve once the problem is eliminated.

196. **Correct Answer: B**
The pulmonary artery pressure, RAP, and PAOP are all elevated, and their values are virtually identical. Heart sounds are muffled, and the BP has converging systolic and diastolic pressures. Pericardiocentesis must be performed immediately.

197. **Correct Answer: A**
MAP formula: $2 \times DPP + SBP = CO$.

198. **Correct Answer: B**
The formula for cardiac index is: $CI = CO/BSA$.

199. **Correct Answer: C**
All of the pulmonary pressures are elevated. The heart cannot pump the fluid out, and the lungs are congested (dyspnea). Edema is a sign of pump failure. The patient will probably develop ascites and hepatomegaly.

200. **Correct Answer: C**
The pulmonary artery pressures are very high. The preexisting pulmonary congestion strained the patient's right heart, causing it to hypertrophy. The pulmonary congestion must be relieved as soon as possible. The patient may potentially become toxic from the oxygen, so you may have to lower the amount of O_2 that is delivered.

201. **Correct Answer: D**
Yolanda received anticoagulation therapy. It is possible that her blood pressure and the anticoagulants combined to cause a bleed. You should notify the physician of any

headaches, change in mentation, change in size of a hematoma, or oozing from the incision site. Lab results must be closely monitored.

202. **Correct Answer: D**
Daniel has the classic signs of sepsis: The PAP, RAP, and PAOP are low; the cardiac output and cardiac index are high. He is running a low-grade temperature. His respiratory rate is increased, and he has subtle changes in mentation.

203. **Correct Answer: C**
Daniel needs copious amounts of fluid and antibiotic therapy.

204. **Correct Answer: C**
Nitroprusside causes vasodilation, reducing afterload. Dobutamine is an inotrope that increases contractility.

BIBLIOGRAPHY

Abraham, W. T., & Hayes, D. L. (2003). Cardiac resynchronization therapy for heart failure. *Circulation, 108*(21), 2596–2603.

Adams-Hamoda, M. G., & Pelter, M. M. (2003). Heart blocks. *American Journal of Critical Care, 12*(1), 77–78.

Ahrens, T. (2006). *Critical care nursing certification.* Columbus, OH: McGraw-Hill.

Albert, N. M. (2003). Cardiac resynchronization therapy through biventricular pacing in patients with heart failure and ventricular dyssynchrony. *Critical Care Nurse, 23*(3 suppl), 2–16.

Allocca, G., Slavich, G., Nucifora, G., Slavich, M., Frassani, R., Crapis, M., et al. (2007). Successful treatment of polymicrobial multivalve infective endocarditis: Multivalve infective endocarditis. *International Journal of Cardiovascular Imaging, 23*(4), 501.

Alpert, J. S. (2003). Defining myocardial infarction: "Will the real myocardial infarction please stand up?" *American Heart Journal, 146*(3), 377–379.

American Association of Critical-Care Nurses. (2004, May). *Practice alert: Pulmonary artery pressure measurement.* Retrieved July 16, 2008, from http://www.aacn.org/WD/Practice/Docs/PAP_Measurement_05-2004.pdf

American Association of Critical-Care Nurses. (2004, August). *Practice alert: ST segment monitoring.* Retrieved July 16, 2008, from http://www.aacn.org/WD/Practice/Docs/ST_Segment_Monitoring_04-2008.pdf

American Association of Critical-Care Nurses. (2006). *Core curriculum for critical care nursing* (6th ed.). Philadelphia: Saunders.

American Association of Critical-Care Nurses. (2007). *AACN certification and core review for high acuity and critical care* (6th ed.). Philadelphia: Saunders.

American Heart Association. (2007). *Guidelines 2005 for cardiopulmonary resuscitation and emergency cardiovascular care.* Retrieved July 16, 2008, from http://circ.ahajournals.org/content/vol112/24_suppl

Anavekar, N. S., McMurray, J. J. V., Velazquez, E. J., Solomon, S. D., Kober, L., Rouleau, J. L., et al. (2004). Relation between renal dysfunction and cardiovascular outcomes after myocardial infarction. *New England Journal of Medicine, 351*(13), 1285–1295.

Anderson, R. H., Razavi, R., & Taylor, A. M. (2004). Cardiac anatomy revisited. *Journal of Anatomy, 205*(3), 159–177.

Antezano, E. S., & Hong, M. (2003). Sudden cardiac death. *Journal of Intensive Care Medicine, 18*(6), 313–329.

Antzelevitch, C., Brugada, P., Borggrefe, M., Brugada, J., Brugada, R., Corrado, D., et al. (2005). Brugada syndrome: Report of the Second Consensus Conference. Endorsed by the Heart Rhythm Society and the European Heart Rhythm Association. *Circulation, 111*(5), 659–670.

Archbold, R. A., & Schilling, R. J. (2004). Atrial pacing for the prevention of atrial fibrillation after coronary bypass graft surgery: A review of the literature. *Heart, 90*, 129–133.

Ariyan, C. E., & Sosa, J. A. (2004). Assessment and management of patients with abnormal calcium. *Critical Care Medicine, 32*(4 suppl), S146–S154.

Aronow, W. S. (2003). Homocysteine: The association with atherosclerotic vascular disease in older persons. *Geriatrics, 58*(2), 22–24, 27–28.

Aurigemma, G. P., & Gassch, W. H. (2004). Clinical practice: Diastolic heart failure. *New England Journal of Medicine, 351*(11), 1097–1105.

Barrett, M. J., Lacey, C. S., Sekara, A. E., et al. (2004). Mastering cardiac murmurs: The power of repetition. *Chest, 126*(2), 470–475.

Barter, P. J., Nicholls, S., Rye, K., Anantharamaiah, G. M., Navab, M., & Fogelman, A. M. (2004). Antiinflammatory properties of HDL. *Circulation Research, 95*(8), 764–772.

Baur, L. H. B. (2008). Three dimensional echocardiography: A valuable tool to assess left atrial function in non-compaction cardiomyopathy! *International Journal of Cardiovascular Imaging, 24*(3), 243.

Berdajs, D., Patonay, L., & Turina, M. I. (2003). The clinical anatomy of the sinus node artery. *Annals of Thoracic Surgery, 76*(3), 732–735.

Birnbaum, Y., & Drew, B. J. (2003). The electrocardiogram in ST elevation acute myocardial infarction: Correlation with coronary anatomy and prognosis. *Postgraduate Medical Journal, 79*(935), 490–504.

Blake, G. J., & Ridker, P. M. (2003). C-reactive protein and other inflammatory risk markers in acute coronary syndromes. *Journal of the American College of Cardiology, 41*(4 suppl S), 37S–42S.

Bollinger, K., & Sader, A. M. (2003). Care and management of the patient with right heart failure secondary to diastolic dysfunction: An advanced practice perspective and case review. *Critical Care Nursing Quarterly, 26*(1), 22–27.

Bolno, P. B., & Kresh, J. Y. (2003). Physiologic and hemodynamic basis of ventricular assist devices. *Cardiology Clinics, 21*(1), 15–27.

Booker, K. J., Holm, K., Drew, B. J., Lanuza, D. M., Hicks, F. D., Carrigan, T., et al. (2003). Frequency and outcomes of transient myocardial ischemia in critically ill adults admitted for noncardiac conditions. *American Journal of Critical Care, 12*(6), 508–516.

Callahan, H. E. (2003). Families dealing with advanced heart failure: A challenge and an opportunity. *Critical Care Nursing Quarterly, 26*(3), 230–243.

Cannon, C. P. (2003). Small molecule glycoprotein IIb/IIIa receptor inhibitors as upstream therapy in acute coronary syndromes. *Journal of the American College of Cardiology, 41*(4 suppl S), 43S–48S.

Canto, J. G., & Iskandrian, A. E. (2003). Major risk factors for cardiovascular disease: Debunking the "only 50%" myth. *Journal of the American Medical Association, 290*, 947–949.

Cardenas, G. A., Lavie, C. J., & Milani, R. V. (2004a). Importance and management of low levels of high-density lipoprotein cholesterol in older adults: Part I: Role and mechanism. *Geriatrics and Aging, 7*(3), 40–45.

Cardenas, G. A., Lavie, C. J., & Milani, R. V. (2004b). Importance and management of low levels of high-density lipoprotein cholesterol in older adults: Part II: Screening and treatment. *Geriatrics and Aging, 7*(3), 41–48.

Carmona, I. T., Dios, P. D., & Scully, C. (2007, Dec.). Efficacy of antibiotic prophylactic regimens for the prevention of bacterial endocarditis of oral origin. *Journal of Dental Research, 86*(12), 1142.

Chen, E. W., Canto, J. G., Parsons, L. S., Peterson, E. D., Littrell, K. A., Every, N. R., et al. (2003). Relation between hospital intra-aortic balloon counterpulsation volume and mortality in acute myocardial infarction complicated by cardiogenic shock. *Circulation, 108*(8), 951–957.

Chiu, C., & Sequeira, I. B. (2004). Diagnosis and treatment of idiopathic ventricular tachycardia. *AACN Clinical Issues, 15*(3), 449–461.

Chobanian, A. V., Bakris, G. L., Black, H. R., Cushman, W. C., Green, L. A., Izzo, J. L. Jr., et al. (2003). The seventh report of the Joint National Committee on Prevention, Detection, Evaluation and Treatment of High Blood Pressure: The JNC 7 report. *Journal of the American Medical Association, 289*(19) 2560–2572.

Chun, A. A., & McGee, S. R. (2004). Bedside diagnosis of coronary artery disease: A systematic review. *American Journal of Medicine, 117*(5), 334–343.

Cianci, P., Lonergan-Thomas, H., Slaughter, M., & Silver, M. A. (2003). Current and potential applications of left ventricular assist devices. *Journal of Cardiovascular Nursing, 18*(1), 17–22.

Coffey, M., Crowder, G. K., & Cheek, D. J. (2003). Reducing coronary artery disease by decreasing homocysteine levels. *Critical Care Nurse, 23*(1), 25–29.

Cohen, M. (2003). The role of low-molecular-weight heparin in the management of acute coronary syndromes. *Journal of the American College of Cardiology, 41*(4 suppl S), 55S–61S.

Colbert, K., & Greene, M. H. (2003). Nesiritide: A new treatment for acutely decompensated congestive heart failure. *Critical Care Nursing Quarterly, 26*(1), 40–44.

Conover, M. B. (2003). *Understanding electrocardiography* (8th ed.). St. Louis, MO: Mosby/Elsevier.

Constantine, G., Shan, K., Flamm, S. D., & Sivananthan, M. U. (2004). Role of MRI in clinical cardiology. *Lancet, 363*(9247), 2162–2171.

Conti, R., Fuster, V., & Badimon, J. J. (2003). Pathogenic concepts of acute coronary syndromes. *Journal of the American College of Cardiology, 41*(4 suppl S), 37S–42S.

Copstead, L., & Banasik, J. L. (2000). *Pathophysiology: Biological and behavioral perspectives* (2nd ed.). Philadelphia: W. B. Saunders/Elsevier.

Coulthwaite, L., & Verran, J. (2007). Potential pathogenic aspects of denture plaque. *British Journal of Biomedical Science, 64*(4), 180.

Coviello, J. S., & Nystrom, K. V. (2003). Obesity and heart failure. *Journal of Cardiovascular Nursing, 18*(5), 360–366.

Crawford, M. H., DiMarco, J. P., & Paulus, W. J. (Eds.). (2004). *Cardiology* (2nd ed.). Philadelphia: Mosby.

Criddle, L. M. (2003). Rhabdomyolysis: Pathophysiology, recognition, and management. *Critical Care Nurse, 23*(6), 14–28.

Cripe, L., Andelfinger, G., Martin, L. J., Shooner, K., & Benson, D. W. (2004). Bicuspid aortic valve is heritable. *Journal of the American College of Cardiology, 44*(1), 138–143.

Crystal, E., & Connolly, S. J. (2004). Atrial fibrillation: Guiding lessons from epidemiology. *Cardiology Clinics, 22*(1), 1–8.

Curley, M. A. Q. (1998). Patient–nurse synergy: Optimizing patients' outcomes. *American Journal of Critical Care, 7,* 64–72.

Darovic, G. O. (2002). *Hemodynamic monitoring: Invasive and noninvasive clinical application* (3rd ed.). Philadelphia: Saunders.

Davidson, M. B., Thakkar, S., Hix, J. K., Bhandarkar, N. D., Wong, A., & Schreiber, M. J. (2004). Pathophysiology, clinical consequences, and treatment of tumor lysis syndrome. *American Journal of Medicine, 116*(8), 546–554.

D'Avila, A., Scanavacca, M., Sosa, E., Ruskin, J. N., Reddy, V. Y. (2003). Pericardial anatomy for the interventional electrophysiologist. *Journal of Cardiovascular Electrophysiology, 14*(4), 422–430.

Deaton, C., Dunbar, S. B., Moloney, M., Sears, S. F., & Ujhelyi, M. R. (2003). Patient experiences with atrial fibrillation and treatment with implantable atrial defibrillation therapy. *Heart and Lung, 32*(5), 291–299.

De Rosa, F. G., Cicalini, S., Canta, F., Audagnotto, S., Cecchi, E., & Di Perri, G. (2007). Infective endocarditis in intravenous drug users from Italy: The increasing importance in HIV-infected patients. *Infection, 35*(3), 154.

Dickerson, R. N., Alexander, K. H., Minard, G., Croce, M. A., & Brown, R. O. (2004). Accuracy of methods to estimate ionized and "corrected" serum calcium concentrations in critically ill multiple trauma patients receiving specialized nutrition support. *Journal of Parenteral and Enteral Nutrition, 28*(3), 133–141.

Diercks, D. B., Shumaik, G. M., Harrigan, R. A., Brady, W. J., & Chan, T. C. (2004). Electrocardiographic manifestations: Electrolyte abnormalities. *Journal of Emergency Medicine, 27*(2), 153–160.

Dimick, J. B., Swoboda, S., Talamini, M. A., Pelz, R. K., Hendrix, C. W., & Lipsett, P. A. (2004). Risk of colonization of central venous catheters: Catheters for total parenteral nutrition vs. other catheters. *American Journal of Critical Care, 12*(4), 328–335.

Drazner, M. H., Rame, J. E., & Dries, D. L. (2003). Third heart sound and elevated jugular venous pressure as markers of the subsequent development of heart failure in patients with asymptomatic left ventricular dysfunction. *American Journal of Medicine, 114*(6), 431–437.

Drew, B. J., Califf, R. M., Funk, M., Kaufman, E. S., Krucoff, M. W., Laks, M. M., et al. (2004). Practice standards for electrocardiographic monitoring in hospital settings. *Circulation, 110*(17), 2721–2746.

Eagle, K. A., Kline-Rogers, E., Goodman, S. G., Gurfinkel, E. P., Avezum, A., Flather, M. D., et al. (2004). Adherence to evidence-based therapies after discharge for acute coronary syndromes: An ongoing prospective, observational study. *American Journal of Medicine, 117*(2), 73–81.

Edwards, D. F. (1999). The Synergy Model: Linking patient needs to nurse competencies. *Critical Care Nurse, 19*(1), 88–98.

Emergency Nurses Association & Newberry, L. (2003). *Sheehy's emergency nursing: Principles and practice* (5th ed.). St. Louis, MO: Mosby/Elsevier.

Enriquez-Sarano, M., Schaff, H. V., & Frye, R. L. (2003). Mitral regurgitation: What causes the leakage is fundamental to the outcome of valve repair. *Circulation, 108,* 253–256.

Epstein, A. E. (2004). An update on implantable cardioverter–defibrillator guidelines. *Current Opinion on Cardiology, 19*(1), 23–25.

Eremeeva, M. E., Gerns, H. L., Lydy, S. L., Goo, J. S., Ryan, E. T., Mathew, S. S., et al. (2007). Bacteremia, fever, and splenomegaly caused by a newly recognized *Bartonella* species: Brief report. *New England Journal of Medicine, 356*(23), 2381.

Everett, T. H., & Olgin, J. E. (2004). Basic mechanism of atrial fibrillation. *Cardiology Clinics, 22*(1), 9–20.

Faybush, E. M., & Fass, R. (2004). Gastroesophageal reflux disease in noncardiac chest pain. *Gastroenterology Clinics of North America, 33*(1), 41–54.

Fields, L. E., Burt, V. L., Cutler, J. A., Hughes, J., Roccella, E. J., & Sorlie, P. (2004). The burden of adult hypertension in the United States 1999 to 2000: A rising tide. *Hypertension, 44*(4), 398–404.

Finkelmeier, B. A. (2000). *Cardiothoracic surgical nursing* (2nd ed.). Philadelphia: Lippincott Williams & Wilkins.

Finta, B., & Haines, D. E. (2004). Catheter ablation therapy for atrial fibrillation. *Cardiology Clinics, 22*(1), 127–145.

Fox, C. S., Evans, J. C., Larson, M. G., Kannel, W. B., & Levy, D. (2004). Temporal trends in coronary heart disease mortality and sudden cardiac death from 1950 to 1999: The Framingham Heart Study. *Circulation, 110*(5), 522–527.

Franklin, K., Goldberg, R. J., Spencer, F., Klein, W., Budaj, A., Brieger, D., et al. (2004). Implications of diabetes in patients with acute coronary syndromes: The Global Registry of Acute Coronary Events. *Archives of Internal Medicine, 164*(13), 1457–1463.

Frey, N., Katus, H. A., Olson, E. N., & Hill, J. A. (2004). Hypertrophy of the heart: A new therapeutic target? *Circulation, 109*(13), 1580–1589.

Frishman, W. H., Sonnenblick, E. H., & Sica, D. A. (Eds.). (2004). *Cardiovascular pharmacotherapeutics* (2nd ed.). New York: McGraw-Hill.

Garber, A. J., Moghissi, E. S., Bransome, Jr., E. D., Clark, N. G., Clement, S., Cobin, R. H., et al. (2004). American College of Endocrinology position statement on inpatient diabetes and metabolic control. *Endocrinology Practice, 10*(1), 37–82.

Goldman, L., & Ausiello, D. (2004). *Cecil textbook of medicine* (22nd ed.). Philadelphia: Mosby.

Goldstein, J. A. (2004). Cardiac tamponade, constrictive pericarditis, and restrictive cardiomyopathy. *Current Problems in Cardiology, 29*(9), 503–567.

Graham, L. (2008). AHA releases updated guidelines on the prevention of infective endocarditis. *American Family Physician, 77*(4), 538.

Greenland, P., Knoll, M. D., Stamler, J., Neaton, J. D., Dyer, A. R., Garside, D. B., et al. (2003). Major risk factors as antecedents of fatal and nonfatal coronary heart disease events. *Journal of the American Medical Association, 290,* 891–897.

Greig, J., O'Sullivan, C. E., Adam, O., Klein, H. H., & Schäfers, H. J. (2007). Intraaortic vegetations and infective endocarditis. *New England Journal of Medicine, 356*(23), 2430.

Grif Alspach, J. (Ed.). (2006). *Core curriculum for critical care nursing* (6th ed.). St. Louis, MO: Saunders.

Grundy, S. M., Cleeman, J. I., Merz, C. N., Brewer, H. B. Jr., Clark, L. T., Hunninghake, D. B., et al. (2004). Implications of recent clinical trials for the National Cholesterol Education Program Adult Treatment Panel III. *Circulation, 110,* 227–239.

Hallstrom, A. P., Ornato J. P., Weisfeldt, M., Travers, A., Christenson, J., McBurnie, M. A., et al. (2004). Public-access defibrillation and survival after out-of-hospital cardiac arrest. *New England Journal of Medicine, 351*(7), 637–646.

Halperin, J. L. & Fuster, V. (2003). Meeting the challenge of peripheral arterial disease. *Archives of Internal Medicine, 28,* 877–878.

Hardin, S. R., & Kaplow, R. (Eds.). (2004). *Synergy for clinical excellence: The AACN Synergy Model for Patient Care.* Boston: Jones and Bartlett.

Haskell, W. L. (2003). Cardiovascular disease prevention and lifestyle interventions: Effectiveness and efficacy. *Journal of Cardiovascular Nursing, 18*(4), 245–255.

Henry, L. B. (2003). Left ventricular systolic dysfunction and ischemic cardiomyopathy. *Critical Care Nursing Quarterly, 26*(1), 16–21.

Hickey, J. V. (2002). *The clinical practice of neurological and neurosurgical nursing* (5th ed.). Philadelphia: Lippincott Williams & Wilkins.

Hill, E. E., Vanderschueren, S., Verhaegen, J., Herijgers, P., Claus, P., Herregods, M. C., et al. (2007). Risk factors for infective endocarditis and outcome of patients with *Staphylococcus aureus* bacteremia. *Mayo Clinic Proceedings, 82*(10), 1165.

Hirsh, J., Heddle, N., & Kelton, J. G. (2004). Treatment of heparin-induced thrombocytopenia: A critical review. *Archives of Internal Medicine, 164*(4), 361–369.

Holmes, E. C. (2003). Outpatient management of long-term assist devices. *Cardiology Clinics, 21*, 91–99.

Horstkotte, D., Follath, F., Gutschik, E., Lengyel, M., Oto, A., Pavie, A., et al. (2004). Guidelines on prevention, diagnosis and treatment of infective endocarditis: Executive summary. The Task Force on Infective Endocarditis of the European Society of Cardiology. *European Heart Journal, 25*(3), 267–276.

Houterman, S., Verchuren, W. M., & Kromhout, D. (2003). Smoking, blood pressure, and serum cholesterol: Effects on 20 year mortality. *Epidemiology, 14*(1), 24–29.

Irwin, M. E. (2004). Cardiac pacing device therapy for atrial dysrhythmias. *AACN Clinical Issues, 15*(3), 377–390.

Jacobs, A. K., Leopold, J. A., Bates, E., Mendes, L. A., Sleeper, L. A., White, H., et al. (2003). Cardiogenic shock caused by right ventricular infarction: A report from the SHOCK registry. *Journal of the American College of Cardiology, 41*(8), 1273–1279.

James, T. N. (2003). Structure and function of the sinus node, AV node and His bundle of the human heart: Part II: Function. *Progress in Cardiovascular Disease, 45*(3), 327–360.

Jessup, M., & Brozena, S. C. (2003). Epilogue: Support devices for end stage heart failure. *Cardiology Clinics, 21*, 135–139.

Jesurum, J. (2004). Protocols for practice: SvO_2 monitoring. *Critical Care Nurse, 24*(4), 73–76.

Kang, N., Smith, W., Greaves, S., & Haydock, D. (2007). Pulmonary-valve endocarditis. *New England Journal of Medicine, 356*(2), 2224.

Kawasaki, T., Akakabe, Y., Yamano, M., Miki, S., Kamitani, T., Kuribayashi, T., et al. (2008). R-wave amplitude response to myocardial ischemia in hypertrophic cardiomyopathy. *Journal of Electrocardiology, 41*(1), 68.

Kellen, J. C. (2004). Implementations for nursing care of patients with atrial fibrillation: Lessons learned from the AFFIRM and RACE studies. *Journal of Cardiovascular Nursing, 19*(2), 128–137.

Keller, K. B., & Lemberg, L. (2004). Prinzmetal's angina. *American Journal of Critical Care, 13*(4), 350–354.

Kern, L. S. (2004). Postoperative atrial fibrillation: New directions in prevention and treatment. *Journal of Cardiovascular Nursing, 19*(2),103–115.

Khot, U. N., Khot, M. B., Bajzer, C. T., Sapp, S. K., Ohman, E. M., Brener, S. J., et al. (2003). Prevalence of conventional risk factors with coronary heart disease. *Journal of the American Medical Association, 290*, 898–904.

Khurana, R. K. (2008). Takotsubo cardiomyopathy in a patient with postural tachycardia syndrome. *Clinical Autonomic Research, 18*(1), 43.

Krahn, A. D., Klein, G. J., Skanes, A. C., & Yee, R. (2003). Use of the implantable loop recorder in evaluation of patients with unexplained syncope. *Journal of Cardiovascular Electrophysiology, 14*(9 suppl), S70–S73.

Krajinovic, V., Andrasevic, A. T., & Barsic, B. (2007). Tricuspidal valve endocarditis due to *Yersinia enterocolitica. Infection, 35*(3), 203.

Krinsley, J. S. (2003). Test-ordering strategy in the intensive care unit. *Journal of Intensive Care Medicine, 18*(6), 330–339.

Lang, C., Sauter, M., Szalay, G., Racchi, G., Grassi, G., Rainaldi, G., et al. (2008). Connective tissue growth factor: A crucial cytokine-mediating cardiac fibrosis in ongoing enterovirus myocarditis. *Journal of Molecular Medicine, 86*(10), 49.

Lefler, L. L., & Bondy, K. N. (2004). Women's delay in seeking treatment with myocardial infarction: A meta-synthesis. *Journal of Cardiovascular Nursing, 19*(4), 251–268.

Lin, J. C., Apple, F. S., Murakami, M. M., & Luepker, R. V. (2004). Rates of positive cardiac troponin I and creatine kinase MB mass among patients hospitalized for suspected acute coronary syndromes. *Clinical Chemistry, 50*(2), 333–338.

Lipson, J. G., Dibble, S. L., & Minarik, P. A. (Eds.). (1996). *Culture and nursing care: A pocket guide.* San Francisco, CA: UCSF Nursing Press.

Lloyd-Jones, D. M., Wang, T. J., Leip, E. P., Larson, M. G., Levy, D., Vasan, R. S., et al. (2004). Lifetime risk for development of atrial fibrillation: The Framingham Heart Study. *Circulation, 110*(9), 1042–1046.

López, J., Revilla, A., Vilacosta, I., Villacorta, E., González-Juanatey, C., Gómez, I., et al. (2007). Definition, clinical profile, microbiological spectrum, and prognostic factors of early-onset prosthetic valve endocarditis. *European Heart Journal, 28*(6), 760.

Maalouf, M., Moon, W., Leers, S., Papasavas, P. K., Birdas, T., & Caushaj, P. F. (2007). Mycotic aneurysm of the infrarenal aorta after drainage of an infected chronic pancreatic pseudocyst: Case report and review of the literature. *American Surgeon, 73*(12), 1266.

Maisch, B., Seferovic, P. M., Ristic, A. D., Erbel, R., Rienmüller, R., Adler, Y., et al. (2004). Guidelines on the diagnosis and management of pericardial diseases executive summary: The Task Force on the Diagnosis and Management of Pericardial Diseases of the European Society of Cardiology. *European Heart Journal, 25*(7), 586–610.

Malinoski, D. J., Slater, M. S., & Mullins, R. J. (2004). Crush injury and rhabdomyolysis. *Critical Care Clinics, 20*(1), 171–192.

McGuire, D. K., Newby, L. K., Bhapkar, M. V., Moliterno, D. J., Hochman, J. S., Klein, W. W., et al. (2004). Association of diabetes mellitus and glycemic control strategies with clinical outcomes after acute coronary syndromes. *American Heart Journal, 147*(2), 246–252.

McKay, R. G. (2003). Ischemic guided versus early invasive strategies in the management of acute coronary syndromes/non-ST-segment elevation myocardial infarction. *Journal of the American College of Cardiology, 41*(4 suppl S), 96S–102S.

McQuillan, K. A., Von Rueden, K. T., Hartsock, R. L., Flynn, M. B., & Whalen, E. (Eds.). (2002). *Trauma nursing: From resuscitation through rehabilitation* (3rd ed.). Philadelphia: W. B. Saunders/Elsevier.

McSweeney, J. C., Cody, M., O'Sullivan, P., Elberson, K., Moser D. K., & Garvin, B. J. (2003). Women's early warning symptoms of acute myocardial infarction. *Circulation, 108*(21), 2619–2623.

Medina, J., & Puntillo, K. (2006). *AACN protocols for practice: Palliative care and end-of-life issues in critical care.* Sudbury, MA: Jones and Bartlett.

Mehta, L. S. R., & Yusuf, S. (2003). Short- and long-term oral antiplatelet therapy in acute coronary syndromes. *Journal of the American College of Cardiology, 41*(4 suppl S), 79S–88S.

Menon, T., Nandhakumar, B., Jaganathan, V., Shanmugasundaram, S., Malathy, B., & Nisha, B. (2008). Bacterial endocarditis due to Group C *Streptococcus. Journal of Postgraduate Medicine, 54*(1), 64.

Mosca, L., Appel, L. J., Benjamin, E. J., Berra, K., Chandra-Strobos, N., Fabunmi, R. P., et al. (2004). Evidence based guidelines for cardiovascular disease prevention in women. *Circulation, 109*(5), 672–693.

Nemes, A., Anwar, A. M., Caliskan, A. K., Soliman, O. I., van Dalen, B. M., Geleijnse, M. L., et al. (2008). Evaluation of left atrial systolic function in noncompaction cardiomyopathy by real-time three-dimensional echocardiography. *International Journal of Cardiovascular Imaging, 24*(3), 237.

Newby, L. K., Goldmann, B. U., & Ohman, E. M. (2003). Troponin: An important prognostic marker and risk-stratification tool in non-ST-segment elevation acute coronary syndromes. *Journal of the American College of Cardiology, 41*(4 suppl S), 31S–36S.

Niebauer, J. (2008). Effects of exercise training on inflammatory markers in patients with heart failure. *Heart Failure Reviews, 13*(1), 39.

Nikolsky, E., Mehran, R., Halkin, A., Aymong, E. D., Mintz, G. S., Lasic, Z., et al. (2004). Vascular complications associated with arteriotomy closure devices in patients undergoing percutaneous coronary procedures: A meta-analysis. *Journal of the American College of Cardiology, 44*(6), 1200–1209.

Nishimura, R. A., Ommen, S. R., & Tajik, A. J. (2003). Hypertrophic cardiomyopathy: A patient perspective. *Circulation, 108,* e133–e135.

Novis, D. A., Jones, B. A., Dale, J. C., Walsh, M. K., & College of American Pathologists. (2004). Biochemical markers of myocardial injury test turnaround time: A College of American Pathologists Q-Probes study of 7020 troponin and 4368 creatine kinase-MB determinations in 159 institutions. *Archives of Pathology and Laboratory Medicine, 128*(2), 158–164.

Olivery, H. E., Compton, L. A., & Barnett, J. V. (2004). Coronary vessel development the epicardium delivers. *Trends in Cardiovascular Medicine, 14*(6), 246–251.

Paelinck, B., & Dendale, P. A. (2003). Images in clinical medicine: Cardiac tamponade in Dressler's syndrome. *New England Journal of Medicine, 248*(23), e8.

Pagana, K. D., & Pagana, J. (2005). *Mosby's manual of diagnostic and laboratory tests* (3rd ed.). St. Louis, MO: Mosby/Elsevier.

Palmer, B. F. (2004). Managing hyperkalemia caused by inhibitors of the renin–angiotensin–aldosterone system. *New England Journal of Medicine, 351*(6), 585–592.

Patel, H., & Pagani, F. D. (2003). Extracorporeal mechanical circulatory assist. *Cardiology Clinics, 21*(1), 29–41.

Paterick, T. E., Paterick, T. J., Nishimura, R. A., & Steckelberg, J. M. (2007). Complexity and subtlety of infective endocarditis. *Mayo Clinic Proceedings, 82*(5), 615.

Patten, R. D., & Soman, P. (2004). Prevention and reversal of LV remodeling with neurohormonal inhibitors. *Current Treatment Options in Cardiovascular Medicine, 6*(4), 313–325.

Paul, S. (2003). Ventricular remodeling. *Critical Care Nursing Clinics of North America, 15*(4), 407–411.

Peel, D. A. (2007). Endocarditis due to a nutritionally variant *Streptococcus:* A lesson in recognition and isolation. *British Journal of Biomedical Science, 64*(4), 175.

Pelter, M. M., Adams, M. G., & Drew, B. J. (2003). Transient myocardial ischemia is an independent predictor of adverse in-hospital outcomes in patients with acute coronary syndromes treated in the telemetry unit. *Heart and Lung, 32*(2), 71–78.

Perez-Lugones, A., McMahon J. T., Ratliff, N. B., Saliba, W. I., Schweikert, R. A., Marrouche, N. F., et al. (2003). Evidence of specialized conduction cells in human pulmonary veins of patients with atrial fibrillation. *Journal of Cardiovascular Electrophysiology, 14*(8), 803–809.

Pope, J. H., Ruthazer R., Kontos, M. C., Beshansky, J. R., Griffith, J. L., & Selker, H. P. (2004). The impact of electrocardiographic left ventricular hypertrophy and bundle branch block on the triage and outcome of ED patients with a suspected acute coronary syndrome: A multicenter study. *American Journal of Emergency Medicine, 22*(3), 156–163.

Prabhakar, N. R., & Peng, Y. J. (2004). Peripheral chemoreceptors in health and disease. *Journal of Applied Physiology, 96*(1), 359–366.

Prahash, A., & Lynch, T. (2004). B-type natriuretic peptide: A diagnostic, prognostic, and therapeutic tool in heart failure. *American Journal of Critical Care, 13*(1), 46–55.

Pyle, W. G., & Solaro, R. J. (2004). At the crossroads of myocardial signaling: The role of Z-discs in intracellular signaling and cardiac function. *Circulation Research, 94*(3), 296–305.

Reinhart, K., Kuhn, H., Hartog, C., & Bredle, D. L. (2004). Continuous central venous and pulmonary artery oxygen saturation monitoring in the critically ill. *Intensive Care Medicine, 30*(8), 1572–1578.

Richard, C., Warszawski, J., Anguel, N., Deye, N., Combes, A., Barnoud, D., et al. (2003). Early use of the pulmonary artery catheter and outcomes in patients with shock and acute respiratory distress syndrome: A randomized controlled trial. *Journal of American Medical Association, 290*(20), 2713–2720.

Robicsek, F., Thubrikar, M. J., Cook, J. W., & Fowler, B. (2003). The congenitally bicuspid aortic valve: How does it function? Why does it fail? *Annals of Thoracic Surgery, 77*(1),177–185.

Roden, D. M. (2004). Drug-induced prolongation of the QT interval. *New England Journal of Medicine, 350*(10), 1013–1022.

Rudisill, P. T., Kennedy, C., & Paul, S. (2003). The use of beta-blockers in the treatment of chronic heart failure. *Critical Care Nurse of North America, 15*(4), 439–446.

Sandham, J. D., Hull, R. D., Brant, R. F., Knox, L., Pineo, G. F., Doig, C. J., et al. (2003). A randomized, controlled trial of the use of pulmonary artery catheters in high-risk surgical patients. *New England Journal of Medicine, 348*(1), 5–14.

Saul, L., & Shatzer, M. (2003). B-type natriuretic peptide testing for detection of heart failure. *Critical Care Nursing Quarterly, 26*(1), 35–59.

Schwarz, K. A., & Elman, C. S. (2003). Identification of factors predictive of hospital readmissions for patients with heart failure. *Heart and Lung, 32*(3), 88–99.

Schwert, D. W., & Vatikus, P. (2003). Drug-eluding stents to prevent re-blocking of coronary arteries. *Journal of Cardiovascular Nursing, 18*(1), 11–16.

Sealey, B., & Lui, K. (2004). Diagnosis and management of vasovagal syncope and dysautonomia. *AACN Clinical Issues, 15*(3), 449–461.

Segal, B. L. (2003). Valvular heart disease, part 2: Mitral valve disease in older adults. *Geriatrics, 58*(10), 26–31.

Shadman, R., Criqui, M. H., Bundens, W. P., Fronek, A., Denenberg, J. O., Gamst, A. C., et al. (2004). Subclavian artery stenosis: Prevalence, risk factors, and association with cardiovascular diseases. *Journal of the American College of Cardiology, 44*(3), 618–623.

Shak, P. K. (2003). Mechanisms of plaque vulnerability and rupture. *Journal of the American College of Cardiology, 41*(4 suppl S), 15S–22S.

Shan, K., Constantine, G., Sivananthan, M., et al. (2004). Role of cardiac magnetic resonance imaging in the assessment of myocardial viability. *Circulation, 109*(11), 1328–1334.

Sharis, P. J., & Cannon, C. P. (2003). *Evidence-based cardiology* (2nd ed.). Philadelphia: Lippincott Williams & Wilkins.

Singer, D. E., Albers, G. W., Dalen, J. E., Go, A. S., Halperin, J. L., & Manning, W. J. (2004). Antithrombotic therapy in atrial fibrillation: the Seventh ACCP Conference on Antithrombotic and Thrombolytic Therapy. *Chest, 126*(3 suppl), 429S–456S.

Skidmore-Roth, L. (2004). *Mosby's 2004 nursing drug reference*. St. Louis, MO: Mosby/Elsevier.

Smeltzer, S., & Bare, B. G. (2003). *Brunner and Suddarth's textbook of medical–surgical nursing* (10th ed.). Philadelphia: Lippincott Williams & Wilkins.

Smith, S. W., Tibbles, C. D., Apple, F. S., & Zimmerman, M. (2004). Outcome of low-risk patients discharged home after a normal cardiac troponin I. *Journal of Emergency Medicine, 26*(4), 401–406.

Sneed, N. V., & Paul, S. C. (2003). Readiness for behavioral changes in patients with heart failure. *American Journal of Critical Care, 12*(5), 444–453.

Sohail, M. R., Uslan, D. Z., Khan, A. H., Friedman, P. A., Hayes, D. L., Wilson, W. R., et al. (2008). Infective endocarditis complicating permanent pacemaker and implantable cardioverter–defibrillator infection. *Mayo Clinic Proceedings, 83*(1), 46.

Sole, M. L., Hartshorn, J., & Lamborne, M. L. (2001). *Introduction to critical care nursing* (3rd ed.). Philadelphia: W. B. Saunders/Elsevier.

Stuart-Shor, E. M., Buselli, E. F., & Carroll, D. L. (2003). Are psychosocial factors associated with pathogenesis and consequences of cardiovascular disease in the elderly? *Journal of Cardiovascular Nursing, 18*(3), 169–183.

Swami, A., & Spodick, D. H. (2003). Pulsus paradoxus in cardiac tamponade: A pathophysiologic continuum. *Clinical Cardiology, 26*(5), 215–217.

Szekendi, M. K. (2003). Compliance with acute MI guidelines lowers inpatient mortality. *Journal of Cardiovascular Nursing, 18*(5), 356–359.

Taubert, K. A. (2008). Endocarditis prophylaxis: An evolution of change. *American Family Physician, 77*(4), 421.

Thohan, V., Torre-Amione, G., & Koerner, M. M. (2004). Aldosterone antagonism and congestive heart failure: A new look at an old therapy. *Current Opinions in Cardiology, 19*(4), 301–308.

Tilley, P., & Petersen, D. (2003). Pulling axis together. *Dimensions of Critical Care Nursing, 22*(5), 210–215.

Timothy, P. R., & Rodeman, B. J. (2004). Temporary pacemakers in critically ill patients: Assessment and management strategies. *AACN Clinical Issues, 15*(3), 305–325.

Tleyjeh, I. M., & Baddour, L. M. (2007). *Staphylococcus aureus* bacteremia and infective endocarditis: Old questions, new answers? *Mayo Clinic Proceedings, 82*(10), 1163.

Topol, E. J. (2003). A guide to therapeutic decision-making in patients with non-ST-segment elevation in acute coronary syndromes. *Journal of the American College of Cardiology, 41*(4 suppl S), 123S–129S.

Topol, E. J. (Ed.). (2004). *Textbook of interventional cardiology* (4th ed.). Philadelphia: Saunders.

Trotman-Dickenson, B. (2003). Radiology in the intensive care unit (Part I). *Journal of Intensive Care Medicine, 18*(4), 198–210.

Trotman-Dickerson, B. (2003). Radiology in the intensive care unit (Part II). *Journal of Intensive Care Medicine, 18*(4), 239–252.

Tsai, T., Chen, H., Hsia, H., Zei, P., Wang, P., & Al-Ahmad, A. (2007). Cardiac device infections complicated by erosion. *Journal of Interventional Cardiac Electrophysiology, 19*(2), 133.

Tung, P., Kopelnik, A., Banki, N., Ong, K., Ko, N., Lawton, M. T., et al. (2004). Predictors of neurocardiogenic injury after subarachnoid hemorrhage. *Stroke, 35*(2), 548–551.

Urden, L. D., Stacy, K. M., & Lough, M. E. (2007). *Thelan's critical care nursing: Diagnosis and management* (5th ed.). St. Louis, MO: Mosby.

Wang, K., Asinger, R. W., & Marriott, H. J. (2003). ST-segment elevation in conditions other than acute myocardial infarction. *New England Journal of Medicine, 349*(22), 2128–2135.

Wessels, M. W., De Graaf, B. M., Cohen-Overbeek, T. E., Spitaels, S. E., de Groot-de Laat, L. E., Ten Cate, F. J., et al. (2008). A new syndrome with noncompaction cardiomyopathy, bradycardia, pulmonary stenosis, atrial septal defect and heterotaxy with suggestive linkage to chromosome 6p. *Human Genetics, 122*(6), 595.

Wiegand, D. J. L., & Carlson, K. K. (Eds.). (2005). *AACN procedure manual for critical care* (5th ed.). Philadelphia: Elsevier.

Wong, W. M., & Fass, R. (2004). Noncardiac chest pain. *Current Treatment Options in Gastroenterology, 7*(4), 273–278.

Woods, S., Sivarajan Froelicher, E. S., & Motzer, S. U. (2000). *Cardiac nursing* (4th ed.). Philadelphia, PA: Lippincott Williams & Wilkins.

Wu, L. A., & Nishimura, R. A. (2003). Images in clinical medicine: Pulses paradoxus. *New England Journal of Medicine, 349*(7), 666.

Yasuma, F., & Hayano, J. (2004). Respiratory sinus arrhythmia: Why does the heartbeat synchronize with respiratory rhythm? *Chest, 125*(2), 683–690.

Zhang, J. (2003). Sudden cardiac death: Implantable cardioverter defibrillations and pharmacological treatments. *Critical Care Nursing Quarterly, 26*(1), 45–49.

Zhang, S., Younis, G., Hariharan, R., Ho, J., Yang, Y., Ip, J., et al. (2004). Lower loop reentry as a mechanism of clockwise right atrial flutter. *Circulation, 109*(13), 1630–1635.

Zile, M. R., Baicu, C. F., & Gaasch, W. H. (2004). Diastolic heart failure: Abnormalities in active relaxation and passive stiffness of the left ventricle. *New England Journal of Medicine, 350*(19), 1953–1959.

Zimetbaum, P. J., Constantine, G., Sivananthan, M., Fisher, J. D., Hafley, G. E., Lee, K. L., et al. (2004). Electrocardiographic predictors of arrhythmic death and total mortality in the multicenter unsustained tachycardia trial. *Circulation, 110*(7), 776–769.

QUESTIONS

1. Brianna is a 26-year-old housewife admitted to your ICU with status asthmaticus. She has been taking Accolate, Allegra and has been using a Proventil HFA rescue inhaler at home. Today Brianna was working in her garden when she could not catch her breath. Her bronchospasms worsened and she was transported to the ED. In the ED, she received albuterol, oxygen, and epinephrine without significant improvement. On auscultation, inspiratory and expiratory wheezing with a prolonged expiratory phase is heard throughout the lung fields. Brianna is using accessory muscles for respiration and is tachycardic and tachypneic. She is placed on 2 L/min oxygen via NC and ABGs drawn. Blood gas results show the following findings: pH 7.52, PaO_2 106 mm Hg, $PaCO_2$ 27 mm Hg, and HCO_3 24 mEq/L. These blood gas results indicate:
   A. Uncompensated respiratory acidosis
   B. Compensated metabolic alkalosis
   C. Compensated metabolic acidosis
   D. Uncompensated respiratory alkalosis

2. Continuing with the scenario from Question 1, what is the most probable cause of Brianna's acid–base imbalance?
   A. An adverse effect of albuterol
   B. A side effect of theophylline
   C. Hyperventilation
   D. Hypoventilation

3. Continuing with the scenario from Questions 1 and 2, the hospitalist now orders Inderal (propranololol) for Brianna. As a nurse, you know that propranolol is contraindicated for asthmatics because
   A. It will exacerbate the tachycardia.
   B. It will lead to a severe respiratory acidosis.
   C. Pneumonia may result.
   D. Bronchospasm may worsen.

4. Continuing with the scenario from Questions 1–3, Brianna's O_2 was increased to 5 L/min via mask. On auscultation, you note that the wheezing is now barely audible. This finding may indicate
   A. Improvement.
   B. A need to lower the O_2.
   C. A need for epinephrine.
   D. A worsening condition.

5. A possible treatment to best improve air flow in status asthmaticus is:
   A. PEEP
   B. Heliox
   C. Norepinephrine
   D. Nebulizer treatment

6. Continuing with the scenario from Questions 1–5, Brianna now needs to be placed on mechanical ventilation. The anesthesiologist uses pancuronium bromide (Pavulon) to paralyze the respiratory muscles. Which of the following drugs will counteract the effects of Pavulon?
   A. Atropine
   B. Narcan
   C. Neostigmine
   D. Regitine

7. Your patient has been diagnosed with pulmonary hypertension. A pulmonary artery catheter is placed and would be expected to show increases in which of the following parameters?
   A. Pulmonary artery pressures
   B. PAOP
   C. PCWP
   D. Left ventricular pressures

8. Type II alveolar cells produce
   A. Macrocytes.
   B. Phagocytes.
   C. Surfactant.
   D. CO_2.

9. If you hear faint breath sounds on the left side of the chest and normal sounds on the right side immediately after your patient has been intubated, what is the most likely cause?
   A. The patient has a tumor.
   B. The physician has intubated the esophagus.
   C. The endotracheal tube is at the carina.
   D. The right mainstem has been intubated.

10. Nathan is a 26-year-old engineer who has been on hemodialysis for 3 years. He missed his last 2 treatments, and now he is lethargic, lacks stamina, and is very edematous. His ABGs show the following results: pH 7.30, $PaCO_2$ 32 mm Hg, HCO_3 17 mEq/L, PaO_2 70 mm Hg. Nathan's results indicate
    A. Metabolic alkalosis.
    B. Respiratory acidosis.
    C. Metabolic acidosis.
    D. Respiratory alkalosis.

11. You ask a fellow nurse to carry a newly drawn ABG specimen to the lab. She does not place the sample on ice. What effect will the lack of icing have on the sample?

A. None.

B. It will invalidate the sample.

C. The pH will rise.

D. The PaO_2 will rise.

12. You are asked to draw an arterial blood gas sample. You prepare a glass syringe with heparin. What effect will the presence of too much heparin have on the sample, if any?

    A. Decrease the bicarbonate level

    B. No effect

    C. Increase the $PaCO_2$

    D. Totally prevent clotting

13. You are attempting to draw an arterial blood gas sample from an arterial line. The syringe requires a lot of force to move the cylinder. What effect will the high friction of the syringe have on blood gas results?

    A. It will put the artery into spasm.

    B. It will increase the $PaCO_2$.

    C. It will decrease the PaO_2.

    D. It will not have any effect on the results.

14. The respiratory therapist arrives to obtain an arterial blood gas sample and asks if the patient has a fever. The possibility of fever will have what effect on the sample?

    A. The HCO_3 will be elevated.

    B. The PaO_2 will rise.

    C. Fever has no effect on ABG findings.

    D. The pH will rise.

15. Familial emphysema is a condition that results in a deficiency in

    A. Adenosine monophosphate.

    B. Ability to produce mucus.

    C. Alveoli.

    D. Serum alpha-antitrypsin.

16. People who have emphysema develop chronic hypoxia. Which potential imbalance would be expected with this condition?

    A. Hypokalemia

    B. Hypochloremia

    C. Decreased bicarbonate levels

    D. Hyponatremia

17. Your patient had an exacerbation of COPD and is now intubated. When the family visits, they are shocked to see the patient this way. No one had told them the condition of their family member had deteriorated so that he required intubation. They try to communicate verbally with the patient, but he does not respond except to gesture. What should the nurse tell family members?

    A. They must leave the room because they are exciting the patient.

    B. The tube used for breathing prevents the patient from speaking.

    C. They must speak with the doctor, who will explain why the patient cannot speak.

    D. The patient is very sick and may die.

18. Carl has been in the ICU for 2 weeks. He was intubated for a time because of his ARDS. Today his nurse informed Carl that he is to be transferred to a progressive care unit. Carl became tachycardic and restless. He stated, "I can't go now. What if something like this happens to me again?" The nurse's best response would be:

    A. "The nurses in the other unit can take care of you."
    B. "We are not very far away if you need to come back."
    C. "Your insurance will not cover another day here."
    D. "You sound concerned about leaving our ICU."

19. Continuing with the scenario in Question 18, a set of blood gases drawn just prior to Carl's transfer shows the following results: pH 7.50, $PaCO_2$ 32 mm Hg, HCO_3 21 mEq/L, PaO_2 86 mm Hg. These results would indicate:

    A. Respiratory acidosis
    B. Respiratory alkalosis
    C. Metabolic acidosis
    D. Metabolic alkalosis

20. Continuing with the scenario in Questions 18 and 19, Carl is finally released from the hospital. He plans to visit his family in Denver. Part of the patient teaching for Carl should include information on the effects of high altitude on his ability to oxygenate effectively. Which of the following changes would be expected on his blood gas results when Carl is in Denver?

    A. The pH will decrease.
    B. No effect is expected.
    C. O_2 saturation would decrease.
    D. PaO_2 would increase.

21. SaO_2 values account for what percentage of oxygen (O_2) carried within the bloodstream?

    A. 2–3%
    B. 10–24%
    C. 97–98%
    D. 100%

22. Hypoxemia is best defined as:

    A. A decrease in oxygen levels at the cellular level
    B. A decrease in oxygen levels in arterial blood
    C. A decrease in oxygen levels in venous blood
    D. A decrease in oxygen levels from the brain

23. Adam, a 50-year-old patient with severe bronchitis, has been treated with a non-rebreather mask for 5 days. He is exhibiting increased distress with chest discomfort, restlessness, a dry hacking cough with dyspnea, and numbness in his extremities. Pulmonary function tests (PFTs) indicate a decreased vital capacity (VC), decreased compliance, and decreased functional residual capacity (FRC). As the nurse caring for this patient, you should:

    A. Prepare for intubation with 100% FiO_2 (fraction of inspired oxygen)
    B. Administer Lasix 40 mg IV
    C. Take the patient for a CT scan and prepare to give tPA
    D. Check the pulse oximeter correlation with an arterial blood gas and decrease the FiO_2

24. Mary, a patient with ARDS, has been ventilated with mechanical ventilation for 4 days. During your assessment, you note a temperature of 100°F, heart rate of 120, respiratory rate of 30, increased cough, and decreased breath sounds on the right side without tracheal deviation. You suspect her symptoms are the result of
    A. Pulmonary edema.
    B. Atelectasis.
    C. Pneumothorax.
    D. Sepsis.

25. As patients age, chest wall compliance decreases. One of the reasons for this change is:
    A. Decreased total lung capacity
    B. Costal cartilage degeneration
    C. Increased arterial oxygen tension
    D. Decreased residual volume

26. The cells that are responsible for forming a barrier for alveoli are:
    A. Macrophages
    B. Type II alveolar epithelial cells
    C. Type I alveolar epithelial cells
    D. Cilia

27. Anatomic dead space is referred to as
    A. Minute ventilation.
    B. Wasted ventilation.
    C. Physiologic dead space.
    D. Conducting airways.

28. The oxyhemoglobin dissociation curve is:
    A. A graphic representation of the relationship between dissolved oxygen and the affinity for oxygen in the hemoglobin molecule
    B. A graphic representation of carbon dioxide content versus oxygen content in arterial blood
    C. A measure of methemoglobin
    D. A way to calculate gas transport across the alveoli

29. If the oxyhemoglobin dissociation curve shifts to the right, one of the factors that will affect this shift is:
    A. A decrease in CO_2
    B. A decrease in pH
    C. A decrease in temperature
    D. A decrease in 2,3-DPG

30. If the oxyhemoglobin dissociation curve shifts to the left, which of the following factors would precipitate this change?
    A. Increased temperature
    B. Increased $PaCO_2$
    C. Increased 2,3-DPG
    D. Increased pH

31. Your patient had a mixed venous sample drawn from his pulmonary artery catheter with a PaO_2 result of 42 mm Hg. This result would indicate
    A. Hypoxia.
    B. Hypoxemia.
    C. A normal value.
    D. Acute respiratory acidosis.

32. Chronic hypoxia usually results in which of the following electrolyte imbalances?
    A. Decreased chloride
    B. Decreased potassium
    C. Decreased calcium
    D. Decreased bicarbonate

33. If you are auscultating lung sounds and you can clearly hear the patient's spoken word through the stethoscope, this is known as:
    A. Egophony
    B. A friction rub
    C. Whispered pectroliloquy
    D. Bronchophony

34. What is the interpretation of the following arterial blood gas results?
    pH: 7.22
    PO_2: 93 mm Hg
    $PaCO_2$: 52 mm Hg
    HCO_3: 23 mEq/L
    A. Uncompensated respiratory acidosis
    B. Compensated metabolic acidosis
    C. Uncompensated metabolic alkalosis
    D. Compensated respiratory acidosis

35. Your patient had 1,250 mL of pleural effusion removed via thoracentesis. He immediately began coughing and became dyspneic. You believe he has developed
    A. A pneumothorax.
    B. Reexpansion pulmonary edema.
    C. A cardiac tamponade.
    D. A hemothorax.

36. Falsely low readings on a pulse oximeter may be due to:
    A. Electronic interference from hemodialysis
    B. Fever
    C. Vascular dyes
    D. Polycythemia

37. Joseph's endotracheal tube cuff has been requiring increasing pressures all shift to maintain a good air seal. The cuff now requires 64 mm Hg. What is the probable cause for the increasing pressure?
    A. Tracheal stenosis
    B. A cuff leak
    C. Tracheal atresia
    D. A wider endotracheal tube is necessary.

38. **Endotracheal cuff pressures should not exceed**
    A. PAOP.
    B. Tracheal capillary filling pressure.
    C. RAP.
    D. Pulmonary artery diastolic pressure.

39. **The respiratory therapist tells you he is covering another unit and cannot perform postural drainage on your patient. He says that your patient needs the left upper lobes drained if possible. The correct position to help this patient is:**
    A. Semi-reclining
    B. Flat with hips elevated
    C. Supine
    D. Flat on left side

40. **The respiratory therapist has just given your patient an aerosol treatment. Which of the following conditions is contraindicated for this treatment?**
    A. Pleural effusions
    B. Head injury
    C. Asthma
    D. Stridor

41. **PEEP is useful in ARDS (acute respiratory distress syndrome) because:**
    A. PEEP decreases cardiac output.
    B. PEEP decreases venous return so lungs drain more effectively.
    C. PEEP prevents barotrauma.
    D. PEEP can open collapsed alveoli.

42. **Patients at risk for thrombosis formation have been classified by a trio of factors known as**
    A. Beck's triad.
    B. Belchod's triad.
    C. Virhow's triad.
    D. Goodman's triad.

43. **PEEP may cause an increase in**
    A. PVR.
    B. SVR.
    C. PAOP.
    D. PAD.

44. **Increased PEEP may cause**
    A. Alveolar collapse.
    B. Hepatomegaly.
    C. Hemothorax.
    D. Increased PAOP.

45. **Signs and symptoms of a pulmonary embolus can include**
    A. A normal EKG or sinus bradycardia.
    B. Pleuritic chest pain, decreased cardiac output.
    C. ABGs that show respiratory acidosis, increased respiratory rate.
    D. Decreased PAS pressure.

46. A patient who is being mechanically ventilated with continuous end-tidal CO_2 (pet CO_2) monitoring develops a pulmonary embolism. An expected change in parameters would include:
    A. Increased PaO_2
    B. Decreased CVP
    C. Decreased pet CO_2
    D. Increased $PaCO_2$

47. On an EKG, an extensive pulmonary embolism may have the following appearance:
    A. Tall, peaked T waves in leads II, III, and AVF
    B. Sinus bradycardia
    C. Inverted T waves in leads V_6–V_9
    D. Complete heart block

48. Dorothy was admitted to the ICU with a fever of 102.3°F, headache, dyspnea, dry cough, and chills. Her lab results indicate a low white blood cell count, low platelets, and increased C-reactive protein levels. Dorothy's history includes a recent trip to a remote Chinese village within the past 2 weeks. You suspect Dorothy may have:
    A. Pneumonia
    B. SARS
    C. Influenza
    D. Pericarditis

49. Which of the following statements is true about pulmonary embolism?
    A. Respiratory acidosis will occur.
    B. Heparin is used to dissolve clots.
    C. Normal D-dimer results can rule out a pulmonary embolism.
    D. Metabolic alkalosis will develop.

50. Myla was admitted to the ICU following a fall from a ladder. She complains of stabbing substernal pain each time she changes her position. She has been diagnosed with pneumomediastinum. A common significant finding with this condition is
    A. Cullen's sign.
    B. Grey-Turner's sign.
    C. Hamman's sign.
    D. Handes's sign.

51. Severe carbon monoxide poisoning occurs when carboxyhemoglobin levels are higher than what percentage?
    A. 10–15%
    B. 20–40%
    C. 40–50%
    D. 50–60%

52. Carbon monoxide has an affinity for hemoglobin thought to be 200–300 times greater than the affinity of oxygen for hemoglobin. Elimination of carbon monoxide occurs via the

A. Kidneys.

B. Liver.

C. Spleen.

D. Lungs.

53. **George lost his home to a fire this morning. He was burned on the chest and neck while trying to put out the fire. He is dyspneic and has soot on his face, and his eyebrows and nares are singed. What is the priority for his treatment?**

A. Maintain cardiac output

B. Airway patency

C. Treat burned areas

D. Obtain ABGs and a carboxyhemoglobin level

54. **Increases in lung compliance occur with**

A. Pulmonary edema.

B. Pleural effusions.

C. Obesity.

D. Emphysema.

55. **Which of the following statements about laryngeal mask airways is true?**

A. A laryngeal mask airway may be inserted by any nurse.

B. A laryngeal mask airway may cause hoarseness after its removal.

C. The patient must have an absent gag reflex.

D. The laryngeal mask airway (LMA) eliminates the risk of aspiration.

56. **Which of the following drugs would be considered a mucolytic agent?**

A. Atropine

B. Terbutaline

C. Acetyl-cysteine

D. Albuterol

57. **Side effects of acetyl-cysteine include**

A. Bronchospasm.

B. Headache.

C. Hypertension.

D. Red urine.

58. **One of the most effective ways to relieve bronchospasm is:**

A. Adrenalin

B. Use of an antihistamine

C. Prednisone

D. A B_2-receptor agonist

59. **Which of the following drugs is a methylzanthine?**

A. Prednisone

B. Theophylline

C. Atropine

D. Accolate

60. To determine if your patient has a genetic predisposition for malignant hyperthermia, which of the following drugs might be used?
    A. Halothane
    B. Caffeine
    C. Accolate
    D. Singular

61. During a cardiac arrest, your patient aspirated gastric contents. Which of the following statements is true regarding this type of aspiration?
    A. If the pH of the material is less than 2.5, necrosis will be minimal.
    B. The patient will always develop ARDS.
    C. Onset of symptoms is gradual.
    D. There is little danger of atelectasis.

62. Roy was admitted for abrupt-onset fever, chills, vomiting, diarrhea, and headache that developed in the past 24 hours. Roy had recently been on a cruise to Barbados. Roy is probably suffering from
    A. A *Pseudomonas* infection.
    B. Influenza.
    C. A *Klebsiella* infection.
    D. Legionnaires' disease.

63. Placement of a central line via a subclavian vein may cause
    A. Cardiac tamponade.
    B. An open pneumothorax.
    C. A tension pneumothorax.
    D. Limb pain.

64. When the resident attempts to place a central line, air is accidentally introduced into the line when the IV tubing becomes disconnected. What is the best position in which to place this patient so as to minimize the venous air embolism?
    A. Reverse Trendelenburg
    B. Right side
    C. Trendelenburg with left decubitus tilt
    D. Left side

65. The definitive study for determination of thrombolic emboli is:
    A. Pulmonary ventilation–perfusion scan
    B. Mixed venous oxygen saturation
    C. Pulmonary angiography
    D. PAWP

66. Risk factors for thrombolic emboli include:
    A. A patient who is 1 week postpartum
    B. Carcinoma
    C. Long bone fractures
    D. Heparin administration

67. A venous air embolism may be caused by
   A. Hemodialysis.
   B. Pulmonary artery catheter.
   C. Radial arterial catheter.
   D. Peritoneal dialysis.

68. Blood gasses you would expect to see with thrombotic emboli are:
   A. pH 7.42, PaO_2 88, $PaCO_2$ 28, HCO_3 22
   B. pH 7.50, PaO_2 74, $PaCO_2$ 52, HCO_3 24
   C. pH 7.32, PaO_2 86, $PaCO_2$ 29, HCO_3 26
   D. pH 7.32, PaO_2 90, $PaCO_2$ 30, HCO_3 24

69. Sandra was admitted for multiple fractures and contusions following a motor vehicle accident this evening. She complains of dyspnea, and petechiae are noted. Sandra probably has
   A. A pulmonary embolus.
   B. Thrombocytopenia.
   C. A venous air emboli.
   D. A fat embolus.

70. The best position for a patient with ARDS is:
   A. Prone
   B. On the right side
   C. On the left side
   D. Supine

71. Fluid therapy in ARDS is directed toward
   A. Keeping a high CO state.
   B. Maintaining a low protein content.
   C. Maintaining hyponatremia.
   D. Maintaining a low circulating fluid volume.

72. Pulmonary hypertension is usually defined by the level of the mean pulmonary artery pressure. A diagnosis of pulmonary hypertension can be made if the MPAP is
   A. 3–5 mm Hg.
   B. 5–9 mm Hg.
   C. 10–20 mm Hg.
   D. Greater than 20 mm Hg.

73. The hallmark sign of asthma is:
   A. PEFR 100–125
   B. FEF 80%
   C. Decreased FEV_1
   D. Wheezing

74. When assessing a patient with a chest tube drainage system, which of the following statements would be correct?
    A. Check for subcutaneous emphysema around the insertion site by auscultation.
    B. If using a Pleur-Evac with auto-transfusion connection, make certain all clamps are open.
    C. The average chest tube size for an adult patient is 20 Fr.
    D. If using a chest tube drainage system with a one-way value and suction, water is required to maintain a seal.

75. The oxyhemoglobin dissociation curve may be shifted to the right by
    A. Alkalosis, hyperthermia, and hypercapnia.
    B. Acidosis, hypercarbia, and hyperthermia.
    C. Acidosis, hypocarbia, and hypothermia.
    D. Alkalosis, hypothermia, and hypercapnia.

76. Which statement about esophageal detection devices (EDDs) is true?
    A. An EDD reduces silent aspiration.
    B. An EDD will have a beige color when gas exchange is adequate.
    C. An EDD is more reliable than a CO_2 detector in a pulseless patient.
    D. A false-positive may result if the patient recently ingested a carbonated beverage.

77. Research has shown that use of normal saline does not thin secretions and may cause which of the following adverse effects?
    A. Anxiety
    B. Depression
    C. Decreased mean arterial pressure
    D. Bronchodilation

78. Complications of PEEP include all of the following *except*
    A. Barotrauma.
    B. Increased cardiac output.
    C. Decreased intracranial pressure.
    D. Sodium and water excretion.

79. In which of the following ventilator modes can the patient breathe spontaneously?
    A. SIMV
    B. CMV
    C. HFV
    D. Oscillator

80. On a ventilator, a high-pressure limit alarm may sound if
    A. The tubing is disconnected.
    B. A leak in a chest tube occurs.
    C. A pneumothorax may have occurred.
    D. The ventilator did not sense a mandatory breath.

81. A side effect of succinylcholine is:
    A. Hypokalemia
    B. Malignant hypothermia
    C. Hypotension
    D. Cardiac arrest

82. Vecuronium (Norcuron) is eliminated primarily via the
    A. Renal glomerulus.
    B. Spleen.
    C. Hepatic/biliary system.
    D. Hoffman elimination.

83. Asthma patients may receive steroids and neuromuscular blocking agents. As a consequence, these patients are at increased risk for
    A. Renal failure.
    B. Hypertension.
    C. Hepatic failure.
    D. Prolonged muscle weakness.

84. The FiO$_2$ for a nasal cannula set at a flow rate of 6 L/min is:
    A. 24%
    B. 30%
    C. 21%
    D. 40%

85. A non-rebreather mask can deliver what percentage of oxygen when the O$_2$ flow rate is 10–15 L/min?
    A. 30–40%
    B. 24–40%
    C. 60–80%
    D. 50–60%

86. Pulse oximetry readings are considered unreliable when oxygen saturation falls below
    A. 60%.
    B. 90%.
    C. 55%.
    D. 70%.

87. A factor that increases pulmonary vascular resistance is:
    A. Prostaglandin therapy
    B. Sepsis
    C. Hypoxia
    D. Hypovolemia

88. A cause of decreased SVO$_2$ would be:
    A. Increased metabolic rate
    B. Sedation
    C. Decreased metabolic rate
    D. Increased cardiac output

89. When an oral ETT is properly positioned in an adult, the centimeter mark will usually be _____ for women at the front teeth.
    A. 14 cm
    B. 21 cm
    C. 23 cm
    D. 25 cm

90. The control variable on a ventilator refers to
    A. The termination of inspiratory time.
    B. The ventilatory patterns.
    C. A preset maximum value.
    D. The variable manipulated to cause inspiration.

91. A common site for the placement of electrodes for a peripheral nerve is on the:
    A. Posterior tibial
    B. Medial nerve
    C. Temporal nerve
    D. Radial nerve

92. Muscles will stop moving in the following order in response to neuromuscular blocking agents:
    A. Abdomen, glottis, extremities, face, eyes
    B. Glottis, extremities, face, abdomen, eyes
    C. Eyes, face, extremities, abdomen
    D. Glottis, intercostals, extremities, neck

93. The usual goal for a patient having neuromuscular blockade during mechanical ventilation is 1 to 2 twitches, indicating _____ to _____ block.
    A. 85%, 90%
    B. 60%, 70%
    C. 40%, 50%
    D. 25%, 40%

94. Analyze the following arterial blood gas results and determine which condition they indicate. Use the provided space to the right side to assist in interpretation by writing acidosis, alkalosis, compensated, or uncompensated.
    pH 7.38
    CO_2 27
    HCO_3 16
    A. Normal
    B. Compensated respiratory acidosis
    C. Compensated metabolic acidosis
    D. Uncompensated respiratory alkalosis

95. Analyze the following arterial blood gas results and determine which condition they indicate. Use the provided space to the right side to assist in interpretation by writing acidosis, alkalosis, compensated, or uncompensated.
    pH 7.46
    CO_2 34
    HCO_3 24
    A. Normal
    B. Compensated respiratory acidosis
    C. Compensated metabolic acidosis
    D. Uncompensated respiratory alkalosis

96. Analyze the following arterial blood gas results and determine which condition they indicate. Use the provided space to the right side to assist in interpretation by writing acidosis, alkalosis, compensated, or uncompensated.
    pH 7.18
    CO_2 40
    HCO_3 15
    A. Normal
    B. Compensated respiratory acidosis
    C. Uncompensated metabolic acidosis
    D. Uncompensated respiratory alkalosis

97. Analyze the following arterial blood gas results and determine which condition they indicate. Use the provided space to the right side to assist in interpretation by writing acidosis, alkalosis, compensated, or uncompensated.
    pH 7.56
    CO_2 25
    HCO_3 34
    A. Uncompensated (mixed) respiratory/metabolic alkalosis
    B. Compensated respiratory acidosis
    C. Compensated metabolic acidosis
    D. Uncompensated respiratory alkalosis

98. Analyze the following arterial blood gas results and determine which condition they indicate. Use the provided space to the right side to assist in interpretation by writing acidosis, alkalosis, compensated, or uncompensated.
    pH 7.42
    CO_2 36
    HCO_3 23
    A. Compensated respiratory acidosis
    B. Normal
    C. Compensated metabolic acidosis
    D. Uncompensated respiratory alkalosis

99. Analyze the following arterial blood gas results and determine which condition they indicate. Use the provided space to the right side to assist in interpretation by writing acidosis, alkalosis, compensated, or uncompensated.
    pH 7.49
    CO_2 30
    HCO_3 22
    - A. Uncompensated metabolic alkalosis
    - B. Compensated respiratory acidosis
    - C. Compensated metabolic acidosis
    - D. Uncompensated respiratory alkalosis

100. Analyze the following arterial blood gas results and determine which condition they indicate. Use the provided space to the right side to assist in interpretation by writing acidosis, alkalosis, compensated, or uncompensated.
    pH 7.37
    CO_2 68
    HCO_3 38
    - A. Uncompensated metabolic alkalosis
    - B. Compensated respiratory acidosis
    - C. Compensated metabolic acidosis
    - D. Uncompensated respiratory alkalosis

101. Analyze the following arterial blood gas results and determine which condition they indicate. Use the provided space to the right side to assist in interpretation by writing acidosis, alkalosis, compensated, or uncompensated.
    pH 7.11
    CO_2 65
    HCO_3 17
    - A. Uncompensated (mixed) respiratory/metabolic acidosis
    - B. Uncompensated metabolic alkalosis
    - C. Compensated metabolic acidosis
    - D. Uncompensated respiratory alkalosis

102. Analyze the following arterial blood gas results and determine which condition they indicate. Use the provided space to the right side to assist in interpretation by writing acidosis, alkalosis, compensated, or uncompensated.
    pH 7.43
    CO_2 31
    HCO_3 20
    - A. Uncompensated metabolic alkalosis
    - B. Compensated respiratory acidosis
    - C. Compensated respiratory alkalosis
    - D. Uncompensated respiratory alkalosis

103. Analyze the following arterial blood gas results and determine which condition they indicate. Use the provided space to the right side to assist in interpretation by writing acidosis, alkalosis, compensated, or uncompensated.

pH 7.51

CO_2 40

HCO_3 35

    A. Uncompensated metabolic alkalosis

    B. Compensated respiratory acidosis

    C. Compensated metabolic acidosis

    D. Uncompensated respiratory alkalosis

104. Analyze the following arterial blood gas results and determine which condition they indicate. Use the provided space to the right side to assist in interpretation by writing acidosis, alkalosis, compensated, or uncompensated.

pH 7.17

CO_2 55

HCO_3 20

    A. Uncompensated metabolic alkalosis

    B. Uncompensated (mixed) respiratory/metabolic acidosis

    C. Compensated metabolic acidosis

    D. Uncompensated respiratory alkalosis

105. Analyze the following arterial blood gas results and determine which condition they indicate. Use the provided space to the right side to assist in interpretation by writing acidosis, alkalosis, compensated, or uncompensated.

pH 7.38

CO_2 38

HCO_3 22

    A. Uncompensated metabolic alkalosis

    B. Compensated respiratory acidosis

    C. Compensated metabolic acidosis

    D. Normal

106. Analyze the following arterial blood gas results and determine which condition they indicate. Use the provided space to the right side to assist in interpretation by writing acidosis, alkalosis, compensated, or uncompensated.

pH 7.30

CO_2 61

HCO_3 25

    A. Uncompensated metabolic alkalosis

    B. Compensated respiratory acidosis

    C. Compensated metabolic acidosis

    D. Uncompensated respiratory acidosis

107. A disadvantage of closed catheter suctioning of a mechanically ventilated patient would be:

    A. The extra weight of the inline tubing

    B. The patient does not receive oxygen during the procedure.

    C. Cost is higher with a single-use catheter.

    D. Cost effective if used sporadically

108. **The function of a stoma stent is:**
    A. To provide the ability for the patient to speak
    B. To prevent aspiration
    C. To avoid translaryngeal intubation
    D. To keep the stoma tract open

109. **Which of the following statements is true regarding the use of laryngeal mask airways (LMA)?**
    A. Nurses routinely insert these airways.
    B. There is a low risk of aspiration.
    C. It is a temporary airway.
    D. The vocal cords must be visualized.

110. **Which of the following statements about silicone or plastic tracheostomy tubes is true?**
    A. The tubes offer a lower cost to the facility.
    B. Wire-reinforced tubes cannot be used in MRI imaging.
    C. Use of a one-way speaking valve is easy to use.
    D. Silicone holds up well to repeated cleaning.

111. **A complication of a tracheostomy tube would be:**
    A. Allows for right mainstem intubation
    B. Increases airway resistance
    C. A permanent scar
    D. The airway is less stable.

112. **A complication/contraindication of a nasal endotracheal tube could be:**
    A. Patient cannot drink
    B. Easy access to right mainstem bronchus
    C. It cannot be used for a patient with a cervical injury.
    D. It may cause otitis.

113. **Your patient has just been intubated. Documentation of the procedure usually would *not* include**
    A. The amount of time the intubator took to complete the task.
    B. Depth of the tube.
    C. Size of the tube.
    D. CXR taken.

114. **Which of the following statements is true regarding the use of capnography to verify endotracheal tube placement?**
    A. ETCO$_2$ is a moderately reliable indicator of correct tube placement.
    B. It is not necessary to auscultate lung sounds when this device is used.
    C. It is a substitute for pulse oximetry.
    D. Placement of the device can be difficult to learn initially.

115. Sinusitis and ventilator-acquired pneumonia (VAP) pose many challenges for the critical care. Which statement is true regarding these conditions?
    A. Good handwashing technique is effective in reducing the incidence of VAP.
    B. Sinusitis can be prevented by using a smaller-diameter endotracheal tube.
    C. Nasogastric tubes are preferred to orogastric tubes.
    D. Oral tubes have a greater incidence of sinusitis.

116. Donald is a 64-year-old male with a significant history of emphysema. He started smoking when he was 5 years old and, up until this admission, he continued to smoke up to 5 packs of cigarettes per day. In addition, he has uncontrolled diabetes and peripheral vascular disease. Three days ago, Donald had a major stroke when he was walking down the stairs. He suffered a broken pelvis and fractured his left radius. He has been comatose since his admission with a flat-line EEG study. His wife has agreed that a do not resuscitate (DNR) order will be issued. She has also agreed to discontinue ventilatory support. His physician recommends that he receive morphine as a comfort measure during this process. Donald's wife has been informed that the morphine will make him more comfortable, but may decrease his ability to ventilate and, in fact, may hasten his demise. This type of ethical dilemma is known as
    A. A null ethical principle.
    B. Double effect.
    C. Slippery slope.
    D. Palliative principle.

117. A patient with acute respiratory failure will benefit from the use of which of the following strategies?
    A. Limiting plateau pressure
    B. Hyperventilation
    C. Lower CO_2 levels
    D. Maintain PEEP less than 5 cm H_2O

118. Mask continuous positive airway pressure (CPAP) should be used with caution if a patient has a
    A. Low functional residual capacity (FRC).
    B. Basilar skull fracture.
    C. Sinusitis.
    D. Pneumonia.

119. An intubated patient who is stable with some residual factors that will affect readiness to wean from the ventilator is said to be in the
    A. Acute stage of weaning.
    B. Pre-wean stage.
    C. Weaning stage.
    D. Chronic weaning stage.

120. Mort was driving his car through an intersection when his vehicle was T-boned by another car. Mort suffered a fractured pelvis and was stabilized in the ED; he was then transferred to your unit to await surgical fixation of the fracture. When auscultating lung sounds, you hear what you believe to be bowel sounds in his chest. Mort also states he has moderate shoulder pain on the left side, and he is mildly tachypneic. Mort will probably be diagnosed with
    A. A fractured scapula.
    B. Diaphragmatic rupture.
    C. Hemothorax.
    D. Bowel rupture.

121. Continuing with the scenario from Question 120, what is the immediate priority for Mort's treatment?
    A. Ensure adequate oxygenation
    B. Immediate surgery
    C. Locate additional injuries
    D. Insert a chest tube

122. Which of the following conditions mandates the use of pain control?
    A. Hemothorax
    B. ARDS
    C. Flail chest
    D. Pulmonary contusion

123. Your patient has a confirmed flail chest. What alteration in acid–base balance would you expect?
    A. Metabolic alkalosis
    B. Metabolic acidosis
    C. Respiratory acidosis
    D. Respiratory alkalosis

124. One of the factors to be considered when assessing a patient for possible aspiration and chemical/aspiration pneumonitis is:
    A. Possibility of using Syrup of Ipecac
    B. pH
    C. Type of infiltrates on CXR
    D. ABG results

125. What is the proper location of a chest tube for evacuation of a hemothorax?
    A. In the second intercostal space, midclavicular line
    B. Second intercostal space, midaxillary line
    C. Fifth intercostal space, midaxillary line
    D. Fifth intercostal space, midclavicular line

126. The hypoxemic type of respiratory failure is defined as
    A. Increased dead air space.
    B. PaO_2 of less than 60 mm Hg while the person is at rest, at sea level, on room air.
    C. ARDS.
    D. COPD.

127. **A term for a patient who has been diagnosed with right ventricular hypertrophy caused by pulmonary hypertension caused by lung disease is known as:**
    A. Hyperplasia
    B. Thrombotic syndrome
    C. Cor pulmonale
    D. ARDS

128. **Multiple-organ dysfunction syndrome (MODS) may be directly caused by**
    A. Venous thrombosis.
    B. Shunting.
    C. Oral estrogen therapy.
    D. Pulmonary embolism.

129. **Pulmonary embolism is actually considered a complication of deep venous thrombosis. To assess for deep venous thrombosis, which of the following signs should be assessed?**
    A. Moses'
    B. Davis'
    C. Corrigan's
    D. Hamman's

130. **Your patient had a pulmonary artery catheter placed to closely monitor fluid status. The physician ordered PAWP pressures q 8 hours. You obtain the initial readings on your shift. The next afternoon, when you attempt another wedge pressure, you notice decreased resistance to the syringe. Which of the following complications may have occurred?**
    A. Syringe malfunction
    B. Embolization
    C. Balloon rupture
    D. This is an expected finding.

131. **A 34-year-old male is admitted to your unit with a history of ETOH use and multiple previous admissions. He is now in severe end-stage hepatic failure. The patient was intubated and sedated, and he was placed in restraints for airway protection. His ventilator settings are as follows:**

Mode	AC
FiO_2	.40
V_t	700
Rate	14

    Vital signs are:

RR	16
BP	140/84
EKG	ST at 112
SpO_2	96%

    The patient's wife visits and you inform her about the need for the restraints and the patient's need to sleep. She acknowledges the information and says she will sit quietly at the patient's bedside. About 5 minutes later, you find the patient extubated

and very agitated. His wife states she released the restraints because she felt they were "Too tight." Your priority in the care of this patient is:

A. Immediate sedation for the agitation

B. Remove the wife from the unit

C. Notify the charge nurse

D. Place a 40% mask on the patient and observe his response

132. An indication for the use of PEEP would be:

A. To reduce mediastinal bleeding post CABG

B. To help assess mean arterial pressure

C. To increase surfactant

D. To help reduce FiO_2

133. PEEP may produce barotrauma at levels

A. Less than 20 cm H_2O.

B. Less than 30 cm H_2O.

C. Greater than 40 cm H_2O.

D. Greater than 20 cm H_2O.

134. Where does the hypoxemic drive to breathe originate?

A. Cerebellum

B. Aortic and carotid arteries

C. Hypothalamus

D. Medulla

135. The functional residual capacity is:

A. The amount of gas that can be forcefully exhaled after maximum inspiration

B. The amount of air left in the lungs after normal expiration

C. The amount of gas normally exhaled after a maximum inhalation

D. The amount of gas left in the lungs after a maximum exhalation

136. Subcutaneous emphysema usually occurs in the area of the

A. Head.

B. Neck.

C. Thorax.

D. Abdomen.

137. Pulse oximetry has *not* been shown to be affected by

A. Dark skin.

B. Elevated bilirubin.

C. Dark nail polish.

D. The presence of hemoglobin.

138. Pulse oximetry should *never* be used

A. To determine oxygen saturation values.

B. During a cardiac arrest.

C. As a determinant for predicting hemoglobin affinity for oxygen.

D. To help determine a patient's activity tolerance.

139. When setting alarm limits for a pulse oximeter, the oxygen saturation limit should be what percentage less than the patient's acceptable baseline?
    A. 2%
    B. 5%
    C. 8%
    D. 10%

140. A SpO_2 value of 95% correlates with which of the following PaO_2 values?
    A. 95 mm Hg
    B. 80 mm Hg
    C. 90 mm Hg
    D. 75 mm Hg

141. What is the minimum number of staff required for use of the Vollman Prone Positioner (VPP) when providing manual pronation therapy for your patient?
    A. 2
    B. 3
    C. 4
    D. 5

142. Which of the following conditions would *not* be considered a contraindication for the use of pronation therapy?
    A. Pregnancy
    B. Weight of 160 kg
    C. Unstable pelvis
    D. Open abdomen

143. Nursing actions that should be performed prior to initiating pronation therapy would include
    A. Secure EKG leads on the anterior chest with tape.
    B. Note the amount of all drainage for colostomies and ileostomies.
    C. Utilize capnography monitoring.
    D. Document existing drainage on any wound dressings.

144. To prevent complications with chest tube drainage systems, the suction level should not be higher than
    A. –20 cm H_2O.
    B. –30 cm H_2O.
    C. –40 cm H_2O.
    D. –50 cm H_2O.

145. Which of the following statements is true regarding chest tube drainage systems?
    A. Drainage of frank blood in amounts greater than 100 ml/hour is not significant.
    B. Drainage tubing should be placed horizontally on the bed and down to the collection chamber.
    C. All drainage tubing should be dependent to the insertion site.
    D. Chest tube drainage from a mediastinal tube should not bubble in the water seal chamber.

146. Steven is a 36-year-old patient originally admitted for treatment of a fractured femur and to rule out a coronary contusion following a skiing accident. While you are giving Steven his discharge teaching, he suddenly complains of pain in his left chest. He immediately becomes tachypneic and tachycardic. You lay Steven back down in the bed and note asymmetrical chest wall excursion and neck vein distension. He has absent breath sounds on the left side, and his heart sounds are muffled. Steven rapidly becomes dyspneic and cyanotic. Steven's condition is likely due to:
    A. Tension pneumothorax
    B. Cardiac tamponade
    C. Pulmonary embolism
    D. Esophageal rupture

147. Continuing with the scenario from Question 146, Steven requires an immediate needle thoracostomy for a left tension pneumothorax. Where will the needle be placed?
    A. Second intercostal space, left midclavicular line
    B. Third intercostal space, left midaxillary line
    C. Fourth intercostal space, left midaxillary line
    D. Fifth intercostal space, left midclavicular line

148. Which of the following would be considered a relative complication for performing a thoracentesis?
    A. Splenomegaly
    B. Coagulation disorder
    C. Previous pneumonectomy
    D. Pleural fluid protein to serum protein ratio greater than 0.5 g/dL

149. Auto-PEEP is
    A. The same as plateau pressure.
    B. The same as static pressure.
    C. A result of inadequate exhalation time.
    D. Decreases the work of breathing.

150. Conditions that increase lung compliance are:
    A. Kyphoscoliosis
    B. Emphysema
    C. ARDS
    D. Pulmonary edema

151. Factors that would decrease lung resistance would include:
    A. Endotracheal tube size
    B. Bronchospasm
    C. Secretions
    D. Albuterol administration

152. Your patient has blood gas results that indicate uncompensated metabolic acidosis. A probable cause for this result could be:
    A. Anxiety
    B. Nasogastric suction
    C. A Neuromuscular disorder
    D. Diabetic ketoacidosis

153. **Your patient has emphysema. During chest percussion, you would expect which of the following types of sounds to occur?**
    A. Flat
    B. Dull
    C. Hyperresonant
    D. Resonant

154. **Gertrude has chronic COPD. She has smoked for several years. What physiological changes would you expect to see in a patient with COPD?**
    A. Clubbed fingers
    B. Splenomegaly
    C. Left ventricular failure
    D. Hypotension

155. **The most common cause of COPD is:**
    A. Pollution
    B. Smoking
    C. Heredity
    D. Occupation

156. **Surya is a 40-year-old construction worker who suffered a flail chest after a fall from a scaffold. At first, he was ventilated using a high-frequency jet ventilator; he is now on an SIMV mode. Today he is being weaned from the ventilator. About 45 minutes after the start of weaning, which change would indicate Surya might fail weaning at this time?**
    A. The minute ventilation is 7 L/min.
    B. His heart rate has increased from 86 to 108.
    C. The SpO_2 is 96%.
    D. His respiratory rate increased by 10 breaths per minute.

157. **Continuing with the scenario from Question 156, Surya is placed back on the ventilator, but is mistakenly placed on IMV mode instead of SIMV mode. He immediately starts to override the ventilator and becomes quite anxious. ABGs are drawn before he is placed back on the correct mode. What would you expect the results to show:**
    A. Respiratory acidosis
    B. Metabolic alkalosis
    C. Respiratory alkalosis
    D. Metabolic acidosis

158. **Continuing with the scenario from Questions 156 and 157, Surya, like many patients with flail chest, was initially placed on a high-frequency jet ventilator because**
    A. It improves removal of CO_2.
    B. It increases tidal volume.
    C. It helps stabilize the chest wall.
    D. It reduces the need for humidification.

159. **Early signs of impending respiratory failure include**
    A. Tachypnea and agitation.
    B. Crackles and cough.
    C. Peripheral cyanosis and tachypnea.
    D. Restlessness and tachycardia.

160. **In ARDS, pulmonary capillaries leak fluid into the pulmonary interstitium. This phenomenon is due to:**
    A. Alveolar-oxygen gradient
    B. Colloid osmotic pressure
    C. A-a gradient
    D. Diffusion

161. **Carbon dioxide is carried in the blood as**
    A. Bicarbonate.
    B. Carbonic acid.
    C. Carbon anhydrase.
    D. Carbonalate-1.

162. **When correctly placed, a chest tube will be in**
    A. The intercostal space.
    B. The pleural space.
    C. The mediastinal space.
    D. The intrapleural space.

163. **Why is prednisone contraindicated in tuberculosis?**
    A. It masks the infection.
    B. It increases edema, leading to dyspnea.
    C. It decreases the effectiveness of isoniazid.
    D. It increases the effectiveness of isoniazid.

164. **Your patient is receiving chemotherapy for lung cancer. His labs show a WBC of 0.7. You anticipate he will receive which medication?**
    A. Epogen
    B. Antibiotics
    C. Plasmaphoresis
    D. Neupogen

165. **After 3 doses of Neupogen, your patient complains of bone pain and muscle aches. What do you tell him?**
    A. These are common side effects of the medication.
    B. His bone cancer has metastasized.
    C. His arthritis has flared up.
    D. He has gout.

166. **Florence is a 50-year-old secretary who was admitted to your unit with non-radiating chest pain. The pain was intermittent and occurred predominately on the right side. Changes of position or deep inhalation did not affect the quality of the pain. Her V/Q scan showed the probability of a pulmonary embolism. Laboratory and physical findings are as follows:**

Current ABGs: pH 7.24, $PaCO_2$ 32, HCO_3 17, PaO_2 97

SpO_2: 0.98

Lactate: 4.4

EKG: ST at 102 with isolated PVC

Cuff BP: 98/60 mm Hg

Skin pale, cool

Temperature: 98.4°F

RR: 26

Breath sounds: crackles, RML, RLL

O_2: 30% via mask

Mentation: Alert, oriented × 4

What is the interpretation of Florence's ABG results?

A. Respiratory acidosis, compensated

B. Metabolic acidosis, compensated

C. Respiratory alkalosis, uncompensated

D. Metabolic acidosis, compensated respiratory alkalosis

167. **Continuing with the scenario from Question 166, what is your overall impression of Florence's oxygenation status?**

A. Oxygenation is adequate; her O_2 and SpO_2 are normal.

B. Oxygenation is inadequate because she needs an FiO_2 of 35%.

C. Oxygenation is adequate; the FiO_2 is irrelevant.

D. Oxygenation is inadequate; the lactate is high, pH and HCO_3 are low.

168. **A 42-year-old female was admitted to your ICU following a fall down some patio stairs. She sustained a fracture of the fourth rib on the right and fractures of the fourth and fifth ribs on the left. The patient was medicated for pain and while visiting with her husband, the patient becomes dyspneic; her respiratory rate increases to 36 from 16. Her trachea is noted to deviate to the left, and diminished breath sounds are heard throughout the left lung fields. You also note crepitus over the site of the fracture on the right side. This patient is probably developing**

A. A pericardial tamponade.

B. A pneumothorax.

C. A hemothorax.

D. A chylothorax.

169. **The high-pressure alarm on your patient's ventilator is sounding. This is probably due to:**

A. An airway cuff leak

B. A poor seal in the circuitry

C. Decreased lung compliance

D. Displacement of the airway

170. **The low-pressure alarm on your patient's ventilator is sounding. What is a possible cause of this alarm?**

A. A leak in the one-way valve of the inflation port

B. The patient biting on his tube

C. Bronchospasm

D. Water in the ventilator circuitry

171. The patient at greatest risk when auto-PEEP is present would be the patient with
    A. Pericardial tamponade.
    B. Status asthmaticus.
    C. A pleural effusion.
    D. Need for a bag-valve mask device.

172. When a patient is being autotransfused, what size filter is commonly used?
    A. 10 µg
    B. 40 µg
    C. 50 µg
    D. 20 µg

173. Your patient has a closed chest tube drainage system. When he turns slightly to the left, a large amount of dark red blood enters the pleural tube. What is the probable cause of this situation?
    A. A ruptured effusion
    B. Erosion into the intercostal vessels
    C. Old blood dumping
    D. A new hemothorax

This concludes the Pulmonary questions.

ANSWERS

1. **Correct Answer: D**

   The pH is elevated, showing alkalosis. The HCO_3 is normal and the $PaCO_2$ is decreased, which indicates respiratory alkalosis.

2. **Correct Answer: C**

   Brianna is probably very anxious and hyperventilating because she is unable to get enough oxygen due to bronchial constriction. Hypoventilation causes a buildup of CO_2, causing respiratory acidosis. This patient has not received theophylline. Albuterol may cause tachycardia, but not an acid–base imbalance.

3. **Correct Answer: D**

   Propranolol may cause bronchospasm and works by blocking beta-adrenergic effects of the sympathetic nervous system (e.g., bronchodilation). Some beta blockers are cardioselective (e.g., atenolol); some newer drugs (e.g., nebivolol) produce cardioselective beta blockade along with vasodilation.

4. **Correct Answer: D**

   It is unlikely the Brianna's condition is improving. The air becomes trapped in the alveoli and excessive mucus is produced. The patient struggles to breathe and exhausts herself. When the wheezing diminishes or stops altogether, it means air is not able to pass through an opening. This condition is a medical emergency, and the patient may be intubated. A lot of controversy surrounds the issue of intubating patients with asthma because this practice may cause barotrauma, hyperinflation, and cardiac compromise.

5. **Correct Answer: B**

   PEEP must be carefully regulated so as not to cause barotrauma or a dynamic hyperinflation; it might improve air flow. Norepinephrine is a vasoconstrictor. Nebulizers may also work, but if the patient's condition is compromised the effectiveness is minimal at best. Heliox is a helium–oxygen mixture that can help with delivery of inhaled medications to decrease the work of breathing.

6. **Correct Answer: C**

   Neostigmine is an enzyme that prevents the breakdown of acetylcholine into its enzyme. It improves impulse transmission. Sometimes neostigmine causes bradycardia and increases bronchial secretions, so atropine may be used in conjunction with Neostigmine to mitigate these undesirable effects. Narcan is an opioid antagonist.

7. **Correct Answer: A**

   PAOP and PCWP are the same thing: Both indicate pressures on the left side of the heart and generally are not affected by pulmonary hypertension. The same would also apply to left ventricular pressures. Since forward blood flow is impeded by the increased resistance in pulmonary hypertension, the pressures on the right side of the heart are affected (Pulmonary artery, RV, and RAP).

8. **Correct Answer: C**

   Surfactant is a lipoprotein and functions by increasing the surface tension of alveoli and allows alveoli to expand and contract. Some residual pressure in the alveoli at the end of respiration is needed to keep the alveoli open (physiologic PEEP). If surfactant production is impaired, the alveoli's ability to exchange O_2 is compromised. Type I cells line the outside of the alveoli.

9. **Correct Answer: D**
The right mainstem bronchus is somewhat wider and has less of an angle off the mainstem bronchus, so it is much more readily intubated.

10. **Correct Answer: C**
More specifically, these ABG results would indicate an uncompensated metabolic acidosis. The pH is low as is the $PaCO_2$.

11. **Correct Answer: B**
The $PaCO_2$ will rise approximately 3–10 mm Hg per hour. The PaO_2 and the pH will decrease.

12. **Correct Answer: A**
The heparin will have dilutional effects and will decrease the bicarbonate level and the $PaCO_2$.

13. **Correct Answer: C**
Using a vacutainer or a high-friction syringe will create a vacuum. When that occurs, dissolved gases come out of solution, which decreases PaO_2 and $PaCO_2$. The increased effort to move the cylinder may cause the artery to spasm and impede obtaining the sample, but will not directly affect the results of the test.

14. **Correct Answer: D**
Most ABG machines are calibrated to 37°C. If the patient has a fever, the oxyhemoglobin dissociation curve will be shifted to the right. More oxygen will be given off to the tissues when fever is present, so the machine must be calibrated to account for the increased temperature.

15. **Correct Answer: D**
A deficiency in serum alpha-antitrypsin is extremely rare—many references estimate the incidence of this condition at only 1–3% in the general population. It is believed that serum alpha-antitrypsis destroys lung tissue through enzymatic action. Usually Caucasians of European descent express this disease, which results from an autosomal recessive trait. Symptoms usually appear when the patient is a teenager and that is a way to assist in the diagnosis, as most cases of emphysema occur in later years of life.

16. **Correct Answer: B**
Chronic hypoxia leads to chronic respiratory acidosis. The kidneys then retain bicarbonate in the form of sodium bicarbonate. The bicarbonate is exchanged for sodium chloride. Ammonia is an acid, and excess amounts must be removed from the body. This is done by releasing ammonium chloride. In chronic hypoxia, there is an increase in bicarbonate levels and a decrease in chloride levels. Other causes of hypochloremia include NG suctioning, vomiting, and diarrhea.

17. **Correct Answer: B**
In this case, communication is clearly the problem. The family should have been informed by someone that the patient needed assistance with breathing and told what to expect in regard to his appearance. In addition, the patient's inability to speak

could have been explained. There are three nontherapeutic responses. The family is clearly distressed, so a simple explanation is best.

18. **Correct Answer: D**

    Therapeutic communication occurs when the patient's feelings are validated. This response allows for the patient to express the concerns he has about the transfer. The other answers are closed and judgmental and do not allow for any expression of feelings on the part of the patient.

19. **Correct Answer: B**

    Carl was quite anxious and tachycardic. His respiratory rate probably was increased because of anxiety and his condition. He would blow off CO_2. His pH is below normal, so it is uncompensated. The HCO_3 is low, indicating alkalosis. The interpretation would be uncompensated respiratory alkalosis.

20. **Correct Answer: C**

    At higher altitudes, there is less atmospheric pressure to force oxygen into the lungs. To compensate, the person must breathe faster. The percentage of oxygen remains the same, but the partial pressure of the oxygen decreases. Both arterial PaO_2 and O_2 saturation decrease as well. The rapid breathing will result in hyperventilation, raising the pH and lowering the $PaCO_2$ levels.

21. **Correct Answer: C**

    The percentage of total oxygen carried within the bloodstream attributed to the SaO_2 is 97–98%. SaO_2 is the arterial saturation of hemoglobin; this percentage corresponds to the percentage of hemoglobin on the red blood cells that carry O_2. Typically this percentage is considered to be normal if it is in the range 93–99%. PaO_2 is the percentage of oxygen within the bloodstream that is free or dissolved in the plasma. This value is considered to be normal if it is in the range 80–100 mm Hg.

22. **Correct Answer: B**

    Hypoxemia is a decreased oxygen level in the arterial blood or a PaO_2 of less than 80 mm Hg. Hypoxia is defined as a decreased oxygen level at the cellular level. Decreased oxygen levels within the veins and the brain refer to a PaO_2 of less than 50 and a $ScVO_2$ of less than 20, respectively.

23. **Correct Answer: D**

    Adam is exhibiting signs and symptoms of oxygen toxicity after 5 days of oxygen therapy at greater than 50% FiO_2. Non-rebreather masks provide a minimum of 60% FiO_2 at 6 L/min. An arterial blood gas would show an increased PaO_2 greater than 100 mm Hg, ruling out respiratory failure ($PaO_2 < 60$), which would require intubation. The dry, hacking cough rules out pulmonary edema and the need for Lasix. Numbness in the extremities results from the overabundance of oxygen radicals in the blood; it is not a neurologic impairment that would indicate the need for a CT scan with possible tPA administration.

24. **Correct Answer: B**

    Four days of high FiO_2 has resulted in a nitrogen wash-out resulting in atelectasis. Nitrogen's high partial pressure is necessary to maintain alveoli inflation. It is important to titrate FiO_2 to maintain saturations within a prescribed range when oxygen therapy is utilized. Pulmonary edema would result in coarse breath sounds. With a unilateral pneumothorax, tracheal deviation would be apparent. Sepsis would not necessarily present with diminished breath sounds, but rather with additional findings of increased purulent secretions, coarse breath sounds, and altered laboratory diagnostic results.

25. **Correct Answer: B**
Sometimes the costal cartilage becomes calcified with age. Vertebrae develop osteoporosis, and a degree of kyphosis can occur. Weight gain is common, and posture is affected. The chest wall compliance decreases, as does vital capacity. Residual volume increases, PaO_2 decreases, and $PaCO_2$ increases.

26. **Correct Answer: C**
Type I cells line the outside of the alveoli; they are easily inflamed by inhaled toxins or heated air. Type I cells maintain the blood–gas interface. Type II cells produce surfactant.

27. **Correct Answer: D.**
Conducting airways are ventilated, but perfusion (gas exchange) does not take place. Wasted ventilation is the amount of ventilation that does not participate in gas exchange.

28. **Correct Answer: A**
The oxyhemoglobin dissociation curve reflects the patient's physiological circumstances and their effect on hemoglobin's affinity for oxygen.

29. **Correct Answer: B**
A shift to the right means hemoglobin has less affinity for oxygen. 2,3-Diphosphoglyceride (2,3-DPG) is needed to help force O_2 off the hemoglobin molecule. Thus, if 2,3-DPG is decreased, the hemoglobin will hang onto the O_2. If the temperature is increased, the tissues need more O_2. If the $PaCO_2$ is elevated, the tissues need more oxygen.

30. **Correct Answer: D**
Here hemoglobin holds onto the oxygen, so the amount of 2,3-DPG is low, CO_2 would be decreased, and temperature would be decreased. Tissues would not need as much O_2.

31. **Correct Answer: C**
The normal value is 35–40 mm Hg, so perfusion is adequate. The mixed venous sample is a way of assessing ventilation and circulation. If the mixed venous PaO_2 is low, then the tissues are extracting a normal amount of oxygen and returning deoxygenated blood to the heart. The sample is drawn from the distal port of the pulmonary artery catheter.

32. **Correct Answer: A**
The kidneys try to correct the imbalance by retaining bicarbonate. Chronic hypoxia results in an increased level of CO_2 (chronic respiratory acidosis). The bicarbonate is exchanged for the chloride so as to maintain a balance.

33. **Correct Answer: D**
Normally, lung sounds are somewhat muffled. Sounds are heard clearly if the lung is consolidated. If a whisper is transmitted, it is unusual and may also indicate consolidation. Egophony is a sound that changes in intensity. For example, if the patient says "E," it is heard as "A."

34. **Correct Answer: A**
The pH shows that the patient's condition is uncompensated and acidotic (< 7.35), the elevated CO_2 indicates that the source is respiratory (> 45 mm Hg), and the

bicarbonate level is normal (22–26 mm Hg). Hence the patient has uncompensated respiratory acidosis.

35. **Correct Answer: B**
Removal of large amounts of pleural fluid (more than 1,000 mL) increases negative intrapleural pressure. Edema occurs when the lung does not reexpand. The patient develops a severe cough and dyspnea. If these symptoms occur during a thoracentesis, the procedure should be stopped.

36. **Correct Answer: C**
Some dyes interfere with the sensor's ability to conduct red and infrared light—specifically, methylene blue, fluroscein, indocyanine green, and indigo carmine.

37. **Correct Answer: D**
Pressures that exceed 60 mm Hg usually mean only one side of the tube is sealed. The trachea is somewhat oval, whereas the tube and cuff are circular. In case of a cuff leak, the pressure would be lower and the patient might be able to speak or make noise with the tube in place.

38. **Correct Answer: B**
Blood flow to the trachea requires approximately 15–25 mm Hg of tracheal filling pressure. If cuff pressure exceeds this amount, complications such as tracheoe-sophageal fistulas may occur. The over-inflated cuff may also cause ischemia and possible necrosis.

39. **Correct Answer: A**
A semi-reclining or upright position will promote upper lobe drainage. Fluid or secretions will collect if the patient lies flat.

40. **Correct Answer: B**
A position in which the head is lower than the body increases intracranial pressure. It is also best to avoid postural drainage in a woman in the last 2–3 months of pregnancy, as the baby will shift toward the lungs and may cause respiratory distress. It is also a good idea to wait an hour after a patient eats before giving aerosol treatment to avoid nausea, vomiting, and possible aspiration.

41. **Correct Answer: D**
Answers A, B, and C are all complications of PEEP. PEEP must be regulated so as not to cause barotrauma, but still keep alveoli from collapsing during expiration.

42. **Correct Answer: C**
Those factors include venous stasis, hypercoagulability of blood, and injury to vascular endothelium. Beck's triad is indicative of cardiac tamponade.

43. **Correct Answer: A**
Any pressure in the thorax decreases preload, cardiac output, and blood pressure. Forward blood flow is impeded by increased pressure in the pulmonary vasculature.

44. **Correct Answer: B**
Because PEEP raises intrathoracic pressure and PVR, blood "backs up" and can cause hepatic congestion. The increased intrathoracic pressure also can compress blood vessels, cause or exacerbate hypovolemia, lead to low cardiac output, and result in a low wedge pressure.

45. **Correct Answer: B**

An acute pulmonary embolism may be associated with right heart failure. The PAS and PVR are elevated. The patient may be having chest pain, dyspnea, tachycardia, hypotension, shock, and possibly coma.

46. **Correct Answer: C**

The patient will have a sudden decrease in the pet CO_2 due to loss of blood flow in the pulmonary vasculature. The decrease in blood flow increases the amount of dead space, with a resultant decrease in the pet CO_2.

47. **Correct Answer: A**

In addition, the EKG may actually be normal, or it may show right-axis deviation, T-wave inversion (leads V_1 and V_4) and ST-segment depression. New-onset atrial fibrillation and RBBB may also occur.

48. **Correct Answer: B**

Severe acute respiratory syndrome (SARS) is a type of community-acquired pneumonia caused by SARS-associated coronavirus. Incubation is usually 2–14 days, and is spread via droplets. SARS is usually acquired in underdeveloped areas. There is no cure and symptoms are treated as they appear. It is incumbent on the nurse to make certain the patient is placed in a negative-pressure isolation room and that an N-95 respirator mask is used.

49. **Correct Answer: C.**

An elevated D-dimer level may be caused by many other conditions. A normal D-dimer level rules out a pulmonary embolism. Hyperventilation will occur subsequent to hypoxemia, so respiratory alkalosis will occur. Heparin does not dissolve existing clots.

50. **Correct Answer: C**

Hamman's sign is a "crunching" sound or a slight clicking sound with each heart sound auscultated over the apex of the heart.

51. **Correct Answer: B**

If carbon monoxide levels exceed 60%, the patient will be comatose and probably die. Smokers often have normal CO levels of 5–10%. By comparison, normal CO levels in nonsmokers are less than 2%.

52. **Correct Answer: D**

In cases of severe carbon monoxide poisoning, hyperbaric therapy must be utilized to force the CO molecule off the hemoglobin; the excess CO is then eliminated by the lungs.

53. **Correct Answer: B**

Airway patency is always a priority. George probably inhaled superheated air and toxins. When burned, most of the products found in a home will give off carbon monoxide. These toxins, as well as the CO, may cause edema of the air passages.

54. **Correct Answer: D**

Answers A, B, and C decrease lung compliance. Other factors that decrease compliance include atelectasis, fibrotic changes, abdominal distention, pain (causes splinting), and flail chest (pain and loss of structure).

55. **Correct Answer: C**

The patient must have an absent gag reflex. The laryngeal mask airway (LMA) cannot be inserted by nurses unless they have specialized training. This device does not usually cause hoarseness because it does not pass through the vocal cords. There is a high risk of aspiration with LMA usage.

56. **Correct Answer: C**

Acetyl-cysteine contains a sulfide group that effectively splits disulfide bonds in mucin molecules; this action reduces the viscosity of the mucus. Atropine is an anticholinergic. Terbutaline and albuterol are B_2 agonists.

57. **Correct Answer: A**

Thinning the mucus may promote excessive coughing with resultant bronchospasm. Additional side effects include rhinorrhea, stomatitus, nausea, and vomiting.

58. **Correct Answer: D**

The B_2-receptor agonists lower cellular calcium levels and relax bronchial smooth muscle. The selective B_2-receptor agonists do not produce cardiac stimulation. The cardiac stimulation can result in tachycardia and reduced cardiac output.

59. **Correct Answer: B**

Theophylline is a methylzanthine, as are caffeine and theobromine. These substances can be found in coffee, tea, and cocoa. This class of drugs, when given in low doses, can stimulate cortical arousal; in higher doses, these drugs can cause insomnia. The methylzanthines can also cause tachycardias and increase production of gastric acid and digestive enzymes. In addition, they inhibit histamine release.

60. **Correct Answer: B**

In malignant hyperthermia, the use of anesthetic agents such as halothane causes muscles to contract and the patient to become hypothermic. Caffeine is used diagnostically because it can contract muscles at higher doses without the danger of depolarizing cell membranes. The antidote for malignant hyperthermia is dantrolene.

61. **Correct Answer: C**

Symptoms have a gradual onset. The patient may develop ARDS, but not always. If the pH is greater than 2.5, very little necrosis will occur. If the pH is less than 2.5, there is the probability of pulmonary edema, necrosis, bleeding, and atelectasis.

62. **Correct Answer: D**

Roy has the classic symptoms of Legionnaires' disease. If left untreated, it may lead to hypotension, acute kidney injury, shock, respiratory failure, and death.

63. **Correct Answer: B**

By definition, an open pneumothorax exists because air enters the pleural cavity from the atmosphere. The hole made into the subclavian vein allows for air to pass from the atmosphere to the pleural cavity.

64. **Correct Answer: C**

Trendelenburg position with left decubitus tilt will minimize the chance of any air migrating through the heart and into the lungs.

65. **Correct Answer: C**

    Pulmonary angiography involves catheterization of the right ventricle, followed by injection of dye into the pulmonary artery. The pulmonary vasculature is easily visualized by this study. The location of the embolus is easily found because the dye trail comes to a sudden end.

66. **Correct Answer: B**

    Neoplasms, obesity, trauma, dysrhythmias, congestive heart failure (CHF), and prolonged immobility are also factors.

67. **Correct Answer: A**

    Other potential causes include central and pulmonary artery catheters, endoscopy, and automatic pressure-driven injectors.

68. **Correct Answer: B**

    The blood gas results show respiratory acidosis with hypoxemia.

69. **Correct Answer: D**

    Fractures—usually long bone fractures—can release free fatty acids which cause vasculitis. Fat globules float around and obstruct the pulmonary vasculature.

70. **Correct Answer: A**

    Prone positioning is the best position to promote drainage and oxygenation. It is often the most difficult position to achieve without proper lifting and safety devices.

71. **Correct Answer: D**

    The fluid volume is kept low to maintain the PAOP (PCWP) at minimal levels. If too much fluid is present, leakage may occur through damaged capillaries into the interstitial space.

72. **Correct Answer: D**

    The patient will also exhibit elevated PVR and pulmonary artery pressures.

73. **Correct Answer: C**

    The forced vital capacity (FVC) is the total amount of gas exhaled as forcefully and rapidly as possible after taking a maximal inspiration. The result should be above 80%. The forced expiratory volume (FEV) is how much gas is exhaled within the first second of effort. This amount should be 75% or more of the predicted normal value. In patients with asthma, this value is decreased because of obstruction.

74. **Correct Answer: B**

    When using an auto-transfusion drainage system, make sure to connect the system per the manufacturer's recommendations. Most connections will be color coded for easy connection. Clamps must remain open to allow for blood collection and to prevent increased intrathoracic pressures. Subcutaneous air should be checked by palpation and borders marked for further monitoring. The average adult-size catheter is 28 Fr or 36 Fr. If a one-way valve system and suction is used, water is not required to maintain a seal because the valve serves this function.

75. **Correct Answer: B**

    Acidosis, hypercarbia, and hyperthermia will all lead to a right shift in the oxyhemoglobin dissociation curve. Hemoglobin in this instance has a decreased affinity for oxygen and enhances tissue uptake of oxygen.

76. **Correct Answer: D**
If a patient has ingested carbonated beverages, the CO_2 production/accumulation within the stomach would lead to inflation of the esophageal detection device (EDD) and a false-positive reading for the ETT placement in the airway. It is best to use auscultation, observation, and improvement in vital signs as primary techniques to confirm ETT placement and to use EDD and CO_2 detectors as secondary methods for confirming placement.

77. **Correct Answer: A**
Normal saline use in tracheal suctioning research has proven that normal saline causes anxiety, increased risk for hospital-acquired pneumonia, and bronchoconstriction. Current recommendations focus on use of dry suctioning, frequent oral care, balanced hydration, and position changes to prevent complications associated with intubation and mechanical ventilation.

78. **Correct Answer: A**
Barotrauma may result if PEEP pressures exceed alveolar tolerance, resulting in alveolar rupture and air trapping. Other complications of excessive PEEP pressures include a decreased cardiac output, increased intracranial pressures, and excessive sodium and water retention.

79. **Correct Answer: A**
Synchronized intermittent mandatory ventilation (SIMV) provides a set frequency of breaths and either volume or pressure. The patient is permitted to breathe spontaneously at his or her own volume between mandatory ventilations. If the spontaneous breath occurs at the same time as a mandatory breath, the ventilator with synchronize with the patient, thereby preventing "stacked" breaths. The other modes of ventilation listed (CMV, HFV, and oscillation) represent full control of settings by the operator.

80. **Correct Answer: C**
Due to increased and changes in thoracic pressure in the presence of a pneumothorax, a high-pressure alarm will sound. In addition, alarms for saturation and possibly heart rate may alarm on the cardiorespiratory monitor. A low-limit alarm may sound if tubing becomes disconnected and a leak in the chest tube occurs.

81. **Correct Answer: D**
Succinylcholine combines with acetylcholine to cause smooth muscle relaxation. Prolonged use may cause a change in blocking action and result in potassium-regulated alterations in electrical activity. Other side effects of succinylcholine include malignant hyperthermia and hypertension or hypotension, hyperkalemia, anaphylaxis, and increased intraocular pressure.

82. **Correct Answer: C**
Norcuron is eliminated via the hepatic/biliary system. This drug should be used with caution in patients with known or suspected hepatic or biliary compromise, such as in individuals with cirrhosis or hepatitis, and may take as much as 2 times as long to clear a patient's system.

83. **Correct Answer: D**
Uncontrolled asthma symptoms during an attack may lead to prolonged and extensive muscle use to maintain independent respirations. Prolonged effort may result in

respiratory failure due to respiratory muscle fatigue. Administration of a neuromuscular blocking agent further inhibits the smooth muscle retractions. Long-term steroid use has been linked to muscle wasting. Ventilatory weaning may be prolonged, as the respiratory muscles must recover from both the disease process and the pharmacologic intervention.

84. **Correct Answer: D**
The nasal cannula is generally considered a low-flow oxygen device unless connected to a high-flow system. If the flow is greater than 4 L/min, the oxygen should be humidified to prevent it from drying out the mucosal membranes.

85. **Correct Answer: C**
If both exhalation ports have one-way valves, then near-100% oxygen delivery may be achieved. To prevent suffocation in patients in case the oxygen becomes disconnected, non-rebreather masks now have only a single one-way valve to prevent/limit inhalation of room air. This system decreases the highest concentration of actual inspired oxygen to 60–80%.

86. **Correct Answer: D**
The accuracy of pulse oximetry may be affected by patient motion, low perfusion, venous pulsation, light, poor probe positioning, edema, anemia, and carbon monoxide levels. It is important to compare pulse oximetry values against arterial blood gas findings to validate values that are less than 70%.

87. **Correct Answer: B**
Sepsis may result in lung tissue injury and, consequently, increased pulmonary vascular resistance (PVR). Prostaglandin and oxygen therapies lead to pulmonary vasodilatation and decrease PVR.

88. **Correct Answer: A**
An increased metabolic rate would increase O_2 uptake by tissues, resulting in a lower value as measured by venous blood gases. The other answers would result in a lower tissue oxygen requirement and, therefore, higher concentrations of oxygen in the bloodstream.

89. **Correct Answer: B**
For women, the average depth for an ETT is 21 cm at the lip when using a 7 to 8 Fr tube. For men, the average depth for an ETT is 23 cm at the lip when using an 8 to 8.5 Fr tube. Assessment documentation should always include both of these values in case the tube should become dislodged at any time during respiratory support.

90. **Correct Answer: D**
Examples of control variables include pressure, volume, and flow. Their values do not change with changes in patient lung compliance or resistance.

91. **Correct Answer: A**
Stimulation of the posterior tibial nerve results in plantar flexion of the great toe. Other locations for peripheral nerve stimulation electrode placement include the ulnar nerve and the facial nerve.

92. **Correct Answer: C**
The progression of muscles to stop movement is as follows: eyes, face, neck, extremities, abdomen, glottis, intercostals, and diaphragm. It is important to recall that muscle movement will return in the reverse order.

93. **Correct Answer: A**

One to two twitches represents 85–90% blockage. Different muscles may respond differently to neuromuscular blocking agents. As muscles of the face will stop movement before the diaphragm, the nurse might check twitches on the face and an extremity rather than just the patient's face.

94. **Correct Answer: C**

This set of values indicates the presence of compensated metabolic acidosis. The pH is between 7.35 and 7.45, so the value is compensated; because it is closer to 7.35, the value is considered acidotic. To determine whether the acidosis is respiratory or metabolic, find the value that represents acidosis—that is, $HCO_3 < 22$ mEq/L.

95. **Correct Answer: D**

This set of values indicates the presence of uncompensated respiratory alkalosis. The pH is greater than 7.45, so the value is uncompensated alkalosis. To determine whether the alkalosis is respiratory or metabolic, find the value that represents alkalosis: $CO_2 < 35$ mm Hg.

96. **Correct Answer: C**

This set of values indicates the presence of uncompensated metabolic acidosis. The pH is less than 7.35, so the value is uncompensated acidosis. To determine whether the acidosis is respiratory or metabolic, find the value that represents acidosis: $HCO_3 < 22$ mEq/L.

97. **Correct Answer: A**

This set of values indicates the presence of an uncompensated (mixed) respiratory/metabolic alkalosis. The pH is greater than 7.45, so the value is uncompensated. To determine whether the acidosis is respiratory or metabolic, find the value that represents alkalosis: $HCO_3 > 26$ mEq/L and $CO_2 < 35$ mm Hg. Thus the cause of the alkalosis is both respiratory and metabolic in nature.

98. **Correct Answer: B**

The pH is between 7.35 and 7.45; the values for CO_2 (between 35 and 45 mm Hg) and HCO_3 (between 22 and 26 mEq/L) are within normal ranges. These ABG results are considered normal.

99. **Correct Answer: D**

This set of values indicates the presence of an uncompensated respiratory alkalosis. The pH is greater than 7.45, so the value is uncompensated alkalosis. To determine whether the alkalosis is respiratory or metabolic, find the value that represents alkalosis: $CO_2 < 35$ mm Hg.

100. **Correct Answer: B**

This set of values indicates the presence of compensated respiratory acidosis. The pH is between 7.35 and 7.45, so the value is compensated; because it is closer to 7.35, the value is considered acidotic. To determine whether the acidosis is respiratory or metabolic, find the value that represents acidosis: $CO_2 > 45$ mm Hg.

101. **Correct Answer: A**

This set of values indicates the presence of an uncompensated (mixed) respiratory/metabolic acidosis. The pH is less than 7.35, so the value is uncompensated acidosis. To determine whether the acidosis is respiratory or metabolic, find the value that represents acidosis: $HCO_3 < 22$ mEq/L and $CO_2 > 45$ mm Hg. Thus the cause of the acidosis is both respiratory and metabolic in nature.

102. **Correct Answer: C**

This set of values indicates the presence of compensated respiratory alkalosis. The pH is between 7.35 and 7.45, so the value is compensated, but since it is closer to 7.45, the value is considered alkalotic. To determine whether the alkalosis is respiratory or metabolic, find the value that represents alkalosis: $CO_2 < 35$ mm Hg.

103. **Correct Answer: A**

This set of values indicates the presence of an uncompensated metabolic alkalosis. The pH is greater than 7.45, so the value is uncompensated. To determine whether the alkalosis is respiratory or metabolic, find the value that represents alkalosis: This would be the HCO_3 at > 26 mEq/L.

104. **Correct Answer: B**

This set of values indicates the presence of an uncompensated (mixed) respiratory/metabolic acidosis. The pH is less than 7.35, so the value is uncompensated acidosis. To determine whether the acidosis is respiratory or metabolic, find the value that represents acidosis: $HCO_3 < 22$ mEq/L and $CO_2 > 45$ mm Hg. Thus the cause of the acidosis is both respiratory and metabolic in nature.

105. **Correct Answer: D**

The pH is between 7.35 and 7.45; the values for CO_2 (between 35 and 45 mm Hg) and HCO_3 (between 22 and 26 mEq/L) are within normal ranges. Thus the ABG findings are considered normal.

106. **Correct Answer: D**

This set of values indicates the presence of uncompensated respiratory acidosis. The pH is less than 7.35, so the value is uncompensated. To determine whether the acidosis is respiratory or metabolic, find the value that represents acidosis: $CO_2 > 45$ mm Hg.

107. **Correct Answer: A**

Answers B, C, and D are characteristics of open catheter suctioning. When a closed system is used, the extra weight can increase tension on the catheter or tubing, which may cause the endotracheal tube to move. Many manufacturers make the inline tubing for both endotracheal and tracheostomy tubes. Nurses must make certain they are using the correct tube for suctioning. Another problem with inline catheters is the extra tubing that hangs out when the catheter is not in use. Patients may easily reach this tubing and extubate themselves or push the catheter down the airway and obstruct air flow.

108. **Correct Answer: D**

Stents can be manufactured in either straight or curved configurations to accommodate the differing nature of air passages. The stent rests against the anterior wall of the trachea and allows for freer passage of air; the patient can breathe spontaneously around the tube.

109. **Correct Answer: C**

The laryngeal mask airway was intended as a temporary airway. It requires minimal training to insert, but it cannot be placed by an RN as a matter of course. The patient must be unconscious and/or without gag reflex. The seal around the mask is a low-pressure seal, so it cannot be used on patients with high peak ventilator pressures. The

LMA is also associated with a significant risk of aspiration. Advantages of this airway are that it is simply blindly inserted into the hypopharynx, does not require visualization of the vocal cords, and does not traumatize the trachea. Patients will not have hoarseness or lose their voice altogether. At best, patients will complain of a mild sore throat.

110. **Correct Answer: B**
The magnet in the MRI will attract the wires in the tube. The silicone or plastic tubes cannot tolerate repeated cleanings. Use of a one-way speaking valve is contraindicated when using a foam cuff because the cuff may lie at an angle to the valve due to its orientation in the airway. The costs of silicone or plastic tracheostomy tubes are actually higher for facilities because the tubes are difficult to keep clean and are labor intensive.

111. **Correct Answer: C**
The tracheal tube provides a more stable airway, can be placed in an ICU setting, and decreases airway resistance. The tube is not near the right mainstem bronchus, so it will not facilitate intubation of the bronchus. A large number of complications can potentially occur with the use of a tracheostomy tube. Some of these complications include tracheal stenosis, tracheal malacia, aspiration, infection, hemorrhage, subcutaneous emphysema, and pneumothorax.

112. **Correct Answer: D**
Because of the direct connection via the eustachian tube, infection in the ear is possible. If a cervical injury has been stabilized, it is certainly possible for a skilled intubator to place the tube. Additional complications of the nasal endotracheal tube include nasal bleeding, sinusitis, accidental esophageal intubation, vocal cord injuries, necrosis, cuff leak or failure, and obstruction.

113. **Correct Answer: A**
Generally, the time it takes for the intubator to complete the task is not documented. If there is an unusual occurrence or a complication, it should be properly documented. The depth of the tube is important to chart because it gives a reference point for any questions about tube migration. The size of the tube may be too small or large, so it would have to be adjusted to the next appropriate size. A chest X ray is performed to confirm tube placement; and the time it is done should be documented. Any medications given during the procedure should be documented as to reason for their administration, patient response, and follow-up such as vital sign measurements or untoward reactions.

114. **Correct Answer: C**
The $ETCO_2$ is not a substitute for pulse oximetry. A pulse oximeter measures the availability of sites on the hemoglobin molecule for oxygen transport versus the percentage of sites occupied. The $ETCO_2$ measures whether gas exchange is taking place at the cellular level. If CO_2 is being given off, it will react with chemically treated paper in the detector. There is no excuse for not auscultating lungs to determine correct ETT placement. If the esophagus has been intubated, the $ETCO_2$ can give a false-positive reading if the patient has consumed a carbonated beverage within the past few hours.

115. **Correct Answer: A**
Sinusitis cannot be prevented simply by using a smaller-diameter ETT. If anything, it will make the patient's work of breathing more difficult, though it will not necessarily contribute to an infectious process. Orogastric tubes are preferred over nasogastric tubes whenever possible. Good handwashing technique has been shown to be effective in reducing all types of hospital-acquired infections.

116. **Correct Answer: B**

Double effect is a type of ethical dilemma that is commonly encountered in health care. In such a case, an action is justified as long as there is no intent to do further harm. Neither the physician nor the wife wants to hasten the patient's death, but they do want to make him more comfortable. It is the intent of the use of the narcotic rather than the use itself that defines the double effect. At least some good is done with the outcome of the discussion and resolution of the dilemma.

117. **Correct Answer: A**

The plateau or alveolar pressure should be limited to 30 cm H_2O. If a higher pressure is maintained, microvascular permeability is increased. The high pressure may also cause a stress fracture of capillary endothelium, epithelium, and basement membranes, potentially causing the lung to completely rupture. If this happens, blood, fluids, proteins, and exudates will leak into the air spaces and the tissue. The reverse is also true and air may leak into the tissues. If the pressure can be maintained at 30 cm H_2O, the CO_2 level may increase, leading to elevated intracranial pressure and respiratory acidosis will result. By slowly reducing tidal volume, the kidneys will be able to compensate for the respiratory acidosis.

118. **Correct Answer: B**

CPAP should be used with caution in patients who have basilar skull fractures. Research has shown that pneumocephalus may occur if a basilar skull fracture exists. CPAP helps by increasing the functional residual capacity and helping to reexpand the alveoli. Patients who have acute cardiogenic pulmonary edema may also benefit from the use of CPAP.

119. **Correct Answer: B**

This patient is in the pre-wean stage. During this stage, interventions and patient care are focused on restoring a patient to baseline status or improving the baseline status. Ventilator settings can be frequently changed to increase patient interaction, change modes, decrease FiO_2, or decrease PEEP. The pre-wean stage in a short-term ventilated patient is often quite brief and can last only a few hours. In a long-term ventilated patient this stage can last up to several months because only minute changes can dramatically alter a patient's condition.

120. **Correct Answer: B**

Abdominal contents have probably entered the thoracic cavity secondary to a diaphragmatic tear. If air also enters the thoracic cavity, it will increase intrathoracic pressure and help to transmit sound. This type of tear usually occurs on the left side of the diaphragm that ruptures—and Mort was injured on that side. It is postulated that the liver, because it is large, protects the right side of the diaphragm. A fractured pelvis usually also results in an almost 50% increased probability of a ruptured diaphragm.

121. **Correct Answer: A**

Mort's condition is a medical emergency. Maintenance of the airway and adequate oxygenation are always a priority. The abdominal contents' excursion into the thoracic cavity, along with the rise in intrathoracic pressure, will cause hemodynamic compromise. Preload will be decreased, the patient will become tachycardic and dyspneic, have uneven diaphragmatic movement (on palpation), and may progress to shock. The shoulder pain on the side of the tear may become quite severe and further hinder respiratory effort. Complications may include bowel obstruction and/or strangulation. The patient may become so unstable that he must be stabilized before surgery can even be considered.

122. **Correct Answer: C**
A flail chest results when two or more adjacent ribs are broken in two or more places, causing the chest wall to become unstable. During normal inspiration, the chest wall moves outward with an increase in negative intrathoracic pressure. In flail chest, the opposite movement—a "paradoxical" movement—of the chest wall is seen. Eventually the result will be atelectasis and alveolar collapse, with possible development of ARDS. To adequately stabilize the fracture, neuromuscular blockade is sometimes used. The patient must be given pain medication and sedation. Also, pain relief is the priority because the work of breathing needs to be reduced. (Just think about any time when you have had a pain in your side and how difficult it was to take a full breath.)

123. **Correct Answer: C**
Flail chest is a very painful condition that limits respiratory effort because of the pain or from analgesia and sedation that may be required. In this situation, CO_2 will increase, PaO_2 will decrease, and the pH will be below 7.35. The patient will develop respiratory acidosis.

124. **Correct Answer: B**
The pH of the aspirate is very important. If the aspirate is acidic, there is an almost immediate production of pulmonary edema owing to the collapse and breakdown of the alveoli, capillaries, and their interface. Atelectasis, possible intra-alveolar hemorrhage, and some interstitial edema may lead to hypoxia. Alkalotic aspirate destroys surfactant, which causes alveolar collapse, leading to hypoxia. Other factors to identify are the type of material aspirated and the amount. Syrup of Ipecac is used for ingestions. ABG findings would be considered more of a diagnostic tool.

125. **Correct Answer: C**
To evacuate fluids, the tube is placed low in the thoracic cavity and utilizes gravity to help clear the fluid. If a hemothorax is not completely removed, an infection may result, which can in turn lead to empyema. When assessing a patient, it is a good idea to ask (if possible) the origin of small scars on the thoracic area. It may take years for a hemothorax to cause a problem.

126. **Correct Answer: B**
In this type of respiratory failure, the $PaCO_2$ may be either decreased or normal. There may be a ventilation/perfusion mismatch (pneumonia, atelectasis) due to an intrapulmonary shunt. Alternatively, there may be increased alveolar dead space (shock, pulmonary embolism). Pulmonary fibrosis may reduce diffusion capacity (COPD, ARDS).

127. **Correct Answer: C**
Cor pulmonale also results from right ventricular failure or dilation secondary to pulmonary hypertension caused by lung disease. The important distinction here is that the patient's condition is not caused by any problem with the left ventricle. Acute cor pulmonale is usually the result of a massive pulmonary embolism that raises the PVR and causes increased preload and strain on the right heart.

128. **Correct Answer: D**

If a pulmonary embolism decreases oxygen availability, the work of breathing increases, as does the respiratory rate. The thoracic respiratory muscles and the diaphragm will increase their demand for oxygen, potentially leading to respiratory muscle fatigue. Oxygen may then be diverted to these muscles, so that less oxygen and nutrients are supplied to other vital organs. These organs may become ischemic and the patient may develop multiple-organ dysfunction syndrome (MODS). Answers A, B, and C may contribute to the formation of a pulmonary embolus.

129. **Correct Answer: A**

Traditionally, we were taught to assess Homan's sign: dorsiflexion of the ankle while bending the knee. If that action elicits pain, the patient has a problem with circulation and possibly DVT. Moses' sign is elicited by pressing the calf toward the tibia; it may also elicit pain. These results are not exclusive to DVT, but may complement a diagnosis.

130. **Correct Answer: C**

When balloons are old and weakened, they tend to rupture easily. The balloons can be made of latex and will disintegrate in the presence of circulating lipoproteins. If the balloon does rupture, it will not wedge and you can attempt to aspirate blood through the inflation port. If you cannot aspirate the blood, the balloon is probably ruptured. Immediately place a piece of tape with a notation that the balloon is ruptured at the port site so the next person will not attempt to use the port and inject air into the pulmonary circulation. Sometimes the balloon shatters into small parts, which become latex or rubber emboli. Another precaution is to determine if the patient has a preexisting latex allergy.

131. **Correct Answer: D**

The airway is always the priority. After placing the mask and notifying the charge nurse, you have other options. If the patient is stable, you can notify the attending physician and determine if he or she wants to reintubate the patient or leave on the mask, change to another form of O_2 delivery and/or FiO_2, draw ABGs, or do nothing. If the patient's condition deteriorates, you may have the option of asking the ED physician to intubate the patient. The wife may have innocently believed she was doing good, but she may also be a facilitator for her husband's drinking and behavior. She would certainly bear close watching if she is allowed to stay on the unit. This multifaceted question allows for different interpretations and requires critical thinking.

132. **Correct Answer: D**

PEEP helps keep alveoli open by raising PaO_2, so it will decrease the need for FiO_2.

133. **Correct Answer: C**

PEEP can produce barotrauma at pressures greater than 40 cm H_2O if that pressure is sustained. Pneumothorax is another complication. CPAP will also cause a pneumothorax.

134. **Correct Answer: B**

In the bifurcation of the internal and external carotid arteries, carotid bodies, and aortic bodies (in the carotid arch) are chemoreceptors. When the supply of oxygen decreases, stimulation of the aortic and/or carotid bodies occurs and, in turn, stimulates cortical activity. The result is adrenal gland secretions (epinephrine, norepinephrine), tachycardia, tachypnea, increased respiratory rate, and increased blood pressure.

135. **Correct Answer: B**
The formula for functional residual capacity is FRC = ERV (expired residual volume) + the RV (residual volume). The normal FRC in healthy lungs is about 2,000–3,000 mL.

136. **Correct Answer: C**
Subcutaneous emphysema usually occurs in the thorax as a result of a pulmonary air leak. This air leak may occur secondary to the patient receiving positive-pressure ventilation or from alveolar rupture from a pneumothorax. The air travels along under the skin and may be easily palpated and may feel like a crackling sensation. Patients who have chest tubes often have at least a small amount of subcutaneous emphysema at the tube insertion site. Sometimes the patient will feel pain when palpation is performed because the air tears the tissue. The free air must be reabsorbed—a process that may take several days.

137. **Correct Answer: A**
Bilirubin is not within the color spectrum that will interfere with pulse oximetry results. Dark nail polish (especially black, brown, blue, and green) will interfere with light transmission and cause an artificial lowered SpO_2. Patients who have bruising under the nails may have SpO_2 values that are artificially decreased.

138. **Correct Answer: B**
During resuscitation, blood pressure and blood flow may vary. The pharmacologic effects of medications such as vasoactive drugs used during resuscitation will compromise SpO_2 values.

139. **Correct Answer: B**
SpO_2 values are not the same as PaO_2 values. A slight drop in SpO_2 is reflective of a major change in PaO_2 values. That relationship is why the alarm limits should never exceed 5% of the acceptable baseline. Also, heart rate alarms can be set in accordance with any EKG limits.

140. **Correct Answer: B**
Pulse oximetry values do not directly correlate with PaO_2. Instead, you must use ABGs to determine PaO_2, the amount of oxygen available to the tissues. SpO_2 only measures the number of hemoglobin-binding sites that are occupied compared to the number of hemoglobin-binding sites available. The following data show the correlation.

Values of Pulse Oximetry	Probable PaO_2
97	100
95	80
94	70
90	60
85	50
75	40
57	30
32	20
10	10

141. **Correct Answer: B**

    One person is positioned on either side of the bed; the third person is at the head of the bed. The person at the head of the bed is responsible for ensuring cervical stability, maintaining the stability and positioning of the endotracheal tube, and managing ventilator tubing, intravenous lines, and any monitoring cables.

142. **Correct Answer: D**

    If the abdomen is open, it is possible to cover the area with synthetic material and use an abdominal binder to help secure the abdomen. Additional contraindications include an unstable spine, unstable chest wall, open chest, bifurcated endotracheal tube, and blood pressure less than 90 mm Hg when the patient is receiving vasoactive medications.

143. **Correct Answer: C**

    Adding a capnography device will help assure appropriate positioning of the endotracheal tube while turning the patient and when the patient is in the prone position. All EKG leads should be removed from the anterior chest wall. All wound dressings should be changed prior to placing the patient prone. All colostomy and ileostomy bags should be emptied because the patient's weight may cause the bags to rupture.

144. **Correct Answer: C**

    Maintaining suction levels at pressures higher than −40 cm /H_2O may cause reexpansion pulmonary edema, pleural air leaks, and lung tissue entrapment. The lung may not be able to expand properly.

145. **Correct Answer: D**

    If a mediastinal chest tube is in place, bubbling in the water seal chamber may indicate a communication between the mediastinal space and the pleural space. The physician should be notified immediately. Some sporadic bubbling will occur when suction is first turned on because fluid must displace air in the collection chamber. Chest tube tubing that is dependent or coiled will allow for the accumulation of drainage. This obstruction may increase the pressure in the lung.

146. **Correct Answer: A**

    These are the classic symptoms of a tension pneumothorax. Air has leaked into the pleural space and, because the thorax is closed, increasing pressure has caused the lung to collapse. Tension pneumothorax is a medical emergency.

147. **Correct Answer: A**

    The needle is placed just above the 3rd rib at the midclavicular line on the affected side. This placement, using the edge of the bone to guide the needle, should lessen the possibility of damaging the artery, vein, and nerve that are located just below each rib. Additional complications could include cellulitis, localized hematoma, pleural infection, and pneumothorax if the patient did not already have a tension pneumothorax.

148. **Correct Answer: D**

    A high pleural fluid to serum protein ratio will cause a fluid shift and result in an effusion. This is a reason for performing a thoracentesis. Contraindications for performing a thoracentesis include: coagulation disorders or patients receiving anticoagulants, abnormal anatomy–normal landmarks cannot be clearly identified, PEEP/CPAP, and splenomegaly. In patients with a pneumonectomy, thoracentesis may damage the remaining lung or drastically change intraplural pressure, possibly leading to collapse of the lung.

149. **Correct Answer: C**

Physiologic PEEP is the amount of positive pressure that remains in the alveoli after exhalation and keeps the alveoli from totally collapsing. Auto-PEEP occurs when the patient is mechanically ventilated and an amount of PEEP remains in the alveoli. The Auto-PEEP is in addition to the physiologic PEEP. Some of the causes of Auto-PEEP are small-diameter endotracheal tubes, bronchospasms, water in the ventilator tubing, high minute ventilation, and high respiratory rates. The patient actually had increased work of breathing because, in order to initiate a breath on the ventilator, they must overcome the set sensitivity and the amount of Auto-PEEP. Corrective measures include use of a large-diameter endotracheal tubes, slower respiratory rates, emptying the water from the ventilatory tubing, using sedatives and/or narcotics, and adjusting the ventilator to shorten inspiratory time to allow for a greater exhalation time.

150. **Correct Answer: B**

Compliance is the ability of the lung and the chest wall to freely move (distensibility). It is the ability of the lung and chest wall to stretch. In emphysema patients you often see the barrel-shaped chest. ARDS, atelectasis, obesity, pulmonary fibrosis, pulmonary edema, kyphoscoliosis, and pneumonia are other conditions that inhibit lung and chest wall movement (compliance).

151. **Correct Answer: D**

Albuterol administration would decrease lung resistance. Resistance means how easy it is to move gases through airways. Albuterol is a bronchodilator which increases the size of the lumen, making it easier for ventilation through the bronchi. Conditions that decrease the size of the bronchi lumen increase resistance.

152. **Correct Answer: D**

A buildup of ketones results from impaired glucose utilization. Additional causes of metabolic acidosis include diarrhea, renal failure, methanol poisoning, aspirin overdose, and lactic acidosis. Nasogastric suction removes chloride and causes metabolic alkalosis.

153. **Correct Answer: C**

Emphysema causes air to become trapped in the lungs. Also, there is less consolidation (density), so sound travels through this area. Percussion is performed to determine whether an area is filled with fluid, air, or solids. The liver would give off a dull sound because it is solid. A total thoracotomy or pneumonia would produce a flat sound because of consolidation.

154. **Correct Answer: A**

Generally, a patient with COPD will be hypoxic and demonstrate right heart failure, not left heart failure. Pulmonary hypertension leads to right heart failure. Chronic hypoxia also causes an increase in the concentration of red blood cells (polycythemia). The clubbing of the fingers has no known etiology, but occurs with chronic COPD.

155. **Correct Answer: B**

Smoking remains the number one cause of COPD. Smoking generates carbon monoxide, and the CO molecules produce a hypoxic state by occupying receptor sites on the hemoglobin molecule (oxygen has a lower affinity for these sites). Smoking causes vasoconstriction and increases afterload. It also leads to bronchoconstriction and decreases the efficiency of cilia and macrophages. Sputum production is increased. Pollution is now a major cause of COPD, and there is a documented increase in all types of allergens. An individual's occupation may certainly be a factor in the etiology of COPD, but that alone will rarely cause the condition.

156. **Correct Answer: B**
An increase in heart rate is an early sign of failure to wean. If PaO_2 levels drop or the minute ventilation is increased to more than 10 L/min, the patient is considered to have failed the attempt at weaning.

157. **Correct Answer: C**
Surya's anxiety probably resulted in hyperventilation and he was overriding the ventilator. Carbon dioxide would be blown off and the pH would fall; as a consequence, the patient would become alkalotic. Flail chest is very painful. It could be the pain that contributed to the failure to wean. If Surya was medicated, the drugs might also hinder his chance of success. Weaning a patient from a ventilator is a delicate balance.

158. **Correct Answer: C**
Small tidal volumes are used and delivered at a high rate. The chest wall does not move as much, which could cause pain and displace the fractures. The chest wall is more stable. Humidification is more critical with this type of ventilator because of the fast rate. Secretions may be thicker and suctioning may have to be done more often.

159. **Correct Answer: D**
Tachycardia is a direct result of carbon dioxide retention, as is restlessness. Cyanosis is a late sign of respiratory failure. Recognition of these signs is important because early treatments such as O_2, aerosols, suctioning, and even repositioning can prevent or mitigate respiratory failure.

160. **Correct Answer: B**
Normally the colloid osmotic pressure is about 10–25 mm Hg higher than the pulmonary capillary wedge pressure (PAOP). Colloid osmotic pressure from proteins and albumin keeps fluid in the intravascular space. If this pressure decreases, fluid leaks from the pulmonary capillaries. This fluid will also leak if the wedge pressure increases.

161. **Correct Answer: A**
Carbon anhydrase is an enzyme that helps convert water and carbon dioxide to bicarbonate. This form of CO_2 comprises about 70% of the total circulating CO_2. Approximately 10% of carbon dioxide is dissolved and becomes arterial $PaCO_2$. About 20% exists as carbaminohemoglobin in hemoglobin.

162. **Correct Answer: B**
When the chest tube is correctly placed in the pleural space, it can drain air or fluid. A tube could be located in the mediastinal space, but it is referred to as a mediastinal tube, not a chest tube.

163. **Correct Answer: C**
Prednisone decreases the effectiveness of isoniazid.

164. **Correct Answer: D**
Neupogen stimulates granulocyte and macrophage proliferation and differentiation as well as some end-cell functions.

165. **Correct Answer: A**

Neupogen stimulates the bone marrow to increase production of macrophages and granulocytes. Bone pain and muscle aches are common side effects of its use.

166. **Correct Answer: D**

The pH indicates a partial compensation, CO_2 is compensated, and HCO_3 is low (metabolic).

167. **Correct Answer: D**

Even with the FiO_2 at 30%, the patient can only maintain her oxygenation. There has been an increase of dead air space secondary to the pulmonary embolus.

168. **Correct Answer: B**

These symptoms are classic indicators of the presence of a pneumothorax. The air must be expelled, usually via a thoracentesis, and chest tubes will be placed. Be alert for hemodynamic compromise. Pain management will be necessary, though be aware of the potential for respiratory depression.

169. **Correct Answer: C**

Diminished lung compliance—as seen with a pneumothorax, pulmonary edema, atelectasis, and ARDS—will cause a high-pressure alarm.

170. **Correct Answer: A**

Any leak or loose connection will cause the alarm to sound as pressure drops.

171. **Correct Answer: B**

The patient with status asthmaticus is at greatest risk because the auto-PEEP may not be detected because of a shortened exhalation period.

172. **Correct Answer: B**

The most common size is 40 µg. This size will greatly reduce the dangers of microembolization.

173. **Correct Answer: C**

Old blood sometimes collects in the pleural cavity, and a change in position may cause it to flow into the tube. If there is any question as to the origin of the blood, check the patient's blood pressure and do a thorough assessment.

BIBLIOGRAPHY

Adhikari, N., Burns, K. E. A., & Meade, M. O. (2004). Pharmacologic therapies for adults with acute lung injury and acute respiratory distress syndrome. *Cochrane Database of Systematic Reviews,* (4), Art No CD004477, pub 2, DOI: 10.1002/14651858.

Agbaht, K., Lisboa, T., Pobo, A., Rodriguez, A., Sandiumenge, A., Diaz, E., et al. (2007). Management of ventilator-associated pneumonia in a multidisciplinary intensive care unit: Does trauma make a difference? *Intensive Care Medicine, 33*(8), 1387–1395.

Ahrens, T. (2006). *Critical care nursing certification.* Columbus, OH: McGraw-Hill.

Ahrens, T., & Sona, C. (2003). Capnography application in acute and critical care. *AACN Clinical Issues, 14,* 123–132.

American Association of Critical Care Nurses. (2004). *Ventilator associated pneumonia (VAP).* Practice alert series. Aliso Viejo, CA: AACN.

American Association of Critical Care Nurses. (2006). *Core curriculum for critical care nursing* (6th ed.). Philadelphia: Saunders.

American Association of Critical Care Nurses. (2007). *AACN certification and core review for high acuity and critical care* (6th ed.). Philadelphia: Saunders.

American Heart Association. (2007). *Guidelines 2005 for cardiopulmonary resuscitation and emergency cardiovascular care.* Retrieved July 18, 2008, from http://circ.ahajournals.org/content/vol112/24_suppl

American Lung Association. (2005). *Lung transplants: Treatments and support.* Retrieved February 2, 2005, from http://www.lungusa.org/site/c.dvLUK9O0E/b.23012/k.A039/Lung_Transplants.htm

American Thoracic Society. (2005). Consensus statement: Guidelines for the management of adults with hospital-acquired, ventilatory-associated, and healthcare-associated pneumonia. *American Journal of Respiratory Critical Care Medicine, 171,* 388–416.

Andenaes, R., Kalfoss, M. H., & Wahl, A. (2004). Psychological distress and quality of life in hospitalized patients with chronic obstructive pulmonary disease. *Journal of Advanced Nursing. 46*(5), 523–530.

Arora, S., Lang, I., Nayyar, V., Stachowski, E., & Ross, D. L. (2007). Atrial fibrillation in a tertiary care multidisciplinary intensive care unit: Incidence and risk factors. *Anesthesia and Intensive Care, 35*(5), 707–713.

Association of Operating Room Nurses. (2007). AORN guideline for prevention of venous stasis. *AORN Journal, 85*(3), 607–624.

Azu, M. C., McCormack, J. E., Huang, E. C., Lee, T. K., & Shapiro, M. J. (2007). Venous thromboembolic events in hospitalized trauma patients. *American Surgeon, 73*(12), 1228–1231.

Bailey, P. H., Colella, T., & Mossey, S. (2004). COPD—intuition or template: Nurses' stories of acute exacerbations of chronic obstructive pulmonary disease. *Journal of Clinical Nursing, 13*(6), 756–764.

Barnes, P. J., & Adcock, I. M. (2003). How do corticoid steroids work in asthma? *Annals of Internal Medicine, 139*(5 pt 1), 359–370.

Berkowitz, D. S., & Coyne, N. C. (2003). Understanding primary pulmonary hypertension. *Critical Care Nursing Quarterly, 26*(1), 28–34.

Bialk, J. L. (2004). Ethical guidelines for assisting patients with end-of-life decision making. *Medsurg Nursing, 13*(2), 87–90.

Bigatello, L. M., Davidson, K. R., & Stelfox, H. T. (2005). Respiratory mechanics and ventilatory waveforms in the patient with acute lung injury. *Respiratory Care, 50,* 235–245.

Booker, R. (2004). The effective assessment of acute breathlessness in a patient. *Nursing Times, 100*(24), 61–63.

Booker, R. (2005). Chronic obstructive pulmonary disease: Non-pharmacological approaches [review]. *British Journal of Nursing, 14*(1), 14–18.

Borges, J. B., Okamoto, V. N., Matos, G. F. J., Caramez, M. P., Arantes, P. R., Barros, F., et al. (2006). Reversibility of lung collapse and hypoxemia in early acute respiratory distress syndrome. *American Journal of Respiratory and Critical Care Medicine, 174*(3), 268–278.

Boron, W. F., & Boulpaep, E. L. (2004). *Medical physiology*. Philadelphia: Saunders.

Boyle, A. H., & Locke, D. L. (2004). Update on chronic obstructive pulmonary disease. *Medsurg Nursing, 13*(1), 42–48.

Burgess, A. W. (2005). Death by catheterization? Sudden, unexpected deaths of older adults are often not questioned. *American Journal of Nursing, 105*(4), 56–59.

Burns, D. M. (2003). Tobacco-related diseases. *Seminars in Oncology Nursing, 19*(4), 244–249.

Burns, S. M. (2003). Working with respiratory waveforms: How to use bedside graphics. *AACN Clinical Issues, 14,* 133–144.

Burns, S. M. (2004). The science of weaning: When and how? *Critical Care Nursing Clinics of North America, 16*(3), 379–386, ix.

Burns, S. M. (Ed.). (2007). *American Association of Critical-Care Nurses (AACN): AACN protocols for practice: Healing environments* (2nd ed.). Sudbury, MA: Jones and Bartlett.

Celli, B. R., MacNee, W., & ATS/ERS Task Force. (2004). Standards for the diagnosis and treatment of patients with COPD: A summary of the ATS/ERS position paper. *European Respiratory Journal, 23,* 932–946.

Chasen, E. R., & Umlauf, M. G. (2003). Nocturia: A problem that disrupts sleep and predicts obstructive sleep apnea. *Geriatric Nursing, 24*(2), 76–81.

Chojnowski, D. (2003). "GOLD" standards for acute exacerbation in COPD. *Nursing Practice, 28*(5), 26–35.

Conner, B., & Meng, A. (2003). Pulmonary function testing in asthma: Nursing applications. *Critical Care Nursing Clinics of North America, 38*(4), 571–583.

Conover, M. B. (2003). *Understanding electrocardiography* (8th ed.). St. Louis, MO: Mosby/Elsevier.

Cooper, S. J. (2004). Methods to prevent ventilator associated lung injury: A summary. *Critical Care Nurse, 20*(6), 358–365.

Copstead, L., & Banasik, J. L. (2000). *Pathophysiology: Biological and behavioral perspectives* (2nd ed.). Philadelphia: Saunders/Elsevier.

Corbridge, S. J., & Corbridge, T. C. (2004). Severe exacerbations in asthma. *Critical Care Nursing Quarterly, 27,* 207–228.

Costello, J., & Hogg, C. T. (2003). CT pulmonary angiogram compared with ventilation–perfusion scan for the diagnosis of pulmonary embolism in patients with cardiorespiratory disease. *Emergency Medicine Journal, 20,* 547–548.

Criner, G. J., Scharf, S. M., Falk, J. A., et al. (2007). Effect of lung volume reduction surgery on resting pulmonary hemodynamics in severe emphysema. *American Journal of Respiratory and Critical Care Medicine, 176*(3), 253–260.

Curley, M. A. Q. (1998). Patient–nurse synergy: Optimizing patients' outcomes. *American Journal of Critical Care, 7,* 64–72.

de Perrot, M., Granton, J., & Fadel, E. (2006). Pulmonary hypertension after pulmonary emboli: An underrecognized condition. *Canadian Medical Association Journal, 174*(12), 1706–1707.

Dells, P. L. (2004). Advances in prostacyclin therapy for pulmonary arterial hypertension. *Critical Care Nurse, 24,* 42–54.

Dossey, B. M., Keegan, L., & Guzzetta, C. (2003). *Holistic nursing: A handbook for practice* (3rd ed.). Sudbury, MA: Jones and Bartlett.

Dueker, C. W. (2004). Immersion in fresh water and survival. *Chest, 126*(6), 2027–2028.

Durbin, C. G. (2005). Applied respiratory physiology: Uses of ventilator waveforms and mechanics in the management of critically ill patients. *Respiratory Care, 50,* 287–293.

Ecklund, M. M., & Kurluk, S. A. (2004). Caring for the bariatric patient with obstructive sleep apnea. *Critical Care Nursing Clinics of North America, 16*(3), 311–317.

Edwards, D. F. (1999). The Synergy Model: Linking patient needs to nurse competencies. *Critical Care Nurse, 19*(1), 88–98.

Eli-Masri, M. M., Williamson, K. M., & Fox-Wasylyshyn, S. M. (2004). Severe acute respiratory syndrome: Another challenge for critical care nurses. *AACN Clinical Issues, 15*(1), 150–159.

Ellstrom, K. (2006). The pulmonary system. In American Association of Critical Care Nurses, *Core curriculum for critical care nursing* (6th ed., pp. 45–183). St. Louis, MO: Saunders.

Emergency Nurses Association & Newberry, L. (2003). *Sheehy's emergency nursing: Principles and practice* (5th ed.). St. Louis, MO: Mosby/Elsevier.

Estabrooks, C. A., Midodzi, W. K., Cummings, G. G., Ricker, K. L., & Giovannetti, P. (2005). The impact of hospital nursing characteristics on 30-day mortality. *Nursing Research, 54*(2), 74–84.

Fedullo, P. F., & Tapson, V. F. (2003). Clinical practice: The evaluation of suspected pulmonary embolism. *New England Journal of Medicine, 349,* 1247–1256.

Fehrenbach, C. (2005). Initiatives to improve outcomes for chronic obstructive pulmonary disease. *Journal of Professional Nursing, 20*(6), 43–45.

Fenstermacher, D., & Hong, D. (2004). Mechanical ventilation: What have we learned? *Critical Care Nursing Quarterly, 27,* 258–294.

Finesilver, C. (2003). Pulmonary assessment: What you need to know. *Progress in Cardiovascular Nursing, 18,* 83.

Finkelmeier, B. A. (2000). *Cardiothoracic surgical nursing* (2nd ed.). Philadelphia: Lippincott Williams & Wilkins.

Fost, S. D., Brotman, D. J., & Michota, F. A. (2003). Rational use of D-dimer measurements to exclude acute venous thromboembolic disease. *Mayo Clinic Proceedings, 78,* 1385–1391.

Frazier, S. C. (2005). Implications of the GOLD report for chronic obstructive pulmonary disease for the home care clinician. *Home Health Nurse, 23*(2), 109–114.

Giulliano, K. K., & Higgins, T. L. (2005). New generation pulse oximetry in the care of critically ill patients. *American Journal of Critical Care, 14,* 26–39.

Goldrick, B. A. (2005). Infection in the older adult: Long-term care poses particular risk. *American Journal of Nursing, 105*(6), 31–34.

Gronkiewicz, C., & Borkgen-Okonek, M. (2004). Acute exacerbation of COPD: Nursing application of evidence-based guidelines. *Critical Care Nursing Quarterly, 27*(4), 336–352.

Guyton, A. C., & Hall, J. E. (2005). *Textbook of medical physiology* (11th ed.). Philadelphia: Saunders.

Hanneman, S. (2004). Weaning from short-term mechanical ventilation. *Critical Care Nurse, 24*(1), 70.

Hardie, J. A., Vollmer, W. M., Buist, A. S., Ellingsen, I., Mørkve, O. (2004). Reference values for arterial blood gases in the elderly. *Chest, 125,* 2053.

Hardin, S. R., & Kaplow, R. (Eds.). (2004). *Synergy for clinical excellence: The AACN Synergy Model for Patient Care.* Sudbury, MA: Jones and Bartlett.

Heinzer, M. M., Bish, C., & Detwiler, R. (2003). Acute dyspnea as perceived by patients with chronic obstructive pulmonary disease. *Clinical Nursing Research, 12*(1), 85–101.

Hickey, J. V. (2002). *The clinical practice of neurological and neurosurgical nursing* (5th ed.). Philadelphia: Lippincott Williams & Wilkins.

Hogg, J. C., Chu, F., Utokaparch, S., Woods, R., Elliott, W. M., Buzatu, L., et al. (2004). The nature of small-airway obstruction in chronic obstructive pulmonary disease. *New England Journal of Medicine, 350,* 2645–2653.

Hughes, J. M. B. (2007). Review series: Lung function made easy: Assessing gas exchange. *Chronic Respiratory Disease, 4*(4), 205–214.

Jesurum, J. (2004). SvO_2 monitoring. *Critical Care Nurse, 24,* 73–76.

Jones, P. W. (2003). Ultrasound-guided thoracentesis: Is it a safer method? *Chest, 123,* 418.

Kaczorowski, D. J., & Zuckerbraun, B. S. (2007). Carbon monoxide: Medicinal chemistry and biological effects. *Current Medicinal Chemistry, 14*(25), 2720–2725.

Kallet, R. H., & Katz, J. A. (2003). Respiratory system mechanics in acute respiratory distress syndrome. *Respiratory Care Clinics of North America, 9,* 297.

Kane, C., & Galanes, S. (2004). Adult respiratory distress syndrome. *Critical Care Nursing Quarterly, 27*(4), 325–335.

Kanervisto, M., Paavilainen, E., & Astedt-Kurki, P. (2003). Impact of chronic obstructive pulmonary disease on family functioning. *Heart and Lung, 32*(6), 360–367.

Katis, P. G. (2005). Atraumatic hemopericardium in a patient receiving warfarin therapy for a pulmonary embolus. *Journal of the Canadian Association of Emergency Physicians, 7*(3), 168–170.

Keenan, S. P., Sinuff, T., Cook, D. J., & Hill, N. S. (2004). Does noninvasive positive pressure ventilation improve outcome in acute hypoxemic respiratory failure: A systematic review. *Critical Care Medicine, 32,* 2516–2523.

King, J. E. (2003). Could my patient have deep vein thrombosis? *Nursing, 33*(9), 24.

Kollef, M. H. (2004). Prevention of hospital-associated pneumonia and ventilatory-associated pneumonia. *Critical Care Medicine, 6,* 1396.

Koschel, M. J. (2004). Pulmonary embolism: Quick diagnosis can save a patient's life. *American Journal of Nursing, 140*(6), 46–50.

Kreamer, K. M. (2003). Getting the lowdown on lung cancer. *Nursing, 33*(11), 36–42.

Kress, T., & Krueger, D. (2004). Identifying carbon monoxide poisoning. *Nursing, 34*(11), 68–69.

Kumar, D., Farrell, T., & Tierney, E. (2007). A frightening complication of general anesthesia for pediatric dental extractions. *Pediatric Surgery International, 23*(6), 613–616.

Lindgren, V. A., & Ames, N. J. (2005). Caring for patients on mechanical ventilation: What research indicates is best practice. *American Journal of Nursing, 105*(5), 50–60.

Lipson, J. G., Dibble, S. L., & Minarik, P. A. (Eds.). (1996). *Culture and nursing care: A pocket guide.* San Francisco, CA: UCSF Nursing Press.

Lomborg, K., Bjorn, A., Dahl, R., & Kirkevold, M. (2005). Body care experienced by people hospitalized with severe respiratory disease. *Journal of Advanced Nursing, 50*(3), 262–271.

Lynes, D., & Kelly, C. (2003). The psychological needs of patients with chronic respiratory disease. *Nursing Times, 99*(33), 44–45.

MacIntyre, N. R. (2004). Evidenced-based ventilator weaning and discontinuation. *Respiratory Care, 49*(7), 830–836.

Majer, S., & Graber, P. (2007). Postpartum pneumomediastinum (Hamman's syndrome). *Canadian Medical Association Journal, 177*(1), 32.

Markou, N. K., Myrianthefs, P. M., & Batopoulos, G. J. (2004). Respiratory failure: An overview. *Critical Care Nursing Quarterly, 27*(4), 353–379.

McQuillan, D. P., Duncan, R. A., & Craven, D. E. (2005). Ventilator-associated pneumonia: Emerging principles of management. *Infections in Medicine, 22*(3), 104–118.

McQuillan, K. A., Von Rueden, K. T., Hartsock, R. L., Flynn, M. B., & Whalen, E. (Eds.). (2002). *Trauma nursing: From resuscitation through rehabilitation* (3rd ed.). Philadelphia: Saunders/Elsevier.

Medina, J., & Puntillo, K. (2006). *AACN protocols for practice: Palliative care and end-of-life issues in critical care.* Sudbury, MA: Jones and Bartlett.

Merrel, P., & Mayo, D. (2004). Inhalation injury in the burn patient. *Critical Care Nursing Clinics of North America, 16*(1), 27–38.

Merritt, S. L., & Berger, B. E. (2004). Obstructive sleep apnea–hypopnea syndrome: Nurses may detect a problem often overlooked by other providers. *American Journal of Nursing, 104*(7), 49–52.

Mullan, B., Snyder, M., Lindgren, B., Finkelstein, S. M., & Hertz, M. I. (2003). Home monitoring for lung transplant candidates. *Progress in Transplantation, 13*(3), 176–182.

Muno, N. (2003). Cardiac bypass without the pump. *RN, 66*(10), 28–32.

Musto, P. K. (2003). General principles of asthma management: Education. *Nursing Clinics of North America, 38*(4), 621–633.

Nilsestuen, J. O., & Hargett K. D. (2005). Using ventilator graphics to identify patient–ventilator asynchrony. *Respiratory Care, 50,* 202–234.

O'Shea Forbes, M. (2007). Prolonged ventilator dependence: Perspective of the chronic obstructive pulmonary disease patient. *Clinical Nursing Research, 16*(3), 231.

Pagana, K. D., & Pagana, J. (2005). *Mosby's manual of diagnostic and laboratory tests* (3rd ed.). St. Louis, MO: Mosby/Elsevier.

Petty, M. (2003). Lung and heart–lung transplantation: Implications for nursing care when hospitalized outside the transplant center. *Medsurg Nursing, 12*(4), 250–259.

Poulose, B. K., Griffin, M. R., Zhu, Y., Smalley, W., Richards, W. O., Wright, J. K., et al. (2005). National analysis of adverse patient safety events in bariatric surgery. *American Surgeon, 71*(5), 406–413

Powers, J., & Daniels, D. (2004). Turning points: Implementing kinetic therapy in the ICU. *Nursing Management, 35*(5 suppl), 1–7.

Pruitt, B., & Jacobs, M. (2005). Caring for a patient with asthma. *Nursing, 35*(2), 48–51.

Ramirez, E. G. (2003). Management of asthma emergencies. *Nursing Clinics of North America, 38*(4), 713–724.

Rance, M. (2005). Kinetic therapy positively influences oxygenation in patients with ALI/ARDS. *Nursing Critical Care, 10*(1), 35–41.

Roberts, J. (2003). The new asthma guidelines: A patient-centered approach to asthma. *Journal of Professional Nursing, 18*(7), 379–382.

Roch, A., Blayac, D., Ramiara, P., Chetaille, B., Marin, V., Michelet, P., et al. (2007). Comparison of lung injury after normal or small volume optimized resuscitation in a model of hemorrhagic shock. *Intensive Care Medicine, 33*(9), 1645–1654.

Rowe, C. (2004). Development of clinical guidelines for prone positioning in critically ill adults. *Nursing Critical Care, 9*(2), 50–57.

Salomez, F., & Vincent, J. L. (2004). Drowning: A review of epidemiology, pathophysiology, treatment and prevention. *Resuscitation, 63*(3), 261–268.

Seidel, H. M. (2003). *Mosby's guide to physical examination* (3rd ed.). St. Louis, MO: Mosby.

Sevransky, J. E., Levy, M. M., & Marini, J. J. (2004). Mechanical ventilation in sepsis-induced acute lung-injury/acute respiratory distress syndrome: An evidence-based review. *Critical Care Medicine, 32,* S548–S553.

Simmons, P., & Simmons, M. (2004). Informed nursing practice: The administration of oxygen to patients with COPD. *Medsurg Nursing, 13*(2), 82–85.

Sims, J. M. (2003). Guidelines for treating asthma. *Dimensions of Critical Care Nursing, 22*(6), 247–250.

Skidmore-Roth, L. (2004). *Mosby's 2004 nursing drug reference.* St. Louis, MO: Mosby/Elsevier.

Smeltzer, S., & Bare, B. G. (2003). *Brunner and Suddarth's textbook of medical–surgical nursing* (10th ed.). Philadelphia: Lippincott Williams & Wilkins.

Sole, M. L., Hartshorn, J., & Lamborne, M. L. (2001). *Introduction to critical care nursing* (3rd ed.). Philadelphia: Saunders/Elsevier.

Spector, N., & Connolly, M. (2003). *Dyspnea: Protocols for practice series.* Aliso Viejo, CA: American Association of Critical Care.

Squara, P. (2004). Matching total body oxygen consumption and delivery: A crucial objective? *Intensive Care Medicine, 30,* 2170–2179.

St. John, R. E. (2003). End-tidal CO_2 monitoring. *Critical Care Nurse, 23,* 83–88.

St. John, R. E. (2004). Airway management. *Critical Care Nurse, 4*(2), 93–96.

Tablan, O. C., Anderson, L. J., Besser, R., Bridges, C., Hajjeh, R., CDC, et al. (2004). Guidelines for preventing health-care–associated pneumonia, 2003: recommendations of CDC and the Healthcare Infection Control Practices Advisory Committee. *MMWR Recommendations and Reports, 53,* 1–36.

Tillie-Leblond, I., Gosset, P., & Tonnel, A. B. (2005). Inflammatory events in severe acute asthma. *Allergy, 60*(1), 23.

Tsangaris, I., Galiatsou, E., Kostanti, E., & Nakos, G. (2007). The effect of exogenous surfactant in patients with lung contusions and acute lung injury. *Intensive Care Medicine, 33*(5), 851–855.

Turpie, A. G. G., Chin, B. S. P., & Lip, G. L. H. (2002). Venous thromboembolism: Pathophysiology, clinical features, and prevention. *British Medical Journal. 325,* 887–890.

United Network for Organ Sharing. (2005). Information for transplant professionals about the lung allocation score system. Retrieved February 20, 2005, from http://www.unos.org/SharedContentDocuments/Lung_pro.pdf

Urden, L. D., Stacy, K. M., & Lough, M. E. (2007). *Thelan's critical care nursing: Diagnosis and management* (5th ed.). St. Louis, MO: Mosby.

U.S. Organ Procurement and Transplantation Network (OPTN). (2005). Scientific Registry of Transplant Recipients (SRTR): OPTN/SRTR annual report. Retrieved February 20, 2005, from http://www.ustransplant.org/annual_Reports/archives/2005/default.htm

Vahid, B., & Marik, P. E. (2007). Severe emphysema associated with cocaine smoking. *Journal of Respiratory Diseases, 28*(11), 485.

Vecchiarine, P., Bohaannon, R. W., Ferullo, J., et al. (2004). Short-term outcomes and their predictors for patients hospitalized with community-acquired pneumonia. *Heart and Lung, 33,* 301–307.

Veronesi, J. F. (2004). Trauma nursing: Blunt chest injuries. *RN, 67*(3), 47–54.

Vollman, K. M. (2004). Prone positioning in the patient who has acute respiratory distress syndrome: The art and science. *Critical Care Nurse Clinics of North America, 16*(3), 431–443.

Walker, S. (2003). Updates in small cell lung cancer treatment. *Clinical Journal of Oncology Nursing, 7*(5), 562–568.

Weir, P. (2004). Quick asthma assessment: A stepwise approach to treatment. *Advanced Nursing Practice, 12*(1), 53–56.

Wiegand, D. J. L., & Carlson, K. K. (Eds.). (2005). *AACN procedure manual for critical care* (5th ed.). Philadelphia: Elsevier.

Wilkins, R. L., Stoller, J. K., & Scanlan, C. L. (2003). *Egan's fundamentals of respiratory care* (8th ed.). St. Louis, MO: Mosby.

Williams, T. A., & Leslie, G. D. (2004). A review of the nursing care of enteral feedings tubes in critically ill adults: Part I. *Intensive and Critical Care Nursing, 20*(6), 330–343.

Williams, T. A., & Leslie, G. D. (2004). A review of the nursing care of enteral feedings tubes in critically ill adults: Part II. *Intensive and Critical Care Nursing, 21*(5), 5–15.

Williamson, J. P., Illing, R., Gertler, P., & Braude, S. (2004). Near-drowning treated with therapeutic hypothermia. *Medical Journal of Australia, 181*(9), 500–501.

Wisniewski, A. (2003). Chronic bronchitis and emphysema: Clearing the air. *Nursing, 33*(5), 46–49.

Woods, S., Sivarajan Froelicher, E. S., & Motzer, S. U. (2000). *Cardiac nursing* (4th ed.). Philadelphia: Lippincott Williams & Wilkins.

Wynne, R., & Botti, M. (2004). Postoperative pulmonary dysfunction in adults after cardiac surgery with cardiopulmonary bypass: Clinical significance and implications for practice. *American Journal of Critical Care, 13,* 384–393.

Yang, J. C. (2005). Prevention and treatment of deep vein thrombosis and pulmonary embolism in critically ill patients. *Critical Care Nursing Quarterly, 28*(1), 72–79.

Yoneyama, T., Yoshida, M., Ohrui, T., Mukaiyama, H., Okamoto, H., Hoshiba, K., et al. (2003). Oral care reduces pneumonia in older patients in nursing homes. *Journal of the American Geriatrics Society, 51,* 1018–1022.

Yusen, R. D., Lefrak, S. S., & Gierada, D. S. (2003). A prospective evaluation of lung volume reduction surgery in 200 consecutive patients. *Chest, 123,* 1026–1037.

Endocrine

QUESTIONS

1. Paula, a 35-year-old housewife, is admitted to the ICU after a cholecystectomy due to her morbid obesity. She has a recent history of gastric bypass surgery for weight loss. You find her confused with slurred speech and diaphoretic. Her BP is 90/40, pulse 120, and blood sugar 28. Your first action should be:
   A. Notify the physician and recheck the blood sugar
   B. Open the intravenous fluid and give the patient orange juice with sugar
   C. Give 1 ampule of D_{50} per hospital policy, notify the physician, and recheck blood sugar in 30 minutes
   D. Recheck the blood sugar results with the hospital lab

2. What is the pathophysiology of acute hypoglycemia?
   A. Oral antihyperglycemic agents
   B. Glucose consumption exceeds glucose production
   C. Insulinoma
   D. Alcoholism

3. What therapies are used to treat acute hypoglycemia (blood sugar less than 50 mg/dL)?
   A. Small, frequent meals; increased carbohydrate consumption
   B. Intravenous D_{50} administration; oral glucose; treat the cause
   C. Increased carbohydrate diet; intravenous glucose
   D. Treat the cause; increased carbohydrate consumption

4. What is the most common precipitating factor in the development of diabetic ketoacidosis (DKA)?
   A. Hypoglycemia only
   B. Hypoglycemia with obesity and family history
   C. Hyperglycemia only
   D. Hyperglycemia with concurrent illness or injury

5. What are some of the signs and symptoms associated with diabetic ketoacidosis (DKA)?
   A. Polyuria, polydipsia, polyphagia, dilute urine
   B. Polyuria, polydipsia, polyphagia, fruity breath, dehydration, marked fatigue
   C. Hyperactivity, confusion, nausea, vomiting
   D. Kussmaul's respirations, dilute urine

6. John has been admitted to the intensive care unit with DKA. His insulin drip is at 5 units per hour. His current blood sugar is 275 and his anion gap is 25. Which changes in his care should you anticipate?
   A. Change intravenous fluid to D_5W and continue the insulin drip
   B. Change intravenous fluids to D_5NS and continue insulin drip
   C. Discontinue insulin drip, start blood sugars every 4 hours
   D. No changes in therapy

7. Which of the following diabetic patients is most likely to develop DKA?
   A. A patient with Type I diabetes who is well controlled on 70/30 insulin
   B. A patient with Type I diabetes who is noncompliant with therapy and has cellulitis of his left leg
   C. A patient with Type II diabetes who has an $HgbA_{1c}$ level of 6.5 and has undergone minor surgery
   D. A patient with Type II diabetes who is noncompliant with therapy and has a mild upper respiratory tract infection

8. Your patient with DKA and a blood glucose of 480 mg/dL also has a potassium level of 6.2. You have started an insulin drip. You know that the insulin drip will
   A. Draw more potassium from the intracellular space.
   B. Draw more potassium from the extracellular space.
   C. Will not change potassium levels.
   D. Move potassium back into the intracellular space.

9. Kayexalate is given for hyperkalemia. What is the mechanism of action of this drug?
   A. Kayexalate causes diarrhea, removing potassium from the gastrointestinal tract.
   B. Kayexalate preserves the sodium pump.
   C. Kayexalate exchanges sodium ions for potassium ions.
   D. Kayexalate moves potassium into the intracellular space.

10. Frank has a crush injury to his right thigh. Why does this injury put Frank at risk for hyperkalemia?
    A. There is a greater risk of hypokalemia.
    B. The patient is at no risk for hyperkalemia.
    C. Cellular destruction leads to increased circulating potassium levels.
    D. Wound infection decreases potassium levels.

11. Which EKG changes are seen with hyperkalemia?
    A. Narrow QRS, peaked T waves and U waves
    B. Widening QRS, peaked T waves, loss of P waves
    C. Wide QRS, normal T waves, U waves
    D. Narrow QRS, normal T waves, rapid rate

12. How does hyperglycemic, hyperosmolar, nonketotic syndrome (HHNS) differ from diabetic ketoacidosis (DKA)?
    A. HHNS has the same onset, higher blood sugars, and more dehydration relative to DKA.
    B. HHNS has a slower onset, lower blood sugars, and less dehydration relative to DKA.
    C. HHNS has a slower onset, much higher blood sugar, and more profound dehydration relative to DKA.
    D. HHNS has the same onset, lower blood sugars, and no dehydration relative to DKA.

13. **Which set of lab results would you anticipate for a patient with hyperglycemic, hyperosmolar, nonketotic syndrome (HHNS)?**
    A. Glucose 550; positive ketones; serum osmolality: 280 mOsm/L
    B. Glucose 1,258; negative ketones; serum osmolality: 375 mOsm/L
    C. Glucose 700; negative ketones; serum osmolality: 270 mOsm/L
    D. Glucose 600; positive ketones; serum osmolality: 240 mOsm/L

14. **Ralph is an 87-year-old retiree found unconscious in his board and care unit. His blood sugar is 1,475, he has negative serum ketones, and his serum osmolality is 340 mOsm/L. What do you anticipate for medical treatment of this condition?**
    A. D_5 ½NS intravenous fluids at 300 mL/h and an insulin drip with sliding-scale coverage
    B. Normal saline at 200 mL/h, subcutaneous insulin with sliding-scale coverage every 4 hours, and monitor potassium
    C. Intravenous fluids with normal saline in high volumes, insulin drip with sliding-scale coverage, monitor electrolyte levels
    D. Normal saline intravenously, bicarbonate drip, monitor electrolytes

15. **What is the difference between Somoygi effect and the Dawn phenomenon?**
    A. They are essentially the same process.
    B. The Dawn phenomenon is nocturnal hypoglycemia; the Somoygi effect is greatly elevated blood sugars in the early morning.
    C. The Somoygi effect is nocturnal hypoglycemia with rebound hyperglycemia; the Dawn phenomenon is increased morning glucose without nocturnal hypoglycemia.
    D. The Dawn phenomenon is morning hypoglycemia; the Somoygi effect is nocturnal hyperglycemia.

16. **Your patient has been diagnosed with Cushing syndrome. Which diagnostic tests do you anticipate?**
    A. Computerized tomography of the brain, chest, and abdomen; 24-hour urine cortisol levels; ACTH serum concentrations
    B. Computerized tomography of the brain, chest, and abdomen; thyroid levels; basic metabolic panel
    C. Serum and urine cortisol levels; thyroid panels; beta naturetic peptide levels
    D. Urine ACTH concentrations; thyroid panel; C-reactive protein level

17. **Which physical symptoms do you expect with Cushing syndrome?**
    A. Moon facies, edema, weight loss
    B. Moon facies, acne, weight loss
    C. Moon facies, purple striae on trunk, buffalo hump
    D. Moon facies, easy bruising, weight loss

18. **Functions of the thyroid gland, adrenal gland, and male and female reproductive glands are regulated by**
    A. The pineal gland of the brain.
    B. The thyroid gland.
    C. The pineal–pituitary axis.
    D. The hypothalamic–pituitary axis.

19. **Where is the pituitary gland located?**
    A. Inferior to the hypothalamus, in the sella turcica of the skull
    B. Superior to the hypothalamus gland, near the optic chiasm
    C. Between the thalamus and hypothalamus in the midbrain
    D. Superior to the pons and brain stem

20. **Which of the following hormones are produced by the anterior pituitary gland?**
    A. GRF, TSH, Substance P
    B. ADH, TSH, FSH
    C. FSH, LH, TSH, ACTH
    D. Vasopressin, oxytocin

21. **Your patient's thyroid-stimulating hormone (TSH) level is 0.001. What condition does this value indicate?**
    A. Hypoactive anterior pituitary function
    B. Hyperactive anterior pituitary function
    C. Hypothyroidism
    D. Hyperthyroidism

22. **Where is the thyroid gland located?**
    A. Just below the hyoid bone
    B. In the throat on either side of the trachea
    C. Above the larynx
    D. Sits on top of the thymus gland

23. **What is an important teaching point for a patient with hypothyroidism?**
    A. Take thyroid medication at the same time every day; there is no need to fast.
    B. Take thyroid medication at the same time every day, 30 minutes before breakfast.
    C. Take thyroid medication each evening before bed.
    D. Take thyroid medication daily with food.

24. **Fred had a thyroidectomy yesterday for thyroid cancer. Today he is delirious, vomiting, hyperthermic, and tachycardic. It is imperative to notify the physician immediately because**
    A. Fred has a postoperative infection.
    B. Fred may have had a cerebrovascular accident.
    C. Fred may have thyrotoxic crisis.
    D. Fred is hypoxic and needs a tracheostomy.

25. **Treatment for a thyrotoxic crisis includes:**
    A. Administration of PTH and symptomatic care
    B. Symptomatic care and wait for symptoms to subside
    C. Synthroid administration and supportive care
    D. No need for treatment; the crisis will resolve spontaneously.

26. **Which feature is unique to the pancreas?**
    A. There are no unique features of the pancreas.
    B. It is both an endocrine and an exocrine gland.
    C. It is the largest gland in the body.
    D. The location and size of the pancreas make it unique.

27. **Where are the parathyroid glands located?**
    A. Anterior to the thyroid gland
    B. Posterior to the thyroid gland
    C. On top of the thyroid gland
    D. Below the thyroid gland

28. **Your patient's calcium level is 11.7 mg/dL. This indicates which problem?**
    A. Hypoparathyroidism
    B. Excessive calcium intake
    C. Hyperparathyroidism
    D. Recent fracture of a long bone

29. **When would you expect to see hypoparathyroidism?**
    A. With trauma
    B. With hypercalcemia
    C. With hypophosphotemia
    D. After thyroid or neck surgery

30. **Where is the pancreas located?**
    A. Right lower quadrant of the abdomen
    B. Right upper quadrant of the abdomen
    C. Left upper quadrant of the abdomen
    D. Left lower quadrant of the abdomen

31. **What is the purpose of testing $HgbA_{1c}$ in diabetes mellitus?**
    A. It is of little help in managing diabetes mellitus.
    B. It measures blood sugars over a 6-month period.
    C. It measures the effectiveness of diabetes mellitus.
    D. It measures red blood cell activity in diabetes mellitus.

32. **Sally is a 24-year-old college student in the intensive care unit for new onset of diabetic ketoacidosis. You are teaching her about diabetes mellitus and $HgbA_{1c}$. Which of the following $HgbA_{1c}$ levels should be Sally's goal for good control of her diabetes mellitus?**
    A. 7–8%
    B. 4–5%
    C. 8–9%
    D. 6–7%

33. **Why are hyperglycemia and hyperlipidemia seen concurrently in diabetes mellitus?**
    A. Very-low-density lipoprotein (VLDL) production increases in response to increased insulin production.
    B. Insulin resistance promotes VLDL production.
    C. Lipid breakdown is hindered by hyperinsulinemia.
    D. Glucose increases cause the liver to increase lipid production.

34. **Which of the following are risk factors in the development of diabetes mellitus?**
    A. Obesity (BMI of 42), blood pressure 160/95, HDL 28, brother with diabetes mellitus
    B. Obesity (BMI of 27), blood pressure 120/70, HDL 42, no family history of diabetes mellitus
    C. Obesity (BMI of 26), Caucasian ancestry, blood pressure 190/100, family history of diabetes mellitus
    D. Obesity (BMI of 40), blood pressure 100/50, HDL 50, no family history of diabetes mellitus

35. **Which hormones are secreted by the Islets of Langerhans?**
    A. Insulin and amylase
    B. Glucagon and amylase
    C. Glucagon and insulin
    D. Insulin and lipase

36. **How is insulin secretion regulated?**
    A. Hormonal, insulin, and neuronal controls
    B. Chemical, hormonal, and neuronal controls
    C. Chemical, glucagon, and insulin controls
    D. Hormonal, exocrine gland secretion, and glucose controls

37. **What is the role of glucophage in the body?**
    A. It acts on the liver to decrease blood sugar.
    B. It acts on the liver to increase blood sugar.
    C. It acts on the pancreas to decrease blood sugar.
    D. It acts on the pancreas to increase blood sugar.

38. **John, a patient with Type I diabetes, asks you why he is so thirsty when his blood sugars rise. What do you tell him?**
    A. Polydipsia is increased urine output caused by high blood sugars.
    B. Polyphagia is seen with increased glucose secondary to extracellular dehydration.
    C. Polydispia is seen with increased glucose because of intracellular dehydration.
    D. Polyphagia in seen with increased appetite that leads to excess thirst.

39. **What level of beta-cell function must be lost before hyperglycemia occurs?**
    A. 60–70%
    B. 25–45%
    C. 50–60%
    D. 80–90%

40. **What is non-alcohol steatohepatitis (NASH)?**
    A. Fatty liver infiltrates seen as a precursor to diabetes mellitus Type II
    B. Fatty liver from Hepatitis B infection
    C. Fatty liver from poor diet
    D. Fatty liver from obesity and excess consumption of dietary fats

41. **Jon, a 41-year-old Type II diabetic, is admitted to the intensive care unit for ACS (acute coronary syndrome). He is NPO for angiography. He calls you, stating that he feels funny. You find him pale, diaphoretic, anxious, and restless. What is your next step?**

A. Check vital signs and temperature

B. Check vital signs, repeat cardiac enzymes, STAT EKG

C. Check vital signs and blood sugar

D. Check vital signs and pulse oximetry reading

42. **Continuing the scenario from Question 41, Jon's blood sugar is 37. What is your next action?**

    A. Do nothing—the intravenous fluid will correct the blood sugar

    B. Notify the physician and give Jon a glass of orange juice with three packets of sugar

    C. Notify the physician and increase the intravenous fluids

    D. Give one ampule of D_{50} intravenously per your hospital protocol and notify the physician

43. **When is gastroparesis seen?**

    A. With alcohol abuse

    B. In long-term diabetes mellitus, either type

    C. With acute pancreatitis

    D. With acute cholecystitis

44. **What are the three major problems associated with macrovascular disease in conjunction with diabetes mellitus?**

    A. Retinopathy, coronary artery disease, cerebrovascular accident

    B. Peripheral neuropathy, coronary artery disease, cerebrovascular accident

    C. Coronary artery disease, cerebrovascular accident, peripheral vascular disease

    D. Diabetic peripheral neuropathy, peripheral vascular disease, cerebrovascular accident

45. **What is the pathophysiology of microvascular disease in diabetes mellitus?**

    A. Increased atherosclerotic plaques on the intima

    B. Changes in the capillary basement membrane causing hypoxia on the cellular level

    C. Vasoconstriction from hyperglycemia

    D. Repeated hypoglycemic events

46. **What is the first sign of renal damage in a patient with diabetes mellitus?**

    A. Proteinuria

    B. Elevated blood urea nitrogen and creatinine levels

    C. Oliguria

    D. Hematuria

47. **Where is renin stored?**

    A. Renal tubule

    B. Loop of Henle

    C. Juxtoglomerular cells of the nephron

    D. Adrenal cortex

48. **Which of the following factors can trigger the renin-angiotensin mechanism?**

    A. Aldosterone, diuretics

    B. Diuretics, decreased renal blood flow

    C. Diuretics, adrenergic blockers

    D. Increased renal blood flow, diuretics

49. What is the correct order of the renin–angiotensin mechanism when there is a decrease in blood flow to the kidneys?
    A. Renin, ACTH, angiotensin I
    B. Increased ADH, renin, angiotensin I, angiotensin II
    C. Renin, angiotensinogen, angiotensin I, angiotensin I converting enzyme, angiotensin II, aldosterone
    D. Renin, aldosterone, angiotensin I, angiotensin I converting enzyme, angiotensin II

50. Where are the catecholamines produced?
    A. Liver
    B. Kidneys
    C. Adrenal cortex
    D. Adrenal medulla

51. Frank is admitted to the intensive care unit for diabetic ketoacidosis. As his nurse, you know his insulin drip will be titrated by sliding scale and his anion gap. What does the anion gap measure?
    A. Estimate of cations and anions
    B. An estimate of unmeasured anions
    C. An estimate of anions in the blood
    D. Estimate of the correction of the acid–base balance

52. Continuing with the scenario from Question 51, Frank has arterial blood gases drawn. Which of the following sets of findings would you expect to see with diabetic ketoacidosis?
    A. pH 7.55; CO_2 22 mm Hg; HCO_3 26 mEq/L
    B. pH 7.36; CO_2 54 mm Hg; HCO_3 33 mEq/L
    C. pH 7.15; CO_2 24 mm Hg; HCO_3 12 mEq/L
    D. pH 7.40; CO_2 41 mm Hg; HCO_3 25 mEq/L

53. Your patient with diabetic ketoacidosis is slowly improving. What do the following arterial blood gases represent for this patient: pH 7.32; CO_2 50 mm Hg; HCO_3 20 mEq/L?
    A. Fully compensated respiratory acidosis
    B. Fully compensated metabolic alkalosis
    C. Partially compensated metabolic acidosis
    D. Partially compensated respiratory acidosis

54. The HCO_3 level for your patient with diabetic ketoacidosis is 10 mEq/L. In addition to the insulin drip, you should anticipate which of following?
    A. Sodium bicarbonate drip with frequent HCO_3 levels
    B. Sodium bicarbonate bolus and repeat every 4–6 hours
    C. Increase the insulin drip to hasten the resolution of the metabolic acidosis
    D. Decrease the insulin drip as the acidosis is resolving

55. David is a 60-year-old male admitted to the intensive care unit for an acute myocardial infarction. He has a schizoaffective disorder for which he has taken lithium for 15 years. You note he has a very high urine output—approximately 800 cc/hour and a SpG of 1.001. What is wrong?

A. He is experiencing the diuretic effect of a low-sodium diet.

B. He has diabetes insipidus from long-term lithium use.

C. Excessive oral fluid intake

D. Neurogenic diabetes insipidus

56. **Mrs. R. is admitted to the intensive care unit with myxedema coma. She is receiving intravenous thyroid replacement therapy when she suddenly develops hypotension, hypoglycemia, nausea, and vomiting. What has happened?**

A. The patient is having an allergic response to the thyroid medication.

B. The patient needs an increased dose of thyroid medication.

C. The patient needs a lower dose of thyroid medication.

D. The patient is experiencing Addisonian crisis.

57. **Genevieve has end-stage renal disease (ESRD) stage IV and is on hemodialysis every Monday, Wednesday, and Friday. Her calcium level is 6.3 mg/dL and her PTH is 70 pg/mL. What is happening to this patient?**

A. Hypoparathyroidism

B. Secondary hypoparathyroidism

C. Secondary hyperthyroidism

D. Hypothyroidism

58. **The anterior pituitary gland controls which of the following glands?**

A. Parathyroid, adrenal medulla, gonads

B. Thyroid, adrenal medulla, gonads

C. Parathyroid, thyroid, gonads

D. Thyroid, adrenal cortex, gonads

59. **What is the function of ADH (antidiuretic hormone)?**

A. Water balance

B. Sodium balance

C. Aldosterone production

D. Potassium balance

60. **What condition would possibly inhibit antidiuretic hormone (ADH) production?**

A. Pituitary tumor

B. Water intoxication

C. Increased serum osmolality

D. Increased potassium level

61. **What symptoms are seen with diabetes insipidus?**

A. Low urine output, hypertension, bradycardia

B. Excessive urine output, hypertension, tachycardia

C. Excessive urine output, hypotension, tachycardia

D. Low urine output, hypotension, tachycardia

62. **Why is diabetes insipidus (DI) common in patients with basilar skull fractures?**

A. Cerebral edema

B. Hematomas, especially epidural hematomas

C. DI is not common in basilar skull fractures.

D. Damage to the sella turcica and, therefore, to the pituitary gland

63. **What is the most common presentation of a patient with syndrome of inappropriate antidiuretic hormone (SIADH)?**
    A. Excessive, dilute urine output
    B. Hypotension
    C. Seizures
    D. Tetany

64. **Hank has been diagnosed with diabetes insipidus. Which of the following sets of lab results could be seen with this condition?**
    A. Serum osmolality 275, sodium 137, urine specific gravity 1.020
    B. Serum osmolality 315, sodium 165, urine specific gravity 1.003
    C. Serum osmolality 283, sodium 119, urine specific gravity 1.015
    D. Serum osmolality 265, sodium 150, urine specific gravity 1.001

65. **Which of the following factors is responsible for the symptoms of hypothyroidism?**
    A. Low levels of T_4 (thyroxine)
    B. Low levels of T_3 (thriothyroxine)
    C. Decreased thyrocalcitonin
    D. Increased thyrocalcitonin

66. **What must be present for calcium to be utilized by the body?**
    A. Increased oral calcium
    B. Increased phosphorus
    C. Euthyroid state
    D. Adequate vitamin D levels

67. **Trousseau's sign is seen with which condition?**
    A. Increased serum calcium
    B. Decreased serum calcium
    C. Decreased serum phosphorus
    D. Hypothyroidism

68. **Which of the following signs may be seen with hypocalcemia?**
    A. Short QT interval
    B. Hyperparathyroidism
    C. Chvostek's sign
    D. Cullen's sign

69. **Which glands regulate thyroid function?**
    A. Posterior pituitary and hypothalamus
    B. Anterior pituitary and thalamus
    C. Anterior pituitary and hypothalamus
    D. Posterior pituitary and thalamus

70. **Which of the following can cause a thyroid storm in a patient with hyperthyroidism?**
    A. Overdose of PTU (propylthyrouricil)
    B. Increased iodine intake
    C. Trauma or infection
    D. Decreased iodine intake

71. **What symptoms are to be expected with thyrotoxic crisis?**
    A. Hypotension, bradycardia
    B. Hyperthermia, bradycardia
    C. Flushing, hypoventilation
    D. Hypertension, hyperthermia

72. **Your patient is in thyrotoxic crisis. Which medication would you give to reduce symptoms?**
    A. Propranolol
    B. Levophed
    C. Adenosine
    D. Digoxin

73. **George is admitted to the intensive care unit in hypertensive crisis. You notice large fluctuations in his blood pressure even though you have not changed his nitroprusside drip. The physician orders a plasma catecholamine level. His fractional epinephrine level is very high. What does this finding indicate?**
    A. Cocaine use
    B. Pheochromocytoma
    C. Adrenal cortex tumor
    D. Hyperthyroidism

74. **Continuing with the scenario from Question 73, part of your patient education for George includes dietary restrictions. Which of the following foods should he avoid?**
    A. Cream cheese
    B. Red meat
    C. Aged cheddar cheese
    D. Chocolate

75. **What is the treatment of choice once a diagnosis of pheochromocytoma is made?**
    A. Diet changes
    B. Antihypertensive medications
    C. Surgical removal of the tumor
    D. Diuretics

This concludes the Endocrine questions.

ANSWERS

1. **Correct Answer: C**
   The most important issue is to increase the blood sugar and notify the physician. Orange juice and sugar should not be given to a new post-op patient. Her gastric bypass and NPO status increase her risk for hypoglycemia. Other causes of acute hypoglycemia include alcohol abuse, insulinoma, medications, and adrenal insufficiency.

2. **Correct Answer: B**
   Lack of food or if the liver is unable to provide glucogenesis cause a drop in blood glucose to less than 50 mg/dL. The other answers are risk factors for hypoglycemia.

3. **Correct Answer: B**
   D_{50}, oral glucose, and treating the cause are the most effective ways to treat acute hypoglycemia. The other answers include increased carbohydrate consumption, which would be prohibited with this condition. The optimal diet would consist of small frequent meals and reduced carbohydrates.

4. **Correct Answer: D**
   DKA is seen with illness or injury such as infection, surgery, trauma, or UTI. DKA is defined as a fasting blood sugar greater than 250 mg/dL to approximately 1,000 mg/dL.

5. **Correct Answer: B**
   Polyuria, polydipsia, and polyphagia are known as the "three P's." The fruity breath results from ketone production when fatty acids are broken down. Dehydration is due to the osmotic diuresis. Fatigue is due to potassium shifting from inside the cells to the intravascular space.

6. **Correct Answer: B**
   Once the blood glucose is less than 300 mg/dL, D_5NS should be added to slow the drop in glucose. Hourly blood glucose levels should be continued. The anion gap should slowly be lowered to less than 20.

7. **Correct Answer: B**
   DKA is more common in insulin-dependent diabetics especially those with an illness or infection such as cellulitis. However, 20–30% of DKA patients have no identified precipitating factors. A patient with well-controlled diabetes is at low risk for DKA. Patients with Type II diabetes are more likely to develop HHNS.

8. **Correct Answer: D**
   Potassium is pulled from the intracellular space due to metabolic acidosis. The insulin drip will help correct the metabolic acidosis, allowing the potassium to return to normal levels.

9. **Correct Answer: C**
   Kayexalate permanently exchanges 1 gram of medication for 1 mEq of potassium. Other therapies include IV insulin, D_{50}, and sodium bicarbonate. These latter therapies allow quick, effective, short-term correction of the potassium level. Hemodialysis and Kayexalate are the only 2 methods that permanently remove excess potassium.

10. **Correct Answer: C**
    Crush injuries cause a massive release of potassium into the bloodstream. There is approximately 135–145 mEq of potassium in each cell.

11. **Correct Answer: B**
Hyperkalemia slows conduction, leading to a widened QRS, peaked T waves, and loss of P waves. If the condition becomes severe, the patient can develop asystole.

12. **Correct Answer: C**
HHNS develops slowly in Type II diabetes, most often in elderly patients or those with undiagnosed diabetes mellitus. The blood sugars are generally more than 600 mg/dL and can exceed 1,500 mg/dL. The other differentiation between HHNS and DKA is the lack of ketones observed with HHNS.

13. **Correct Answer: B**
Blood sugars over 600 mg/dL with negative serum ketones and a serum osmolality greater than 310 mOsm/L are typical of HHNS. The pH is usually greater than 7.3; the BUN (blood urea nitrogen) may be elevated as well. Osmolality is the best predictor of survivability, rather than the blood sugar levels.

14. **Correct Answer: C**
Normal saline should be given in large volumes until the depletion is corrected; D_5NS may then be administered once blood glucose is in the 250–300 mg/dL range. An insulin drip would be established at approximately 15 units per hour with hourly glucose monitoring. Frequent electrolyte monitoring would also be done. If the patient was given D_5 ½NS too early in the course of treatment, it could lead to cerebral edema.

15. **Correct Answer: C**
The Somoygi effect is nocturnal hypoglycemia with rebound hyperglycemia. It is more common in Type 1 diabetics, especially children. The dawn phenomenon consists of morning hyperglycemia without nocturnal hypoglycemia caused by growth hormone secretion in the early morning hours.

16. **Correct Answer: A**
Cushing syndrome is usually seen with Cushing disease. It is important to rule out tumors of the pituitary gland, chest (small-cell cancer of the lung), and adrenal tumors, as well as pheochromcytomas. These tumors cause excessive ACTH production, leading to the physical changes seen with Cushing syndrome (e.g., moon facies, buffalo hump, truncal obesity, and purple striae on the abdomen).

17. **Correct Answer: C**
Numerous physical changes occur with Cushing syndrome or Cushing disease, including thinning hair, acne, moon facies, increased body hair, buffalo hump on the upper back, purple striae on the trunk, truncal obesity with thin extremities, and easy bruising.

18. **Correct Answer: D**
The hypothalamic–pituitary axis releases a number of hormones that inhibit or release several other hormones that affect body functions.

19. **Correct Answer: A**
The pituitary gland is inferior to the hypothalamus and sits in the sella turcica of the sphenoid bone. The other locations are incorrect. The correct order is the thalamus, hypothalamus, infidibulum, and pituitary gland.

20. **Correct Answer: C**
The anterior pituitary gland produces numerous hormones, including TSH, LH, FSH, ACTH, and melanocyte-stimulating hormone. Substance P is a hormone released by

the hypothalamus. Vasopressin and oxytocin are hormones released by the posterior pituitary gland.

21. **Correct Answer: D**
This lab value indicates hyperthyroidism or thyrotoxicosis. Causes may include goiter, Graves disease, thyroid carcinoma, and TSH-secreting pituitary adenoma. Hyperthyroidism without toxicosis is most often related to excessive intake of thyroid hormones.

22. **Correct Answer: B**
The thyroid gland is located below the larynx on either side of the trachea.

23. **Correct Answer: B**
Thyroid medications should be taken on an empty stomach 30 minutes before breakfast. Other teaching points include the need for regular follow-up labs for TSH and T_4 and the symptoms of myxedema and hyperthyroidism. Taking thyroid medication in the evening can lead to insomnia.

24. **Correct Answer: C**
Thyrotoxic crisis is a rare but serious problem in post-thyroidectomy patients, undertreated hyperthyroidism, cardiopulmonary disease, and hemodialysis patients.

25. **Correct Answer: A**
Treatment of thyrotoxic crisis includes PTH to decrease thyroid-stimulating hormone and thyroid hormones plus symptomatic care.

26. **Correct Answer: B**
The pancreas is both an endocrine gland (it secretes glucagon and insulin) and an exocrine gland (it secretes amylase and lipase).

27. **Correct Answer: B**
The parathyroid glands are located posterior to the thyroid gland and may consist of 4 to 6 small glands. The parathyroid glands produce parathyroid hormone (PTH) that regulates serum calcium, magnesium, and phosphorus levels. PTH also stimulates the kidney to produce bioavailable vitamin D.

28. **Correct Answer: C**
Hyperparathyroidism can be either primary or secondary in nature. Primary hyperparathyroidism is the excess secretion of parathyroid hormone (PTH) and may be related to a breakdown of the feedback system to the glands or overgrowth of the gland. Secondary hyperparathyroidism is generally related to a chronic disorder such as chronic renal failure or a malabsorption state.

29. **Correct Answer: D**
Hypoparathyroidism is usually caused by damage to the parathyroid gland. This damage leads to increased phosphotemia and lowered calcium levels.

30. **Correct Answer: C**
The pancreas is located in the left upper quadrant of the abdomen and sits behind the stomach, near the spleen and duodenum.

31. **Correct Answer: C**
$HgbA_{1c}$ measures the effectiveness of diabetes mellitus therapy. Hemoglobin and glucose have an affinity for each other, joining together to form a glycolated hemoglobin molecule. The $HgbA_{1c}$ level rises and falls in direct correlation with blood sugars. The

American College of Endocrinologists recommends HgbA$_{1c}$ levels of less than 6.5%; the American Diabetes Association recommends HgbA$_{1c}$ levels of less than 7%. Patients with HgbA$_{1c}$ levels of less than 6% are considered nondiabetic.

32. **Correct Answer: D**
    An HgbA$_{1c}$ of 6 –7% will mean Sally's glucose was 100–150 mg/dL over a 3-month period. A range of 4–5% is normal, 7–8% and 8–9% (or more) are indicative of poorly controlled diabetes mellitus.

33. **Correct Answer: B**
    Insulin resistance predisposes the patient to elevated blood glucose and increased insulin production. Very-low-density lipoprotein (VLDL) production increases with hyperinsulinemia.

34. **Correct Answer: A**
    Risk factors for the development of diabetes mellitus include blood pressure greater than 140/90, a first-degree relative with diabetes mellitus, nonwhite ancestry; obesity (BMI greater than 30), and high-density lipoprotein (HDL) levels less than 35.

35. **Correct Answer: C**
    Beta cells of the Islets of Langerhans secrete glucagon and insulin. Amylase and lipase are enzymes that are produced by the exocrine pancreas, along with trypsin, chymotrypsin, and carboxypeptidase.

36. **Correct Answer: B**
    Insulin secretion is controlled by chemicals such as glucose and amino acids; hormones such as gastrointestinal hormones; prostaglandin; and neuronal responses such as sympathetic response to increased glucose.

37. **Correct Answer: B**
    Glucagon is produced by the alpha cells of the pancreas.

38. **Correct Answer: C**
    Polydipsia (excessive urinary output) is caused by the osmotic pressure in the body's attempt to correct hemoconcentration. This dehydration leads to stimulation of the thirst center by the hypothalamus.

39. **Correct Answer: D**
    Approximately 80–90% of the beta-cell function of the Islets of Langerhans is lost before hyperglycemia occurs.

40. **Correct Answer: A**
    Non-alcohol steatohepatitis (NASH) is observed as fatty liver infiltrates and is often seen with insulin resistance, obesity, and increased triglyceride levels. NASH may progress to cirrhosis if no lifestyle changes are made.

41. **Correct Answer: C**
    Jon is most likely experiencing a hypoglycemic event due to his NPO status. The other options are not wrong, but the question asks about a diabetic that is NPO.

42. **Correct Answer: D**
    The most important action is to raise Jon's blood sugar safely using intravenous administration of D$_{50}$. It would also be prudent to recheck his blood sugar in one

hour. The physician must be notified. To do nothing for a patient with hypoglycemia is negligence.

43. **Correct Answer: B**
    Gastroparesis is a visceral neuropathy that occurs with long-term or uncontrolled diabetes mellitus. The hallmark of this condition is decreased gastric motility. Other visceral neuropathies include cranial nerve pain, Bell's palsy, urinary retention, sexual dysfunction, decreased cardiac reflexes, orthostatic hypotension, and radiculopathies.

44. **Correct Answer: C**
    Coronary artery disease, cerebrovascular accident, and peripheral vascular disease are the 3 major problems associated with macrovascular disease and are seen in type 2 diabetes mellitus. Mortality or morbidity in these patients is due to macrovascular changes. Diabetes leads to early atherosclerosis and atherosclerotic heart disease. The other problems listed (retinopathy, peripheral neuropathy, and diabetic nephropathy) are microvascular diseases.

45. **Correct Answer: B**
    Prolonged hyperglycemia thickens the capillary basement membrane. This thickening leads to decreased blood flow, hypoxia, and a lack of nutrients at the cellular level. The eyes and kidneys are the organs most susceptible to this process.

46. **Correct Answer: A**
    Proteinuria is the first sign of renal dysfunction. It is a reliable symptom, especially when the proteinuria is prolonged. Continued proteinuria usually brings a life expectancy of less than 10 years. The exact pathophysiology is not fully understood, but glomerular destruction is known to allow proteins to leak into the filtrate.

47. **Correct Answer: C**
    Renin is stored in a crystalline form in the juxtoglomerular cells of the kidneys. When the kidneys perceive a decreased blood flow, the sympathetic response triggers the release of renin, which converts angiotensinogen to angiotensin I, a mild vasoconstrictor. If the problem is not resolved, the lungs release angiotensin I converting enzyme to create angiotensin II, a powerful vasoconstrictor. Angiotensin II triggers the release of aldosterone from the adrenal glands. The increased aldosterone production causes sodium and water retention, thereby increasing the blood pressure.

48. **Correct Answer: B**
    Anything that causes a perceived drop in renal blood flow triggers the renin–angiotensin mechanism. Renin release can also be triggered by sodium and volume depletion, such as that seen with diuretic use.

49. **Correct Answer: C**
    The kidneys perceive a drop in blood flow leading to the release of renin from the juxtoglomerular cells of the nephron. This stimulates the release of angiotensinogen, which in turn stimulates the release of angiotensin I. If the blood pressure is not corrected, the lungs release angiotensin I converting enzyme, which in turn causes the secretion of angiotensin II. Angiotensin II causes the release of aldosterone from the adrenal glands, increasing retention of sodium and water and leading to increased blood pressure.

50. **Correct Answer: D**
   The adrenal medulla produces 75–85% of the catecholamine epinephrine and 25% of norepinephrine from phenylalanine.

51. **Correct Answer: B**
   The anion gap measures anions not generally measured in routine lab tests. It is an estimate of the degree of lactic acidosis. The formula for figuring the anion gap is Na – (HCO_3 + Cl). The normal range is 10–20 mEq/L. With diabetic ketoacidosis, the anion gap is greater than 30 mEq/L.

52. **Correct Answer: C**
   These ABG findings demonstrate uncompensated metabolic acidosis. The body has depleted the HCO_3 trying to correct the acidosis. The ABG is uncompensated because the pH is low and the CO_2 is elevated. Answer A is acute respiratory alkalosis; answer B is respiratory acidosis with metabolic alkalosis; and answer D is a normal ABG. Normal values for ABGs are pH 7.35–7.45; CO_2 35–45 mm Hg; HCO_3 22–27 mEq/L.

53. **Correct Answer: C**
   With the pH near-normal (7.35–7.45), increased CO_2, and near-normal HCO_3 the body has tried to correct the acidosis. As the condition resolves, the ABGs should continue to improve.

54. **Correct Answer: A**
   A sodium bicarbonate drip should be anticipated to replace the diminished HCO_3. This will help resolve the metabolic acidosis. Boluses would be given only if the pH was very low. The insulin drip will not directly correct the abnormal HCO_3.

55. **Correct Answer: B**
   This patient has nephrogenic diabetes related to lithium use. The lithium causes insensitivity to vasopressin in the renal tubule, making the tubule incapable of absorbing water. Treatment involves administration of hydrochlorothiazide or indomethicin.

56. **Correct Answer: D**
   Subclinical adrenal insufficiency may coexist with myxedema. The treatment of choice is intravenous hydrocortisone therapy.

57. **Correct Answer: B**
   This patient has secondary hyperparathyroidism. In end-stage renal disease (ESRD), vitamin D synthesis is decreased thus causing hypocalcemia. The calcium is also bound to phosphorus, further reducing the calcium levels. This decrease stimulates the parathyroid glands to secrete parathyroid hormone in an attempt to correct the calcium levels.

58. **Correct Answer: D**
   The anterior pituitary or adenohypophysis controls the function of the thyroid gland with thyroid-stimulating hormone (TSH), the adrenal cortex with antidiuretic hormone (ADH), and the gonads with luteinizing hormone (LH) or interstitial cell-stimulating hormone (ICSH).

59. **Correct Answer: A**
   Antidiuretic hormone deals with thirst and water balance. It is produced by the posterior pituitary gland. When the plasma becomes concentrated or there is a reduced

blood volume, the posterior pituitary gland releases ADH, causing water retention and concentration of urine. ADH is regulated by a feedback mechanism in the pituitary gland.

60. **Correct Answer: A**
Antidiuretic hormone is controlled by a negative feedback system. Production is decreased when the osmoreceptors of the hypothalamus recognize hemodilution or hemoconcentration and adjust ADH production accordingly.

61. **Correct Answer: C**
Diabetes insipidus is caused by low ADH levels, and water absorption is greatly reduced. The hypotension and tachycardia are due to volume depletion.

62. **Correct Answer: D**
The pituitary gland sits in the sella turcica at the base of the skull and can be easily damaged with any head trauma. An anterior basilar skull fracture is the most common fracture leading to diabetes insipidus.

63. **Correct Answer: C**
Seizures are one of the most common presenting symptoms of syndrome of inappropriate antidiuretic hormone (SIADH). SIADH causes hemodilution and a relative decrease in serum sodium levels. Once the sodium falls below 120, the patient is a great risk for seizures. Excessive urine output and hypotension are symptoms of diabetes insipidus.

64. **Correct Answer: B**
The volume loss in diabetes insipidus occurs through hemoconcentration with excess fluid loss. The kidneys are unable to concentrate urine.

65. **Correct Answer: A**
The decreased T_4 leads to hypothyroid symptoms of cold, dry skin, hair loss, periorbital edema, and possible thyroid enlargement.

66. **Correct Answer: D**
Calcium cannot be utilized by the body without adequate vitamin D levels. Fifteen minutes of daylight on the skin without use of sunblock allows the body to create its own vitamin D. An increased phosphorus level would bind the calcium, making it unavailable.

67. **Correct Answer: B**
Trousseau's sign, known as carpal-pedal spasm, is seen with decreased calcium levels. Hypocalcemia can occur with end-stage renal disease (increased phosphorus) and decreased vitamin D levels. It is also seen in patients who receive 3 or more units of red blood cells that are treated with calcium citrate.

68. **Correct Answer: C**
Chvostek's sign is seen with hypocalcemia; it is elicited by tapping the cheek over the zygomatic arch and causes facial twitching. The QT interval would be prolonged with hypocalcemia. Cullen's sign is ecchymosis around the umbilicus and is often seen the pancreatitis.

69. **Correct Answer: C**
The anterior pituitary gland secretes thyroid-stimulating hormone (TSH), and the hypothalamus regulates the anterior pituitary gland with thyrotropin-releasing hormone (TRH).

70. **Correct Answer: C**

    Injury or infection as well as manipulation of the thyroid gland can trigger a thyroid storm and thyrotoxicosis.

71. **Correct Answer: D**

    Thyrotoxic crisis symptoms include hypertension, hyperthermia, flushing, tachycardia (especially atrial tachyarrhythmia), high-output heart failure, nausea and vomiting, psychosis, and delirium. Treatment includes supportive care and medications to block catecholamine effects.

72. **Correct Answer: A**

    Propranolol (Inderal) would be used for this patient. It is a beta blocker and would decrease the effects of the sympathetic stimulation of thyrotoxic crisis. It controls heart rate, hypertension, and oxygen consumption.

73. **Correct Answer: B**

    A pheochromocytoma is a tumor of the adrenal medulla. These tumors are rarely malignant, but they do cause release of large amounts of catecholamines such as dopamine, epinephrine, and norepinephrine. Hypertension with pheochromocytoma can be triggered by foods such as cheese, alcohol, yogurt, and caffeine.

74. **Correct Answer: C**

    Hypertension with pheochromocytoma can be triggered by foods such as cheese, alcohol, yogurt, and caffeine. It is important to give the patient a list of foods to avoid. Crises often occur after life events where these foods might be consumed.

75. **Correct Answer: C**

    The best option for treating pheochromocytoma is surgical removal of the tumor. Alpha-adrenergic blockers or beta-adrenergic blockers may be used to treat hypertension until surgery can be performed.

BIBLIOGRAPHY

Ahrens, T. (2006). *Critical care nursing certification*. Columbus, OH: McGraw-Hill.

American Association of Critical Care Nurses. (2006). *Core curriculum for critical care nursing* (6th ed.). Philadelphia: Saunders.

American Association of Critical Care Nurses. (2007). *AACN certification and core review for high acuity and critical care* (6th ed.). Philadelphia: Saunders.

American Heart Association. (2007). *Guidelines 2005 for cardiopulmonary resuscitation and emergency cardiovascular care*. Retrieved July 21, 2008, from http://circ.ahajournals.org/content/vol112/24_suppl

Boyle, P. J. (2007). Diabetes mellitus and macrovascular disease: Mechanisms and mediators. *American Journal of Medicine: Optimizing Cardiovascular Outcomes in Diabetes Mellitus, 120*(9B), S12.

Brimioulle, S., Orellana-Jimenez, C., Aminian, A., & Vincent, J. L. (2008). Hyponatremia in neurological patients: Cerebral salt wasting versus inappropriate antidiuretic hormone secretion. *Intensive Care Medicine, 34*(1), 125–131.

Burns, S. M. (Ed.). (2007). *American Association of Critical-Care Nurses (AACN): AACN Protocols for practice: Healing environments* (2nd ed.). Sudbury, MA: Jones and Bartlett.

Conover, M. B. (2003). *Understanding electrocardiography* (8th ed.). St. Louis, MO: Mosby/Elsevier.

Copstead, L., & Banasik, J. L. (2000). *Pathophysiology: Biological and behavioral perspectives* (2nd ed.). Philadelphia: Saunders/Elsevier.

Curley, M. A. Q. (1998). Patient–nurse synergy: Optimizing patients' outcomes. *American Journal of Critical Care, 7,* 64–72.

Dossey, B. M., Keegan, L., & Guzzetta, C. (2003). *Holistic nursing: A handbook for practice* (3rd ed.). Sudbury, MA: Jones and Bartlett.

Dunn, J. P., & Jagasia, S. M. (2007). Case study: Management of type 2 diabetes after bariatric surgery. *Clinical Diabetes, 25*(3), 112–114.

Edwards, D. F. (1999). The Synergy Model: Linking patient needs to nurse competencies. *Critical Care Nurse, 19*(1), 88–98.

Eldin, W. S., Ragheb, A., Klassen, J., & Shoker, A. (2008). Evidence for increased risk of prediabetes in the uremic patient. *Nephron, 108*(1), c47–c55.

Emergency Nurses Association & Newberry, L. (2003). *Sheehy's emergency nursing: Principles and practice* (5th ed.). St. Louis, MO: Mosby/Elsevier.

Feldman, B. J., Rosenthal, S. M., Vargas, G. A., & Gitelman, S. E. (2005). Nephrogenic syndrome of inappropriate antidiuresis (NSIAD): A paradigm for activating mutations causing endocrine dysfunction. *New England Journal of Medicine, 352*(18), 1884–1890.

Finkelmeier, B. A. (2000). *Cardiothoracic surgical nursing* (2nd ed.). Philadelphia: Lippincott Williams & Wilkins.

Gaines, K. K. (2004). Desmopressin (DDAVP(r)) for enuresis, diabetes insipidus. *Urologic Nursing, 24*(6), 520–523.

Gale, S. C., Sicoutris, C., Reilly, P. M., Schwab, C. W., & Gracias, V. H. (2007). Poor glycemic control is associated with increased mortality in critically ill trauma patients. *American Surgeon, 73*(5), 454–460.

Hardin, S. R., & Kaplow, R. (Eds.). (2004). *Synergy for clinical excellence: The AACN Synergy Model for patient care*. Sudbury, MA: Jones and Bartlett.

Haskal, R. (2007). Current issues for nurse practitioners: Hyponatremia. *Journal of the American Academy of Nurse Practitioners, 19*(11), 563–579.

Hickey, J. V. (2002). *The clinical practice of neurological and neurosurgical nursing* (5th ed.). Philadelphia: Lippincott Williams & Wilkins.

Inoue, T., & Node, K. (2007). Statin therapy for vascular failure. *Cardiovascular Drugs and Therapy, 21*(4), 281–295.

Jane, J. A., Edward, M. L., & Laws, R. (2006). Neurogenic diabetes insipidus. *Pituitary, 9*(4), 327–329.

Johnson, A. L., & Criddle, L. M. (2004). Pass the salt: Indications for and implications of using hypertonic saline. *Critical Care Nurse, 24*(5), 36–38, 40–44, 46 passim.

Lath, R. (2005). Hyponatremia in neurological diseases in ICU. *Indian Journal of Critical Care Medicine, 9*(1), 47–51.

Lipson, J. G., Dibble, S. L., & Minarik, P. A. (Eds.). (1996). *Culture and nursing care: A pocket guide.* San Francisco, CA: UCSF Nursing Press.

Livingstone, C., & Rampes, H. (2006). Lithium: A review of its metabolic adverse effects. *Journal of Psychopharmacology, 20*(3), 347–355.

McQuillan, K. A., Von Rueden, K. T., Hartsock, R. L., Flynn, M. B., & Whalen, E. (Eds.). (2002). *Trauma nursing: From resuscitation through rehabilitation* (3rd ed.). Philadelphia: Saunders/Elsevier.

Medina, J., & Puntillo, K. (2006). *AACN protocols for practice: Palliative care and end-of-life issues in critical care.* Sudbury, MA: Jones and Bartlett.

Musch, W., Hedeshi, A., & Decaux, G. (2004). Low sodium excretion in SIADH patients with low diuresis. *Nephron, 96*(1), 11–18.

Oksanen, T., Skrifvars, M. B., Varpula, T., Kuitunen, A., Pettilä, V., Nurmi, J., et al. (2007). Strict versus moderate glucose control after resuscitation from ventricular fibrillation. *Intensive Care Medicine, 33*(12), 2093–2100.

Pagana, K. D., & Pagana, J. (2005). *Mosby's manual of diagnostic and laboratory tests* (3rd ed.). St. Louis, MO: Mosby/Elsevier.

Paydas, S., Araz, F., & Balal, M. (2008). SIADH induced by amiodarone in a patient with heart failure. *International Journal of Clinical Practice, 62*(2), 337.

Sata, A., Hizuka, N., Kawamata, T., Hori, T., & Takano, K. (2006). Hyponatremia after transsphenoidal surgery for hypothalamo-pituitary tumors. *Neuroendocrinology, 83*(2), 117–122.

Skidmore-Roth, L. (2004). *Mosby's 2004 nursing drug reference.* St. Louis, MO: Mosby/Elsevier.

Smeltzer, S., & Bare, B. G. (2003). *Brunner and Suddarth's textbook of medical–surgical nursing* (10th ed.). Philadelphia: Lippincott Williams & Wilkins.

Sobel, B. E. (2007). Optimizing cardiovascular outcomes in diabetes mellitus. *American Journal of Medicine: Optimizing Cardiovascular Outcomes in Diabetes Mellitus, 120*(9B), S3.

Sole, M. L., Hartshorn, J., & Lamborne, M. L. (2001). *Introduction to critical care nursing* (3rd ed.). Philadelphia: Saunders/Elsevier.

Sommerfield, A. J., Wilkinson, I. B., Webb, D. J., & Frier, B. M. (2007). Vessel wall stiffness in type 1 diabetes and the central hemodynamic effects of acute hypoglycemia. *American Journal of Physiology: Endocrinology and Metabolism, 293*(5), E1274.

Su, H., Sun, X., Ma, H., et al. (2007). Acute hyperglycemia exacerbates myocardial ischemia/reperfusion injury and blunts cardioprotective effect of GIK. *American Journal of Physiology: Endocrinology and Metabolism, 293*(3), E629.

Sugimoto, A. K. (2007). No elevation of blood urea level in a dehydrated patient with central diabetes insipidus. *QJM, 100*(12), 800.

Thomas, G., Rojas, M. C., Epstein, S. K., Balk, E. M., Liangos, O., & Jaber, B. L. (2007). Insulin therapy and acute kidney injury in critically ill patients: A systematic review. *Nephrology, Dialysis, Transplantation, 22*(10), 2849–2855.

Toprak, O., Cirit, M., Ersoy, R., Uzüm, A., Ozümer, O., Çobanoğlu, A., et al. (2005). New-onset type II diabetes mellitus, hyperosmolar non-ketotic coma, rhabdomyolysis and acute renal failure in a patient treated with sulpiride. *Nephrology, Dialysis, Transplantation, 20*(3), 662–663.

Urden, L. D., Stacy, K. M., & Lough, M. E. (2007). *Thelan's critical care nursing: Diagnosis and management* (5th ed.). St. Louis, MO: Mosby.

Venkataraman, S., Munoz, R., Candido, C., & Feldman-Witchel, S. (2007). The hypothalamic–pituitary–adrenal axis in critical illness. *Reviews in Endocrine & Metabolic Disorders, 8*(4), 365–373.

Wiegand, D. J. L., & Carlson, K. K. (Eds.). (2005). *AACN procedure manual for critical care* (5th ed.). Philadelphia, PA: Elsevier.

Woods, S., Sivarajan Froelicher, E. S., & Motzer, S. U. (2000). *Cardiac nursing* (4th ed.). Philadelphia: Lippincott Williams & Wilkins.

Yeates, K. E., & Morton, A. R. (2006). Vasopressin antagonists: Role in the management of hyponatremia. *American Journal of Nephrology, 26*(4), 348–355.

Hematology/Immunology

QUESTIONS

1. You are working in the capacity of a charge nurse in the ICU. Your patient population is comprised of recent surgical patients and 2 patients waiting for lung transplants. As a critical care nurse, you are aware that the chain of infection includes which of the following components?
   A. Understaffing
   B. Having all transplant patients in strict isolation
   C. Use of non-alcohol-based hand washes
   D. Having bag-valve masks in each patient room

2. Cyclosporine has significant adverse effects which include:
   A. Hypotension
   B. Hepatotoxicity
   C. Acute pancreatitis
   D. Hypokalemia

3. An antirejection drug classified as antimetabolite would be:
   A. Cyclosporine
   B. Terralimus
   C. Prednisolone
   D. Imuran

4. Your patient was admitted for observation following placement of a coronary stent. You note that the patient received Reo Pro during the procedure. As a nurse, you know the patient must be monitored for
   A. Increased bleeding for 48 hours because Aggrastat is used with Reo Pro.
   B. Aggrastat toxicity.
   C. HITS, bleeding at sheath insertion site.
   D. Coagulopathies.

5. A patient can be presensitized and is more likely to undergo organ rejection if he or she has a history of
   A. Multiple pregnancies.
   B. Small or reduced lumens in the bile ducts.
   C. Destruction of small airways.
   D. Cytomegalovirus (CMV) infections.

6. Which of the following conditions is an absolute contraindication for a single-lung, double-lung, or heart–lung transplant?
   A. Previous cardiothoracic surgery
   B. Kidney disease
   C. Liver diseases
   D. Psychiatric illness

7. The most common cause of DIC is:
   A. Carcinomas
   B. Surgery
   C. Sepsis
   D. Vasculitis

8. Mrs. C was a direct admit to your unit from her physician's office following sudden epistaxis with severe headache. She is now obtunded. During your initial assessment, you note gingival bleeding, generalized ecchymosis, and petechial hemorrhages on both legs. You suspect Mrs. C. may have:
   A. DIC
   B. Pulmonary emboli
   C. A fat embolism
   D. ITP

9. Patients who undergo renal transplants often have electrolyte imbalances. Which of the following values would likely occur?
   A. Serum K^+: 6.9 mEq/L
   B. Sodium bicarbonate: 12 mEq/L
   C. Serum Na: 156 mEq/L
   D. Serum Ca: 7.3 mEq/L

10. Your heart transplant patient suddenly exhibits sinus bradycardia. You anticipate administration of:
    A. Atropine
    B. Digoxin
    C. Indocin
    D. Epinephrine

11. Factor VIII deficiency is also known as:
    A. Hemophilia B
    B. Sickle cell anemia
    C. Aplastic anemia
    D. Von Willebrand's disease

12. Your patient received platelet transfusions. It is important to closely monitor the patient and perform a 1- or 2-hour post-transfusion platelet count. You must carefully assess the patient for
    A. Hematuria.
    B. Fever.
    C. Petechiae.
    D. Ecchymosis.

13. **The blood component that contains factor VIII is:**
    A. FFP
    B. PRBCs
    C. Salt-poor albumin
    D. Cryoprecipitate

14. **A fluid that causes decreased platelet aggregation and possible allergic reactions is:**
    A. Dextran
    B. Hetastarch
    C. Lactated Ringer's
    D. D_5/Isolyte M

15. **Which of the following medications is specific for cryptococcal meningitis?**
    A. Amphotericin B
    B. Rifampin
    C. Famvir
    D. Acyclovir

16. **When patients receive multiple transfusions, they are susceptible to increased**
    A. Potassium levels.
    B. BUN and creatinine levels.
    C. Bilirubin and amylase levels.
    D. Sodium and magnesium levels.

17. **Adam was injured at work and has been fairly sedentary since his accident. He has now developed DVT and has been on a heparin drip for 3 days. Which lab value would indicate that Adam is maintaining a therapeutic level of heparin?**
    A. His Cullen's sign is negative.
    B. The platelet count has returned to 100,000 mm^3.
    C. Activated partial thromboplastin time of 45 seconds
    D. Resolution of oozing around IV insertion sites

18. **Your patient has been diagnosed with immune thrombocytopenic purpura (ITP). Which of the following laboratory values would be expected for this patient?**
    A. Elevated PT and PTT
    B. Capillary fragility test result of 0.5
    C. Platelet count of 11,000
    D. Positive anti-RH immunosuppression

19. **Your patient has been diagnosed with hemolytic anemia. She has been in the ICU for 3 days. You believe her condition was caused by**
    A. An inappropriate TPN solution.
    B. Reduced folate deficiency.
    C. Bone marrow aspiration.
    D. Intra-aortic balloon counterpulsation (IABP).

20. **A medication that may cause hemolytic anemia is**
    A. Phenobarbital.
    B. Quinidine.
    C. Furosemide.
    D. Captopril.

21. **As a critical care nurse, you know that Mrs. Z's abrupt-onset of DIC may be due to a previously undiagnosed cause. Some of these causes could include:**
    A. Viral infection
    B. Abdominal aneurysm and hepatic cirrhosis
    C. Influenza
    D. Trauma

22. **The blood component that carries factor VIII, factor XIII, and fibrinogen is:**
    A. FFP
    B. PRBC
    C. Salt-poor albumin
    D. Cryoprecipitate

23. **In the critical care setting, patients with DIC are at a high risk of developing**
    A. Deficiencies in vitamin K and folate.
    B. An increased fibrinogen level.
    C. A decreased D-dimer (less than 300).
    D. Dependency on heparin to maintain hemostasis.

24. **Possible causes of thrombocytopenia in critical care could be:**
    A. Portal hypertension
    B. MI
    C. Latex
    D. Low-protein diet

25. **Type II HIT patients are at great risk for developing**
    A. Generalized bleeding.
    B. Thrombosis.
    C. Pericarditis.
    D. Limb amputation.

26. **Nursing interventions by the critical care nurse should include which of the following actions to minimize risk to a patient with HIT?**
    A. Avoid the use of heparin flushes
    B. Assess the need for manual blood pressure measurements
    C. Monitor platelet counts
    D. Observe for petechiae

27. **What is the most common cause of a fatal transfusion reaction?**
    A. Immunocompromised recipient
    B. Mismatched blood
    C. Volume overload
    D. Severe hyperkalemia

28. Rejection of a transplanted organ usually occurs as a result of
    A. Cellular immunity.
    B. Humoral immunity.
    C. Delayed hypersensitivity reaction.
    D. Complement cascade.

29. Harry is a 34-year-old patient who was envenomated by a rattlesnake on the left forearm this afternoon while gardening. His entire left arm is ecchymotic. The best course of treatment would be:
    A. Clotting factors and antivenin
    B. Clotting factors and heparin
    C. IV at 150 ml/hour and antivenin
    D. IV at 150 ml/hour and heparin

30. Alec is a 26-year-old who was thrown from a horse onto a fence and suffered abdominal trauma with a splenic rupture. While awaiting surgery in the ICU, because the operating rooms were full, he received 12 units of PRBCs. As an ICU nurse, you know that Alec should also receive
    A. Potassium.
    B. Whole blood.
    C. Platelets.
    D. Heparin.

31. Organ rejection that occurs 3 to 5 days post transplant, is antibody mediated, with fever and oliguria is known as:
    A. A chronic rejection
    B. Acute rejection
    C. Accelerated acute rejection
    D. Hyperacute rejection

32. A snakebite will result in activation of the
    A. Fibrinolytic system.
    B. Antithrombin system.
    C. Intrinsic cascade.
    D. Extrinsic cascade.

33. Quincy had a renal transplant about 1 year ago. He was admitted to your unit for severe flu-like symptoms. Which sign or symptom would lead you to suspect that Quincy is having an acute rejection episode?
    A. Pelvic pain
    B. Hypotension
    C. Increased urine output
    D. Decreased urine osmolality

34. An antirejection agent that is used for induction therapy for lung transplants and lowers the number of circulating T cells is known as:
    A. Daclizumab
    B. Muromonab
    C. A polyclonal antibody
    D. Paroxetine

35. **Back pain or abdominal pain with itching can be indicators of acute rejection in which organ?**
    A. Pancreas
    B. Lung
    C. Kidney
    D. Liver

36. **Following heart–lung transplants, Prostiglandin (PGE₁) is used to**
    A. Provide inotropic support.
    B. Augment the heart rate.
    C. Promote pulmonary vasodilation.
    D. Promote wound healing.

37. **Ben ingested shellfish and is having an anaphylactic reaction. He has received epinephrine via Epi-pen and intravenously. He is now intubated because he had severe airway obstruction due to swelling. Epinephrine is given in anaphylaxis because:**
    A. Epinephrine will prevent localized edema.
    B. Epinephrine promotes temporary changes in ST segments.
    C. Epinephrine prevents third space fluid loss.
    D. Epinephrine promotes bronchodilation and inhibits additional mediator release.

38. **Why is DIC usually fatal if untreated?**
    A. Exsanguination
    B. Intracranial hemorrhage
    C. Myocardial infarction
    D. Cerebral thrombosis

39. **Oat cell carcinomas are primarily found in**
    A. Central airways.
    B. Genital area.
    C. Bronchial wall.
    D. The pancreas.

40. **Hemoglobin is phagocytized primarily in the**
    A. Liver.
    B. Spleen.
    C. Kidneys.
    D. Lungs.

41. **Acute posthemorrhagic anemia develops after**
    A. Rapid loss of erythrocytes.
    B. The spleen is damaged.
    C. Iron levels decrease by more than 15%.
    D. Bone marrow is damaged.

42. **The most prevalent type of anemia is:**
    A. Chronic
    B. Acute
    C. Pernicious
    D. Iron-deficiency

43. **Patient teaching for a patient with Thalassemia would include:**
    A. Keep limbs flat to avoid a stasis ulcer.
    B. Avoid oral stimulants (i.e., smoking).
    C. Eat fewer, larger high-protein meals.
    D. Use warm water to cleanse the skin.

44. **A decrease in the available number of erythrocytes caused by bone marrow production failure is:**
    A. Chronic anemia
    B. Aplastic anemia
    C. Hemolytic anemia
    D. Pernicious anemia

45. **High blood viscosity and low oxygen tension are the cause of which of the following types of anemia?**
    A. Pernicious
    B. Aplastic
    C. Sickle cell
    D. Hemolytic

46. **Your patient was admitted for low H and H, epistaxis, and bleeding into the diaphragm. She is bleeding from the gums, even with only the lightest stimulus. Petechiae are noted on her chest and arms. Her platelet count is less than 100,000. Her probable diagnosis is:**
    A. Aplastic anemia
    B. ITP
    C. Hemolytic anemia
    D. Pernicious anemia

47. **How does low-molecular-weight heparin (LMWH) differ from unfractionated heparin?**
    A. LMWH is more difficult to administer than unfractionated heparin.
    B. There are more side effects with LMWH than with unfractionated heparin.
    C. LMWH is more stable than unfractionated heparin.
    D. Unfractionated heparin is easier to administer than LMWH.

48. **Clopidogrel may interfere with the metabolism of which of the following drugs?**
    A. Phenobarbitol
    B. Phenytoin
    C. Cimetidine
    D. Estrogen

49. **Ethacrynic acid works on the body by**
    A. Inhibiting the aldosterone mechanism.
    B. Blocking carbonic anhydrase.
    C. Increasing osmotic pressure.
    D. Inhibiting reabsorption of Na and Cl.

50. Diuretics that are classified as carbonic anhydrase inhibitors would be:
    A. Methazolamide
    B. Mannitol
    C. Urea
    D. Metolazone

51. Which of the following is a potential complication of loop diuretics?
    A. Hypercalcemia
    B. Increase in BUN
    C. Hypokalemia
    D. Hypertension

52. Mannitol would be classified as which type of diuretic?
    A. Loop
    B. Thiazide
    C. Osmotic
    D. Potassium-sparing

53. Which of the following is an effect of Nesiritide?
    A. Vasoconstriction
    B. Decreased wedge pressure
    C. Anemia
    D. Decrease cardiac output

54. Which of the following is an adverse effect of Epogen?
    A. Hypertension
    B. Increased iron
    C. Decreased thrombosis
    D. Decreased BUN

55. Your renal patient needs to have a radiologic procedure that requires contrast dye. He has no allergies. Which of the following medications administered prior to the test would be effective on this patient?
    A. Bicarbonate
    B. NSAIDs
    C. BNP
    D. Mucomyst

56. Which of the following is a normal value for intracellular potassium (K^+)?
    A. 4.5 mEq/L
    B. 140 mEq/L
    C. 45 mEq/L
    D. 104 mEq/L

57. A normal value for bicarbonate (HCO_3) in the intravascular space would be:
    A. 11 mEq/L
    B. 45 mEq/L
    C. 24 mEq/L
    D. 80 mEq/L

58. Which hormone would be released if your patient's CVP suddenly rose from 6 to 17?
    A. BNP
    B. Aldosterone
    C. ANP
    D. ADH

59. Which of the following solutions would be used to expand the intravascular volume?
    A. Hypertonic saline
    B. D_5W
    C. 0.45 NS
    D. 0.9% NS

60. If your patient has a decreased extracellular fluid volume, which of the following hemodynamic profiles would be indicative of this condition?
    A. Decreased CO, CVP, decreased SVR
    B. Increased CVP, CO, PAP, decreased SVR
    C. Decreased SVR, MAP, CVP, increased CO
    D. Decreased CVP, PAP, MAP, CO, increased SVR

61. Sam was aggressively treated with 0.3% hypertonic saline for profound hyponatremia. Now, Sam is having tremors, LOC changes, and paresthesias. Sam is probably developing
    A. ICU psychosis.
    B. Hyponatremia veridans.
    C. Osmotic demyelinization syndrome.
    D. Red cell sequestration.

62. George is a 17-year-old who has not been eating correctly for about 2 weeks because he is stressed out about asking a girl to the prom. He eats a diet of cereals, pastas, and high-caloric, high-sugar foods. Today, George collapsed at work after becoming dyspneic. His EKG shows sinus tachycardia without ectopy, he is pale, somewhat irritable, and complains of a headache. His initial diagnosis is folic acid deficiency. Tomorrow George is scheduled for more tests to determine if there is an underlying disease process. You suspect that he simply has a dietary deficiency and prepare to instruct him about foods that contain high amounts of folic acid. These foods would include:
    A. Green beans
    B. Fish
    C. Oranges
    D. Peanut butter

63. Which of the following cell types would be considered a non-granular leukocyte?
    A. Eosinophil
    B. Neutrophil
    C. Basophil
    D. Monocyte

64. Cellular humoral immunity is mediated by
    A. T lymphocytes.
    B. Eosinophils.
    C. B lymphocytes.
    D. Killer cells.

65. All of the clotting factors in blood are synthesized in the liver *except*
    A. VIII and XIII.
    B. V and IX.
    C. IX and III.
    D. IIa and IXa.

66. Which of the following drugs is useful in the treatment of DIC to inhibit fibrinolysis?
    A. Heparin
    B. Cryoprecipitate
    C. Amicar
    D. Prednisone

67. Teresa is 40 years old and has a history of hemolytic anemia. She was admitted today for chest pain, fever, and heart failure. These symptoms would indicate Teresa is probably suffering from
    A. A myocardial infarction.
    B. Pulmonary edema.
    C. DIC.
    D. Hemolytic crisis.

68. Immune mediated HITT usually begins about _____ after the initiation of heparin therapy.
    A. 48 hours
    B. 72 hours
    C. 4 days
    D. 5–7 days

69. The diagnosis of immune thrombocytopenic purpura may be made by:
    A. Thrombin time
    B. Platelet antibody screen
    C. PTT
    D. PT

70. Your patient has immune thrombocytopenic purpura that has worsened and become refractory to treatment, including plasmaphoresis and injections of gamma globulin and glucocorticoid therapy. The patient will be undergoing a splenectomy. One of the preoperative treatments to expect is:
    A. Interferon
    B. Anti-Rh immunoglobulin
    C. *Haemophilus influenzae* type B vaccination
    D. Colchicine

71. **Blood component replacement therapy for DIC may include all but which of the following treatments?**
    A. FFP
    B. Cryoprecipitate
    C. Amicar
    D. Platelets

72. **A transfusion reaction that usually occurs within 5 to 30 minutes of the start of the transfusion is known as:**
    A. Acute intravascular hemolytic
    B. Febrile
    C. Allergic
    D. Acute extravascular hemolytic

73. **Walter is a 76-year-old gentleman who was admitted for end-stage mesothelioma. Which of the following occupations is more likely to be associated with a diagnosis of mesothelioma?**
    A. Bricklayer
    B. Gardener
    C. Office manager
    D. Shipbuilder

74. **Pernicious anemia results from a lack of**
    A. Vitamin B_6.
    B. Vitamin A.
    C. Vitamin B_{12}.
    D. Vitamin E.

This concludes the Hematology/Immunology questions.

ANSWERS

1. **Correct Answer: A**
   When areas are understaffed, the risk of nosocomial infection is increased. Standards of care, such as suctioning, turning patients, and use of aseptic technique are frequently not met.

2. **Correct Answer: B**
   Other adverse effects include nephrotoxicity, hypertension, hyperkalemia, leg cramps, headache, seizures, and development of neoplasms.

3. **Correct Answer: D**
   Antimetabolites interfere with RNA and DNA synthesis and inhibit T- and B-lymphocyte proliferation.

4. **Correct Answer: C**
   Reo Pro may affect platelet function for as long as 48 hours. It places the patient at risk for HITS because Reo Pro is frequently used with heparin and aspirin. Aggrastat and Integrilin are also inhibitors, but usually affect platelet function up to only 8 hours.

5. **Correct Answer: A**
   Other possible causes are transfusions, previous organ transplants, and blood-type incompatibilities. Answers B, C, and D are the results of organ rejection—not the causes.

6. **Correct Answer: D**
   Patients with a history of psychiatric illness may be unable to comprehend or follow through with a complicated postoperative medication regimen.

7. **Correct Answer: C**
   Sepsis is the most common cause of DIC because endotoxins stimulate production of tissue factor and the extrinsic pathway is activated. If the process continues, thrombi in capillaries can lead to hypoperfusion and metabolic acidosis, causing free-radical formation and damage to tissues. Tissue factor is released, resulting in DIC. Answers A, B, and D are also causes of DIC.

8. **Correct Answer: A**
   Disseminated intravascular coagulation is an overstimulation of the clotting cascade. Both the intrinsic and extrinsic pathways are activated at the same time, which causes an acceleration of the clotting process. When the clots lyse, the fibrin split products are anticoagulants. Eventually, all of the clotting factors are used up and no further clots can form. Heparin is sometimes used to interrupt the clotting cycle.

9. **Correct Answer: B**
   Potassium, sodium, and bicarbonate levels are decreased due to diuresis following a transplant.

10. **Correct Answer: D**
    A transplanted heart is denervated and does not respond to atropine. Epinephrine or isoproteranol may be of use.

11. **Correct Answer: D**
    Hemophilia A and B are factor IX deficiencies.

12. **Correct Answer: B**

    Fever usually causes increased destruction of platelets. Answers A, C, and D are signs and symptoms.

13. **Correct Answer: D**

    Cryoprecipitate means it is quick frozen. It contains large amounts of factor VIII. Cryoprecipitate does have disadvantages: It is expensive, and newer recombinant factor VIII products are available. There is also the risk of transmission of hepatitis A, hepatitis C, hepatitis G, and HIV.

14. **Correct Answer: A**

    Sometimes Dextran causes acute tubular necrosis because it is made of polymers of high-molecular-weight polysaccharides.

15. **Correct Answer: A**

    This form of meningitis is caused by a fungus, and amphotericin B is an antifungal. Rifampin is an antibacterial medication, and famvir and acyclovir are antivirals.

16. **Correct Answer: A**

    When blood is transfused, sometimes the cells lyse and the intracellular potassium is released. This can also occur as the cells strike the floating ball in the infusion chamber. It is sound practice to monitor electrolytes after every 2 units of blood given. Remember to monitor the patient for dysrhythmias.

17. **Correct Answer: C**

    The activated partial thromboplastin time of 45 seconds is correct because therapeutic results are standardized at 2–2½ times the normal time for the patient's blood to clot (20–30 seconds).

18. **Correct Answer: C**

    ITP usually occurs after a viral infection. The first symptom may be purpura and petechiae on the distal extremities. The PT and PTT are normal because they test for nonplatelet parts of the coagulation pathway. The result of the capillary fragility test will be greater than 1. Anti-RH immunoglobulin is a treatment for the disease. Continually monitor for signs and symptoms of intracranial hemorrhage.

19. **Correct Answer: D**

    Usually at about the third day following admission, ICU patients develop anemias. A reduced folate level would lead to megaloblastic anemia. Bone marrow aspiration is a diagnostic procedure, and TPN solutions would not lead to anemia. The IABP could indeed cause cells to lyse, as could prosthetic heart valves, heart–lung bypass, and bacterial endotoxins.

20. **Correct Answer: B**

    Phenobarbital may actually cause aplastic anemia, furosemide may cause a generalized anemia. Captopril causes pancytopenia. In addition, quinidine, procainamide, and acetaminophen may cause hemolytic anemia.

21. **Correct Answer: B**

    Additional causes include progressive gram-negative bacterial infections and malignancies such as prostate cancer. Trauma may result in a bacterial infection.

22. **Correct Answer: D**

    Cryoprecipitate, as mentioned previously, does carry these factors. There is a risk of disease transmission and transfusion reactions.

23. **Correct Answer: A**

    DIC often leads to malnutrition and nutritional deficits.

24. **Correct Answer: A**

    Other potential causes include sepsis, viral infection, burns, and radiation therapy. Medications such as thiazides, furosemide, penicillins, sulfonamides, ranitidine, and heparin may cause thrombocytopenia. Chemotherapy is another cause.

25. **Correct Answer: B**

    HIT is sometimes called "white clot syndrome." Thrombi are primarily venous in origin and can lead to DVT, pulmonary emboli, thrombotic stroke, limb ischemia, and myocardial infarction.

26. **Correct Answer: A**

    HIT is an acronym for "heparin-induced thrombocytopenia."

27. **Correct Answer: B**

    Mismatched blood causes a hemolytic reaction resulting in systemic cellular lysis. The overwhelming destruction of cells cannot be corrected rapidly enough by the bone marrow.

28. **Correct Answer: A**

    The function of T cells is cellular immunity. These cells recognize the transplanted organ cells as foreign resulting in a mounted attack leading to organ rejection. Immunosuppressive drugs suppress this normal response.

29. **Correct Answer: A**

    Rattlesnakes envenomate their victims with an enzyme called hyaluronidase, which breaks down the hyaluronic acid barriers on cells. The cells lyse, and their exudative products enter the bloodstream. Treatment is very similar to that for a patient with DIC because fibrin split products (anticoagulants) are released. The patient may require multiple vials of antivenin.

30. **Correct Answer: C**

    PRBCs contain no platelets, and platelets must be given to aid in hemostasis.

31. **Correct Answer: C**

    That is the standard definition of this type of rejection.

32. **Correct Answer: D**

    Damage to the tissues and vessels initiates the extrinsic cascade. Thromboplastin and factor VII are released and are activated in the presence of calcium.

33. **Correct Answer: A**

    The transplanted kidney is placed in the pelvic area. Pelvic pain is an ominous sign. Patients who have undergone kidney transplants should be educated to notify their physicians immediately if they suffer from pelvic pain, as it is a symptom of rejection.

34. **Correct Answer C:**
    Polyclonal antibodies are also used for episodes of acute rejections. Answers A and B are monoclonal antibodies also used for induction therapy and they alter the T cells so they cannot recognize antigens. Paroxetine (Paxil) is an antidepressant.

35. **Correct Answer: D**
    Additional indicators would include elevated liver enzymes, elevated bilirubin, jaundice, and elevated ammonia levels (a late sign). The itching is a result of bilirubin deposits in the skin.

36. **Correct Answer: C**
    Prostiglandin relaxes the smooth muscles within the pulmonary airways and leads to vasodilation within arteries. Inotropic support is usually accomplished with epinephrine. Heart rate is usually augmented with isoproterenol. Wound healing is promoted with a single, small dose of methylprednisolone.

37. **Correct Answer: D**
    Epinephrine counteracts the bronchoconstrictive and vasodilator actions of histamine by stimulating alpha, $beta_1$, and $beta_2$ receptors. Epinephrine is also useful in treating hayfever and urticaria.

38. **Correct Answer: B**
    DIC involves the depletion of clotting factors, so the patient becomes thrombocytopenic.

39. **Correct Answer: C**
    This is a small-cell carcinoma. On CXR a central mass will be seen. This type of carcinoma readily spreads to the brain, bone, liver, and adrenal glands, so the patient's prognosis is very poor.

40. **Correct Answer: A**
    Hemoglobin is comprised of two parts. The first part is "heme," which causes the reddish color and contains iron and porphyrin. The second part is a protein called "globin." Hemoglobin combines with oxygen to form oxyhemoglobin. Hemoglobin also binds with CO_2 and carries it to alveoli to be expired. When the hemoglobin is phagocytized, it breaks down into the heme and globin. The iron in the hemoglobin is processed and reused to manufacture new hemoglobin. The porphyrin converts to bilirubin and is excreted in urine and feces.

41. **Correct Answer: A**
    Acute posthemorrhagic anemia may be the result of hemorrhage, cancerous lesion, an ulcerative lesion that erodes an arterial wall, trauma to a major vessel, or rupture of an aneurysm. After hemorrhage, plasma is lost and vasoconstriction takes place. The concentration of erythrocytes is increased because the volume is low. In other words, the amount of cells is not diluted in the usual amount of fluid, so the count is artificially high. It can take as long as 6 weeks for hemoglobin levels to return to normal.

42. **Correct Answer: D**
    Iron-deficiency anemia is the most frequently occurring anemia seen around the world. It can be caused by an iron-poor diet or an excessive loss of iron. Trauma is a primary cause of acute loss and can result from bleeding. Blood donations, menses, GI

bleeding, malabsorption syndromes, pica, and excessive diarrhea are other potential causes of this type of anemia. If you view the erythrocytes, they appear kind of "puny": They are pale from lack of hemoglobin and tend to be smaller.

43. **Correct Answer: B**

In thalassemia, which is a type of anemia, the erythrocytes (known as "target cells") are very thin and fragile. The serum bilirubin is very elevated, so you should caution the patient against scratching. Cool water and lotion may be used for skin care. Oral stimulants could lead to vasoconstriction. The integrity of the skin is weakened, so careful positioning is paramount. The patient may require ongoing transfusions. Multiple transfusions may actually lead to too much iron, which may then have to be chelated out.

44. **Correct Answer: B**

Approximately 50% of all cases of aplastic anemia are caused by toxins; the other 50% have an unknown cause. Potential causes include radiation (X rays, radioactive isotopes, radium), benzene, streptomycin, carbon tetrachloride, DDT, chloramphenicol, and sulfonamides. Many types of pesticides other than DDT are thought to contribute to aplastic anemia.

45. **Correct Answer: C**

Sickle cell anemia occurs primarily in the African American population. Affected individuals are homozygous for HgS and have more HgS than HgA. This causes some of the cells to form a "sickle" shape—curved with rough edges. A crisis can occur when the low oxygen tension (postulated) causes a proliferation of these cells. The sharp edges of these cells travel through the microcirculation and damage capillaries. Even a simple event like cold weather can precipitate massive sickling. Other identified factors include dehydration, vomiting, diarrhea, high altitude, excessive exercise, and stress. When these cells break apart, they occlude the microcirculation and lead to lower oxygen tension, which initiates more sickling. This is a very painful time for the patient, and oxygen, pain management, and fluids are very important.

46. **Correct Answer: B**

Idiopathic thrombocytopenia purpura is the result of a low platelet count. Sometimes platelets are destroyed early and systematically. The cause is thought to be an autoimmune response. Hemorrhages may occur in the brain, which may lead to stroke and increased intracranial pressure.

47. **Correct Answer: C**

LMWH (Lovenox) is so stable and predictable that PTT's are not required. It is also easy to administer at home.

48. **Correct Answer: B**

Plavix will interfere with phenytoin, tamoxifen, tolbutamide, fluvastin, toresemide, and warfarin. It also may affect nonsteroidal anti-inflammatory drugs (NSAIDs). Plavix does not seem to affect estrogen, cimetidine, or phenobarbitol.

49. **Correct Answer: D**

Ethacrynic acid is a loop diuretic that prevents reabsorption of Na and Cl at the ascending loop of Henle (in the medulla of the kidney). Loop diuretics include furosemide, torsemide, bumetanide, and ethacrynic acid. As a group, they have vasodilatory effects on renal vasculature.

50. **Correct Answer: A**

Additional carbonic anhydrase inhibitors include dichlorphenamide and acetazolamide sodium. This type of diuretic blocks carbonic anhydrase and promotes excretion of water, Na^+, K^+, and bicarbonate. Potential complications include hypokalemia and hyperchloremic acidosis.

51. **Correct Answer: C**

Because of the high volume of urine excreted, additional complications may include hypocalcemia, dilutional hyponatremia, hyperglycemia, and hypochloremic acidosis.

52. **Correct Answer: C**

Mannitol and urea are osmotic diuretics. The action is to increase osmotic pressure of the filtrate. This will attract water and electrolytes and prevent reabsorption. Unfortunately, these agents can cause a rebound volume expansion, hyponatremia, and hyponatremia. Mannitol may be used in lieu of sodium bicarbonate to manage hemoglobinuria and myoglobinuria secondary to rhabdomyolysis or severe crush injury. If large volumes of fluid are also used, this may reduce or prevent renal tubular obstruction.

53. **Correct Answer: B**

Nesiritide is synthetic brain natriuetic peptide (BNP) used in the management of heart failure associated with prerenal azotemia. The BNP causes vasodilation, decreased systemic resistance (SVR), decreased wedge pressure (PCWP or PAOP), increased cardiac output (or cardiac index), diuresis, and decreased renin–angiotensin activity.

54. **Correct Answer: A**

Epogen and Procrit are recombinant versions of erythropoietin, and they are used to correct anemia that can occur with chronic renal failure. Adverse effects include clotting at the site of vascular access, depletion of iron, and increased levels of potassium, creatinine, and BUN.

55. **Correct Answer: D**

Mucomyst (N-acetylcysteine or NAC) is used to help reduce renal failure or worsening of symptoms caused by contrast media. The contrast media can sometimes cause contrast-induced neuropathy. Mucomyst has antioxidant properties that may counteract the reactive oxygen species that occur when the contrast media causes tubular epithelial cell toxicity.

56. **Correct Answer: B**

Intracellular fluid contains high concentrations of potassium, magnesium, proteins, phosphates, and sulfates.

57. **Correct Answer: C**

Bicarbonate in the interstitial spaces contains about 3 mEq/L more than that found in the intravascular space, which averages 24 mEq/L of bicarbonate.

58. **Correct Answer: C**

Atrial natriuretic peptide (ANP) is released by the atria in response to fluid overload. ANP increases excretion of sodium and water from the kidneys. This results in lowering the blood pressure. When the sodium and water are excreted, this decreases the release of antidiuretic hormone (ADH) and aldosterone.

59. **Correct Answer: A**

D_5W will be distributed equally between the intravascular and extravascular spaces. The hypertonic saline will expand the intravascular volume only. Other solutions used for volume replacement would include Dextran (hetastarch) and Hextend. These are synthetic colloidal solutions.

60. **Correct Answer: D**

If all the fluid is extracellular fluid, the systemic vascular resistance is increased. Because the fluid in the intravascular space is low, all the other parameters are decreased.

61. **Correct Answer: C**

Treatment should have occurred at a slower pace to prevent shrinkage and lysis of brain cells. If this condition is discovered early enough, fluid and electrolyte replacement can be slowed. If permanent damage is done, the patient may develop quadriparesis, flaccidity, and other neurological deficits. Seizure precautions should be implemented.

62. **Correct Answer: D**

Additional foods that are high in folic acid include red beans, broccoli, asparagus, liver, and beef.

63. **Correct Answer: D**

Monocytes and lymphocytes are classified as agranulocytes. The monocyte is the largest leukocyte, but comprises a small amount of the total cell WBC count. When monocytes mature, they become tissue macrophages and work as phagocytes. When a phagocyte lives in the liver, it is called a Kupffer cell. When it is in the lungs, it is called an alveolar macrophage. When a phagocyte is found in the connective tissues, it is called a histiocyte.

Macrophages contain lysosomal enzymes and chemicals that can destroy bacteria. If the macrophage is activated by an antigen, it will secrete monokines, which control communication between all the cells involved in an immune response.

64. **Correct Answer: C**

The B lymphocytes originate and mature in bone marrow. These lymphocytes form antibodies (immunoglobulins) that formulate a response to a specific antigen that bound itself to the B cells' receptor sites. The B cell forms a specific antibody for that particular antigen. Five different types of immunoglobulins are available: IgG, IgA, IgM, IgE, and IgD. After the antibodies are synthesized, the specific antibody can attach to its antigen and set off the reaction to allow for phagocytosis. The cells retain a "memory" for the specific antigen and if another exposure occurs, the response will be quicker and stronger.

65. **Correct Answer: A**

All factors except VIII and XII are synthesized in the liver, which explains why liver injuries can bleed so much and are so dangerous. While we were researching and confirming this question, we found out that the factors in the clotting cascades were numbered by order of discovery, not by order of use. Just FYI!

66. **Correct Answer: C**

Aminocaproic acid (Amicar) interferes with plasmin and inhibits fibrinolysis. Synthetic antithrombin III inhibits thrombin and can be very useful in treating DIC.

67. Correct Answer: D

Patients who have hemolytic anemia may not have any problems until they are exposed to a major stressor like infection, trauma, surgery, or a psychological stressor such as divorce. In such circumstances, the patient may be overwhelmed, causing hemolysis to accelerate. This process may cause tissue hypoxia and ischemia and eventually progress to necrosis and infarction. Treatment is supportive and targeted to presenting symptoms.

68. Correct Answer: D

If a severe reaction develops, the patient will have chest pain due to cardiac ischemia, neurologic impairment, LOC changes, and paresthesias because of cerebral ischemia. The patient may develop pulmonary emboli, dypsnea, extremity pain, and pallor as a result of thrombosis, and possible arterial thrombosis. This condition usually takes 5 to 7 days to manifest, but can take much less time for symptoms to appear.

69. Correct Answer: B

The PT, PTT, and thrombin time are normal with ITP because these tests only measure nonplatelet factors in the coagulation cascade. The platelet antibody screen measures the presence of IgG and IgM antiplatelet antibodies.

70. Correct Answer: C

Interferon is not applicable in this scenario. Answers B and D are treatments for ITP that have probably been tried prior to the decision to perform a splenectomy. The patient may also be vaccinated for pneumococcal and meningococcal organisms to lower the risk of postoperative infection.

71. Correct Answer: C

Amicar is used to inhibit fibrinolysis. Although it is used in the treatment of DIC, Amicar may transform a simple bleeding issue into DIC. Amicar must be used in combination with heparin.

DIC is usually treated with FFP, cryoprecipitate, and platelets. Cryoprecipitate contains more than 5 to 10 times more fibrinogen than FFP. A good rule of thumb is to give 10 units of cryoprecipitate for every 3 units of FFP. If the patient is actively bleeding, platelets are commonly administered.

72. Correct Answer: A

The patient may experience chills, fever, tachycardia, hypotension, hematuria, and back pain, and may exhibit additional signs of shock. The extravascular hemolytic reaction may manifest as fever, low H and H (even after transfusion), and elevated bilirubin.

73. Correct Answer: D

Mesothelioma is a cancer of the mesothelium. Most cases begin in the pleura or peritoneum. Mesothelioma is a relatively rare cancer, with approximately 2,000 new cases of mesothelioma diagnosed in the United States each year. It occurs more often in men than in women, and the risk of developing this disease increases with age. Symptoms of mesothelioma may not appear until 30 to 50 years after exposure to asbestos. An increased risk of developing mesothelioma has been found among shipyard workers, people who work in asbestos mines and mills, producers of asbestos products, workers in the heating and construction industries, and other trade people.

Symptoms of mesothelioma include dyspnea, pleural effusions, weight loss, and abdominal pain and swelling due to an excess of fluid in the abdomen. Other symptoms of peritoneal mesothelioma may include bowel obstruction, clotting disorders, anemia, and fever. Symptoms with metastases may include pain, dysphagia, or swelling of the neck or face.

Asbestos has been widely used in many industrial products, including cement, duct linings, sound insulation, brake linings, roof shingles, flooring products, textiles, and thermal insulation. If tiny asbestos particles float in the air, especially during the manufacturing process, they may be inhaled or swallowed, and can cause serious health problems. In addition to mesothelioma, exposure to asbestos increases the risk of lung cancer, asbestosis, and cancers of the trachea, larynx, and kidney. Smoking does not appear to increase the risk of mesothelioma, but the combination of smoking and exposure increases a person's risk of developing bronchial cancer.

While we were researching this topic, we discovered a sobering piece of information: More than 110,000 schools in the U.S. still contain some form of asbestos.

74. **Correct Answer: C**
Pernicious anemia results from a lack of protein intrinsic factor in the stomach that helps the body absorb vitamin B_{12}. The stress on the heart from the resultant hypoxia can cause heart murmurs, tachycardias, arrhythmias, hypertrophy, and heart failure. A lack of vitamin B_{12} raises the homocysteine level, and the high levels of homocysteine add to the buildup of fatty deposits. A lack of vitamin B_{12} can damage nerve cells and cause problems such as paresthesias in the hands and feet, leading to problems with ambulation and balance. Memory loss, visual disturbances, and confusion may develop. This type of anemia was named "pernicious" because it often proved fatal before the cause was discovered to be a lack of vitamin B_{12}.

BIBLIOGRAPHY

Aberg, F., Koivusalo, A. M., Hockerstedt, K., & Isoniemi, H. (2007). Renal dysfunction in liver transplant patients: Comparing patients transplanted for liver tumor or acute or chronic disease. *Transplant International, 20*(7), 591–599.

Ahrens, T. (2006). *Critical care nursing certification.* Columbus, OH: McGraw-Hill.

American Association of Critical Care Nurses. (2006). *Core curriculum for critical care nursing* (6th ed.). Philadelphia: Saunders.

American Association of Critical Care Nurses. (2007). *AACN certification and core review for high acuity and critical care* (6th ed.). Philadelphia: Saunders.

American Heart Association. (2007). Guidelines 2005 for cardiopulmonary resuscitation and emergency cardiovascular care. Retrieved July 21, 2008, from http://circ.ahajournals.org/content/vol112/24_suppl

Aster, R. H., & Bougie, D. W. (2007). Drug-induced immune thrombocytopenia: Current concepts. *New England Journal of Medicine, 357*(6), 580–587.

Barroso, J., Wells Pence, B., Salahuddin, N., Harmon, J. L., & Leserman, J. (2008). Physiological correlates of HIV-related fatigue. *Clinical Nursing Research, 17*(1), 5.

Bhullar, I. S., Braman, R., & Block, E. F. J. (2007). Recombinant factor VII as an adjunct to control of hemorrhage from chest trauma in a Jehovah's Witness. *American Surgeon, 73*(8), 818–819.

Biagini, E., Spirito, P., Leone, O., Picchio, F. M., Coccolo, F., Ragni, L., et al. (2008). Heart transplantation in hypertrophic cardiomyopathy. *American Journal of Cardiology, 101*(3), 387.

Bonatti, H., Dougerty, M., Martin, K., Hinder, R. A., Nguyen, J. H., & Haddad, M. A. (2007). Whipple procedure for chronic pancreatitis in a Jehovah's Witness. *American Surgeon, 73*(9), 935–936.

Burns, S. M. (Ed.). (2007). *American Association of Critical-Care Nurses (AACN): AACN protocols for practice: Healing environments* (2nd ed.). Sudbury, MA: Jones and Bartlett.

Caliskan, M., Erdogan, D., Gullu, H., Tok, D., Bilgi, M., & Muderrisoglu, H. (2007). Low serum bilirubin concentrations are associated with impaired aortic elastic properties, but not impaired left ventricular diastolic function. *International Journal of Clinical Practice, 61*(2), 218–224.

Campbell, M. S., Constantinescu, S., Furth, E. E., Reddy, K. R., & Bloom, R. D. (2007). Effects of hepatitis C-induced liver fibrosis on survival in kidney transplant candidates. *Digestive Diseases and Sciences, 52*(10), 2501–2507.

Chierakul, W., Tientadakul, P., Suputtamongkol, Y., Wuthiekanun, V., Phimda, K., Limpaiboon, R., et al. (2008). Activation of the coagulation cascade in patients with leptospirosis. *Clinical Infectious Diseases, 46*(2), 254.

Clark, N., Witt, D., Delate, T., Trapp, M., Garcia, D., Ageno, W., et al. (2008). The clinical consequence of subtherapeutic anticoagulation: The Low INR Study (LINeRS). *Journal of Thrombosis and Thrombolysis, 25*(1), 127–128.

Cohney, S. J., Walker, R. G., Haeusler, M. N., Francis, D. M., & Hogan, C. J. (2007). Blood group incompatibility in kidney transplantation: Definitely time to re-examine! *Medical Journal of Australia, 187*(5), 306–308.

Conover, M. B. (2003). *Understanding electrocardiography* (8th ed.). St. Louis, MO: Mosby/Elsevier.

Copstead, L., & Banasik, J. L. (2000). *Pathophysiology: Biological and behavioral perspectives* (2nd ed.). Philadelphia: Saunders/Elsevier.

Curley, M. A. Q. (1998). Patient–nurse synergy: Optimizing patients' outcomes. *American Journal of Critical Care, 7,* 64–72.

Danes, A. F., Cuenca, L. G., Rodriguez Bueno, S., Mendarte Barrenechea, L., & Montoro Ronsano, J. B. (2008). Efficacy and tolerability of human fibrinogen concentrate administration to patients with acquired fibrinogen deficiency and active or in high-risk severe bleeding. *Vox Sanguinis, 94*(3), 221–226.

Delclaux, C., Zerah-Lancner, F., Bachir, D., Habibi, A., Monin, J. L., Godeau, B., et al. (2005). Factors associated with dyspnea in adult patients with sickle cell disease. *Chest, 128*(5), 3336–3344.

Dhaliwal, G., Cornett, P. A., & Tierney, L. M. (2004). Hemolytic anemia. *American Family Physician, 69*(11), 2599–2606.

Domen, R. E., & Hoeltge, G. A. (2003). Allergic transfusion reactions: An evaluation of 273 consecutive reactions. *Archives of Pathology & Laboratory Medicine, 127*(3), 316–320.

Dossey, B. M., Keegan, L., & Guzzetta, C. (2003). *Holistic nursing: A handbook for practice* (3rd ed.). Sudbury, MA: Jones and Bartlett.

Douketis, J. D., Gu, S. Z., Schulman, S., Ghirarduzzi, A., Pengo, V., & Prandoni, P. (2007). The risk for fatal pulmonary embolism after discontinuing anticoagulant therapy for venous thromboembolism. *Annals of Internal Medicine, 147*(11), 766–774.

Drent, G., De Geest, S., & Haagsma, E. B. (2006). Prednisolone noncompliance and outcome in liver transplant recipients. *Transplant International, 19*(4), 342–343

Dvorak, C. C., & Cowan, M. J. (2008). Hematopoietic stem cell transplantation for primary immunodeficiency disease. *Bone Marrow Transplantation, 41*(2), 119–126.

Dwyer, J. (2008). Developing the duty to treat: HIV, SARS, and the next epidemic. *Journal of Medical Ethics, 34*(1), 7.

Eby, C. S., Harris, J. K., Gage, B. F., Ridker, P. M., Goldhaber, S. Z., & Birman-Deych, E. (2008). Pharmacogenetic factors affecting INR control during warfarin initiation. *Journal of Thrombosis and Thrombolysis, 25*(1), 98.

Edwards, D. F. (1999). The Synergy Model: Linking patient needs to nurse competencies. *Critical Care Nurse, 19*(1), 88–98.

El-Husseini, A., Sabry, A., Zahran, A., & Shoker, A. (2007). Can donor implantation renal biopsy predict long-term renal allograft outcome? *American Journal of Nephrology, 27*(2), 144–151.

Emergency Nurses Association & Newberry, L. (2003). *Sheehy's emergency nursing: Principles and practice* (5th ed.). St. Louis, MO: Mosby/Elsevier.

Ezidiegwu, C. N., Lauenstein, K. J., Rosales, L. G., Kelly, K. C., & Henry, J. B. (2004). Febrile non-hemolytic transfusion reactions: Management by premedication and cost implications in adult patients. *Archives of Pathology & Laboratory Medicine, 128*(9), 991–995.

Finkelmeier, B. A. (2000). *Cardiothoracic surgical nursing* (2nd ed.). Philadelphia: Lippincott Williams & Wilkins.

Goldstein, G., Toren, A., & Nagler, A. (2007). Transplantation and other uses of human umbilical cord blood and stem cells. *Current Pharmaceutical Design, 13*(13), 1363–1373.

Gurm, H. S., & Eagle, K. A. (2008). Use of anticoagulants in ST-segment elevation myocardial infarction patients: A focus on low-molecular-weight heparin. *Cardiovascular Drugs and Therapy, 22*(1), 59–69.

Halkes, P., & Algra, A. (2007). Anticoagulants, aspirin and dipyridamole in the secondary prevention of cerebral ischaemia: Which is the best for which patient? *Cerebrovascular Diseases: S1, 24*, 107–111.

Hardin, S. R., & Kaplow, R. (Eds.). (2004). *Synergy for clinical excellence: The AACN Synergy Model for Patient Care.* Boston, MA: Jones and Bartlett.

Hedner, U., & Brun, N. C. (2007). Recombinant factor VIIa (rFVIIa): Its potential role as a hemostatic agent. *Neuroradiology, 49*(10), 789–793.

Heparin-induced thrombocytopenia: A quick review of recent studies. (2007). *Journal of Respiratory Diseases, 28*(9), 396.

Hickey, J. V. (2002). *The clinical practice of neurological and neurosurgical nursing* (5th ed.). Philadelphia: Lippincott Williams & Wilkins.

Hirohata, A., Nakamura, M., Waseda, K., Honda, Y., Lee, D. P., Vagelos, R. H., et al. (2007). Changes in coronary anatomy and physiology after heart transplantation. *American Journal of Cardiology, 99*(11), 1603.

Ishibashi, H., Takashi, O., Hosaka, M., Sugimoto, I., Takahashi, M., Nihei, T., et al. (2005). Heparin-induced thrombocytopenia complicated with massive thrombosis of the inferior vena cava after filter placement. *International Angiology, 24*(4), 387–390.

James, A. H. (2007). Prevention and management of venous thromboembolism in pregnancy. *American Journal of Medicine: Management of Venous Thromboembolism, 120*(10B), S26.

Kamoun, M., & Grossman, R. A. (2008). Kidney-transplant rejection and anti-MICA antibodies. *New England Journal of Medicine, 358*(2), 196; author reply, 196.

Khan, B. A., Deel, C., & Hellman, R. N. (2006). Tumor lysis syndrome associated with reduced immunosuppression in a lung transplant recipient. *Mayo Clinic Proceedings, 81*(10), 1397–1399.

Krentz, A. J., & Wheeler, D. C. (2005). New-onset diabetes after transplantation: A threat to graft and patient survival. *Lancet, 365*(9460), 640–642.

Krishnamoorthy, P., Alyaarubi, S., Abish, S., Gale, M., Albuquerque, P., & Jabado, N. (2006). Primary hyperparathyroidism mimicking vaso-occlusive crises in sickle cell disease. *Pediatrics, 118*(2), 786–787.

Kuznetsov, A. V., Schneeberger, S., Seiler, R., Brandacher, G., Mark, W., Steurer, W., et al. (2004). Mitochondrial defects and heterogeneous cytochrome c release after cardiac cold ischemia and reperfusion. *American Journal of Physiology: Heart and Circulatory Physiology, 286*(5), H1633-1641.

Labbé, E., Herbert, D., & Haynes, J. (2005). Physicians' attitude and practices in sickle cell disease pain management. *Journal of Palliative Care, 21*(4), 246–251.

Leichtman, A. B. (2007). Balancing efficacy and toxicity in kidney-transplant immunosuppression. *New England Journal of Medicine, 357*(25), 2625–2627.

Levi, M., & Cate, H. T. (1999). Disseminated intravascular coagulation. *New England Journal of Medicine, 341*(8), 586–592.

Lipson, J. G., Dibble, S. L., & Minarik, P. A. (Eds.). (1996). *Culture and nursing care: A pocket guide.* San Francisco, CA: UCSF Nursing Press.

Lisman, T., & Leebeek, F. W. G. (2007). Hemostatic alterations in liver disease: A review of pathophysiology, clinical consequences, and treatment. *Digestive Surgery, 24*(4), 250–258.

Marik, P. E. (2006). Adrenal-exhaustion syndrome in patients with liver disease. *Intensive Care Medicine, 32*(2), 275–280.

McNally, P. (2001). *GI/liver secrets* (2nd ed.). Philadelphia: Hanley & Belfus/Elsevier.

McQuillan, K. A., Von Rueden, K. T., Hartsock, R. L., Flynn, M. B., & Whalen, E. (Eds.). (2002). *Trauma nursing: From resuscitation through rehabilitation* (3rd ed.). Philadelphia: Saunders/Elsevier.

Medina, J., & Puntillo, K. (2006). *AACN protocols for practice: Palliative care and end-of-life issues in critical care.* Sudbury, MA: Jones and Bartlett.

Mitka, M. (2007). Dual antithrombotic therapy's increased risks not always offset by benefit. *Journal of the American Medical Association, 298*(13), 1504.

Mongardon, N., Bruneel, F., Henry-Lagarrigue, M., Legriel, S., Revault d'Allonnes, L., Guezennec, P., et al. (2007). Shock during heparin-induced thrombocytopenia: Look for adrenal insufficiency! *Intensive Care Medicine, 33*(3), 547–548.

Neff, G. W., Kemmer, N., Kaiser, T. E., Zacharias, V. C., Alonzo, M., Thomas, M., et al. (2007). Combination therapy in liver transplant recipients with hepatitis B virus without hepatitis B immune globulin. *Digestive Diseases and Sciences, 52*(10), 2497–2500.

Norris, W. E. (2004). Acute hepatic sequestration in sickle cell disease. *Journal of the National Medical Association, 96*(9), 1235–1239.

Olson, J. D., Brandt, J. T., Chandler, W. L., Van Cott, E. M., Cunningham, M. T., Hayes, T. E., et al. (2007). Laboratory reporting of the international normalized ratio: Progress and problems. *Archives of Pathology & Laboratory Medicine, 131*(11), 1641–1647.

Orens, J. B. (2007). Lung transplantation for pulmonary hypertension. *International Journal of Clinical Practice, 61*(s158), 4–9.

Pagana, K. D., & Pagana, J. (2005). *Mosby's manual of diagnostic and laboratory tests* (3rd ed.). St. Louis, MO: Mosby/Elsevier.

Prasad, V. K., & Kurtzberg, J. (2008). Emerging trends in transplantation of inherited metabolic diseases. *Bone Marrow Transplantation, 41*(2), 99–108.

Ratnovsky, A., Elad, D., Izbicki, G., & Kramer, M. R. (2006). Mechanics of respiratory muscles in single-lung transplant recipients. *Respiration, 73*(5), 642–650.

Rizzi, E. B., Schininá, V., Rovighi, L., Cristofaro, M., Bordi, E., Narciso, P., et al. (2008). HIV-related pneumococcal lung disease: Does highly active antiretroviral therapy or bacteremia modify radiologic appearance? Review of. *AIDS Patient Care & STDs, 22*(2), 105.

Shorr, A. K., Helman, D. L., Davies, D. B., & Nathan, S. D. (2004). Sarcoidosis, race, and short-term outcomes following lung transplantation. *Chest, 125*(3), 990–996.

Silverborn, M., Ambring, A., Nilsson, F., Friberg, P., & Jeppsson, A. (2006). Vascular resistance and endothelial function in cyclosporine-treated lung transplant recipients. *Transplant International, 19*(12), 974–981.

Skidmore-Roth, L. (2004). *Mosby's 2004 nursing drug reference.* St. Louis, MO: Mosby/Elsevier.

Smeltzer, S., & Bare, B. G. (2003). *Brunner and Suddarth's textbook of medical–surgical nursing* (10th ed.). Philadelphia: Lippincott Williams & Wilkins.

Smith, W. R., Penberthy, L. T., Bovbjerg, V. E., McClish, D. K., Roberts, J. D., Dahman, B., et al. (2008). Daily assessment of pain in adults with sickle cell disease. *Annals of Internal Medicine, 148*(2), 94–101.

Sole, M. L., Hartshorn, J., & Lamborne, M. L. (2001). *Introduction to critical care nursing* (3rd ed.). Philadelphia: Saunders/Elsevier.

Stewart, S. (2007). Pulmonary infections in transplantation pathology. *Archives of Pathology & Laboratory Medicine, 131*(8), 1219–1231.

Swanson, K., Dwyre, D. M., Krochmal, J., & Raife, T. J. (2006). Transfusion-related acute lung injury (TRALI): Current clinical and pathophysiologic considerations. *Lung, 184*(3), 177–185.

Tien, H., Nascimento, B., Callum, J., & Rizoli, S. (2007). An approach to transfusion and hemorrhage in trauma: Current perspectives on restrictive transfusion strategies. *Canadian Journal of Surgery, 50*(3), 202–209.

Toso, C., Al-Qahtani, M., Alsaif, F. A., Bigam, D. L., Meeberg, G. A., James Shapiro, A. M., et al. (2007). ABO-incompatible liver transplantation for critically ill adult patients. *Transplant International, 20*(8), 675–681.

Unkle, D. W. (2007). Heparin-induced thrombocytopenia. *Orthopaedic Nursing, 26*(6), 383–387.

Urden, L. D., Stacy, K. M., & Lough, M. E. (2007). *Thelan's critical care nursing: Diagnosis and management* (5th ed.). St. Louis, MO: Mosby.

Villar, E., Boissonnat, P., Sebbag, L., Hendawy, A., Cahen, R., Trolliet, P., et al. (2007). Poor prognosis of heart transplant patients with end-stage renal failure. *Nephrology, Dialysis, Transplantation, 22*(5), 1383–1389.

Wiegand, D. J. L., & Carlson, K. K. (Eds.). (2005). *AACN procedure manual for critical care* (5th ed.). Philadelphia: Elsevier.

Williams, S., Wynn, G., Cozza, K., & Sandson, N. B. (2007). Cardiovascular medications. *Psychosomatics, 48*(6), 537–547.

Woods, S., Sivarajan Froelicher, E. S., & Motzer, S. U. (2000). *Cardiac nursing* (4th ed.). Philadelphia: Lippincott Williams & Wilkins.

Yasunaga, H. (2007). Risk of authoritarianism: Fibrinogen-transmitted hepatitis C in Japan. *Lancet, 370*(9604), 2063–2067.

Yip, N. H., Lederer, D. J., Kawut, S. M., Wilt, J. S., D'Ovidio, F., Wang, Y., et al. (2006). Immunoglobulin G levels before and after lung transplantation. *American Journal of Respiratory and Critical Care Medicine, 173*(8), 917–921.

Zhang, D., Zhang, F., Zhang, Y., Gao, X., Li, C., Ma, W., et al. (2007). Erythropoietin enhances the angiogenic potency of autologous bone marrow stromal cells in a rat model of myocardial infarction. *Cardiology, 108*(4), 228–236.

QUESTIONS

1. **A sympathetic response to a stimulus results in**
   A. Heightened awareness, increased blood pressure, bronchial constriction, and increased glucogenesis.
   B. Dilated pupils, bronchial relaxation, increased gastric motility, and normal urine output.
   C. Vasodilatation, increased blood pressure, decreased gastric secretions, and pupils at 3 mm.
   D. Increased respiratory depth, increased heart rate, decreased gastric motility, and sphincter dilation.

2. **Spinal shock is defined as**
   A. Areflexia at or below the spinal cord injury.
   B. Hyperreflexia and spasticity after spinal cord injury.
   C. Areflexia that rises above the site of injury.
   D. Spasticity below injury site.

3. **Fred, an 18-year-old male, was injured while skateboarding and has a T8 spinal cord injury. He has been diagnosed with spinal shock. The critical care nurse knows the symptoms of spinal shock include**
   A. Areflexia, autonomic dysfunction, loss of sensation, and eliminatory dysfunction.
   B. Areflexia, peripheral vasodilatation, decreased SVR, and loss of sensation.
   C. Areflexia, heightened sensation, and cardiovascular shock.
   D. Areflexia, bowel and bladder dysfunction, and bradycardia.

4. **Neurogenic shock differs from spinal shock in which of the following ways?**
   A. It is a less severe form of shock with spinal cord injury that causes a brief decrease in blood pressure.
   B. It is a more severe form of shock that causes cardiovascular collapse in patients with a spinal cord injury above T6.
   C. It is a more severe form of shock that increases the likelihood of paralysis and death.
   D. It is a more severe form of shock that occurs within hours after a spinal cord injury and causes increased sympathetic outflow.

5. **Cerebral aneurysms are most often found in**
   A. Internal carotid arteries.
   B. Bifurcations of the anterior–posterior Circle of Willis.
   C. The temporal artery.
   D. Vertebral arteries.

6. **The most common first symptom of a rupturing cerebral aneurysm is**
   A. Fever.
   B. Nuchal rigidity.
   C. Nausea and vomiting.
   D. An explosive headache, often described as "the worst headache of my life."

7. **Arteriovenous malformations (AVMs) are**
   A. Commonly found misshapen blood vessels.
   B. More common in women than men.
   C. A complex tangle of misshapen blood vessels susceptible to hemorrhage.
   D. Never seen in children.

8. **Nursing management of a patient with a cerebral aneurysm includes**
   A. Ambulation, monitoring of vital and neurologic signs.
   B. Glasgow Coma Scale assessments and monitoring for cerebral vascular spasm.
   C. Maintaining normal intracranial pressure.
   D. Maintaining systolic blood pressure less than 120 mm Hg.

9. **The hallmark of encephalopathy of any cause is**
   A. An altered mental state.
   B. Liver failure.
   C. Renal failure.
   D. Infection.

10. **Treatment of encephalopathy includes**
    A. Antibiotics.
    B. High-dose steroids.
    C. Treating the underlying cause.
    D. Electrolyte replacement.

11. **Diagnostic tests for a patient with encephalopathy could include**
    A. BMP, CRP, CXR.
    B. Blood tests, CSF evaluation, EEG.
    C. EEG, Dilantin levels.
    D. Lumbar puncture, renal ultrasound.

12. **Tom C., a 25-year-old baseball player, is admitted to the ICU after being struck by a baseball bat during a game. He has blunt force trauma to the left side of his head. Nursing management of this patient includes frequent assessments. The critical care nurse knows which of the following is the most sensitive indicator of Tom's status?**
    A. Vital signs
    B. Glasgow Coma Scale score
    C. Level of consciousness
    D. Intracranial pressure monitoring

13. Susan was an unrestrained passenger in a motor vehicle accident. She is admitted to the neuro ICU for observation with a basilar skull fracture. Which of the following signs differentiate a fracture of the middle fossa?
    A. Rhinorrhea
    B. Raccoon's eyes
    C. Battle's sign
    D. Subconjunctival hemorrhage

14. While assessing a patient with a basilar skull fracture, the ICU nurse notices a stain on the patient's pillow. The stain is a small amount of blood encircled by a pale yellow stain. This stain is called
    A. Halo sign.
    B. Battle's sign.
    C. Grey-Turner's sign.
    D. Ludwig's sign.

15. The most accurate method of measuring intracranial pressure is
    A. A subarachnoid bolt.
    B. Intraventriculosotomy.
    C. An epidural catheter.
    D. A subdural catheter.

16. Normal intracranial pressure is
    A. 0–5.
    B. 4–15.
    C. 16–20.
    D. 20–40.

17. Where should the transducer for any type of intracranial pressure monitoring system be placed?
    A. In the foramen ovale
    B. In the aqueduct of Sylvius
    C. In the foramen of Monroe
    D. In the fourth ventricle

18. What is the effect of Cushing syndrome in a patient with increased intracranial pressure?
    A. Increased systolic blood pressure, widening pulse pressure, bradycardia
    B. Elevated blood pressure, narrow pulse pressure, tachycardia
    C. Bradycardia, low blood pressure, narrow pulse pressure
    D. Tachycardia, increased systolic blood pressure, widening pulse pressure

19. When should a lumbar puncture be done on a patient with increased intracranial pressure?
    A. Once the patient has had a CT or MRI scan
    B. Always, to check intracranial pressure
    C. On a case-by-case basis
    D. Never

20. Which of the following decreases intracranial pressure?
    A. CO_2 retention
    B. PaO_2 less than 50 mm Hg
    C. Increased cerebrospinal fluid absorption
    D. Increased metabolic activity

21. Mrs. G. has a closed head injury secondary to a fall. As a critical care nurse, you know that _____ is the most important indicator of neurologic deterioration in this patient.
    A. Blood pressure
    B. Cranial nerve testing
    C. Level of consciousness
    D. Glasgow Coma Scale score

22. Mrs. G., a patient with a closed head injury, has a Foley catheter. In 1 hour, her urine output increases from 30 mL/h to 1,000 mL of very pale, clear urine. The ICU nurse knows this condition is probably
    A. A volume shift from the 3rd space.
    B. Syndrome of inappropriate antidiuretic hormone.
    C. Diabetes insipidus.
    D. Diuresis from steroids.

23. As a critical care nurse, you know the treatment of diabetes insipidus includes
    A. Fluid restriction.
    B. Intravenous replacement to cover the increased urine output.
    C. Diuretics.
    D. Demeclocycline.

24. What is the "Triple H" therapy for cerebral aneurysm rupture?
    A. Hypertension, hypervolemia, hemodilution
    B. Hypertension, hypovolemia, hemodilution
    C. Hypovolemia, hypotension, hemoconcentration
    D. Hemoconcentration, hypertension, hypervolemia

25. Why is it important to stop seizure activity in status epilepticus?
    A. Oxygen depletion is due to an impeded airway.
    B. There is an increased risk of cerebrovascular accident.
    C. Continued seizure activity causes lactic acidosis and cerebral edema.
    D. Injury risk increases with continued seizures.

26. Communicating hydrocephalus is caused by which mechanism?
    A. Closed head injury
    B. Subarachnoid hemorrhage
    C. Epidural bleed
    D. Cerebrovascular accident

27. **What is the formula for calculating cerebral perfusion pressure (CPP)?**
    A. CPP = SBP – MAP – ICP
    B. CPP = MAP – ICP
    C. CPP = ICP – MAP
    D. CPP = MAP – CVP – ICP

28. **The goal for cerebral perfusion pressure (CPP) is a pressure of**
    A. 50–80 mm Hg.
    B. 20–40 mm Hg.
    C. 10–20 mm Hg.
    D. 70–90 mm Hg.

29. **Which of the cranial nerves (CN) are affected by a basilar skull fracture?**
    A. I, VII, VIII
    B. I, II, III
    C. I, V, VIII
    D. II, III, VIII

30. **Your patient with a head injury has developed nystagmus. Nystagmus may be defined as**
    A. Eyes deviated to the side of the injury.
    B. A convergent gaze.
    C. A rhythmic tremor or shaking of the eyes.
    D. A divergent gaze.

31. **Your patient who has oat-cell lung cancer has decreased urinary output of less than 10 ml per hour. This may be caused by**
    A. Dehydration.
    B. Syndrome of inappropriate antidiuretic hormone.
    C. Diabetes insipidus.
    D. Third spacing.

32. **What are the most common causes of syndrome of inappropriate antidiuretic hormone (SIADH)?**
    A. Bronchogenic (oat cell) carcinoma, pneumonia, head injury
    B. Pneumonia, COPD, tuberculosis
    C. Brain tumors, pneumonia, polycystic kidney disease
    D. Polycystic kidney disease, cerebrovascular accident, oat-cell carcinomas

33. **Spinal reflexes indicate**
    A. Functional upper motor neurons.
    B. Nonfunctional lower motor neurons.
    C. Nonfunctional upper motor neurons.
    D. Functional lower motor neurons.

34. **In what manner is the spinothalamic tract tested?**
    A. Deep tendon reflexes
    B. Babinski reflex
    C. Pinprick or monofilament testing
    D. Patellar tendon reflex

35. **What is one cause of autonomic hyperreflexia?**
    A. Diarrhea
    B. Suctioning
    C. Constipation
    D. Warm breeze

36. **What is autonomic hyperreflexia?**
    A. A malfunction of the autonomic nervous system seen with head injury
    B. A malfunction of the autonomic nervous system seen with spinal cord injury
    C. A malfunction of the autonomic nervous system seen with pituitary tumor removal
    D. A malfunction of the autonomic nervous system seen with epidural bleeds

37. **The critical care nurse should anticipate which of the following treatments for the syndrome of inappropriate antidiuretic hormone (SIADH)?**
    A. Fluid replacement, potassium chloride, declomycin
    B. Fluid restriction, diuretics, sodium replacement, declomycin
    C. Declomycin, vasopressin, diuretics
    D. Fluid restriction, potassium chloride, diuretics

38. **What is seen with a normal response to the "doll's eyes" maneuver?**
    A. Disconjugate gaze with head turn
    B. Conjugate gaze in the opposite direction as the head is turned
    C. Conjugate gaze in the same direction as the head is turned
    D. Nystagmus with head turning

39. **What does the Glasgow Coma Scale measure?**
    A. Verbal response, orientation, activity
    B. Eye opening, motor response, verbal response
    C. Eye opening, orientation, motor response
    D. Verbal response, orientation, eye opening

40. **Which Glasgow Coma Scale score indicates coma?**
    A. 8–10
    B. 6–7
    C. 5–6
    D. 4–5

41. **Susan P., an 18-year-old female, was injured in a motor vehicle accident. She now exhibits decerebrate posturing. As the ICU nurse, you will anticipate which symptoms?**
    A. One arm flexed, one arm flaccid, legs flaccid
    B. Both arms fully extended and internally rotated, legs flaccid
    C. Both arms fully extended and internally rotated, legs fully extended with toes pointed
    D. Flaccid arms and legs extended

42. **Felix is an SICU patient with a gunshot wound to his T11–T12 spine. Upon assessment, you find motor paralysis on the same side as the gunshot wound but loss of pain and temperature sensation on the opposite side. This is called**

A. Grey–Turner syndrome.

B. Cushing syndrome.

C. Syndrome X.

D. Brown–Sequard syndrome.

43. **Your ICU patient suddenly develops right pupil dilation. What does this change indicate?**

    A. Basilar skull fracture

    B. Uncal herniation

    C. Brain stem herniation

    D. Cerebral vascular accident

44. **What is the most common bacterium causing meningococcal meningitis?**

    A. *Streptococcus pneumoniae*

    B. *Neisseria meningitidis*

    C. *Staphylococcus aureus*

    D. *Haemophilius influenzae*

45. **What is the hallmark symptom of meningococcal meningitis?**

    A. Headache

    B. Petechiae

    C. Malaise

    D. Vomiting

46. **Bilateral ascending muscle weakness is suggestive of which of the following illnesses?**

    A. Guillain–Barré syndrome

    B. Chronic fatigue syndrome

    C. Tetanus

    D. *Clostridium botulinum* infection

47. **A positive Babinski or Plantar reflex indicates**

    A. A reflex elicited with a reflex hammer to the Achilles tendon.

    B. Normal neurologic functioning.

    C. An upper motor neuron lesion of the pyramidal tract.

    D. A lower motor neuron lesion of the pyramidal tract.

48. **What is the proper technique for eliciting a Babinski reflex?**

    A. Stroke the sole of the foot from side to side.

    B. Stroke the sole of the foot along the lateral sole from the heel up toward the toes and across the ball of the foot.

    C. Strike the heel and the ball of the foot.

    D. Strike the Achilles tendon with a reflex hammer.

49. **Cerebrospinal fluid is formed in what location?**

    A. Lateral ventricles

    B. Choroid plexus

    C. Subarachnoid space

    D. Arachnoid villi

50. What volume of cerebrospinal fluid is produced each day?
    A. 1,000–1,200 mL
    B. 600–700 mL
    C. 400–800 mL
    D. 800–900 mL

51. George B., a 55-year-old man with meningitis, is having a lumbar puncture. As the critical care nurse, you know the cerebrospinal fluid (CSF) should be
    A. Hazy with a glucose level of 85.
    B. Clear with RBCs present.
    C. Clear and colorless with less than 45 mg/dL of protein.
    D. Clear and colorless with a white blood cell count greater than 150 cells/mm².

52. While performing a neurologic examination, the ICU nurse knows that the 6 cardinal eye directions for assessing eye movement are
    A. Testing CN II, III, and IV.
    B. Testing CN III, IV, and VI.
    C. Testing CN II, V, and VII.
    D. Testing CN V, VI, and VII.

53. Your patient was an unrestrained driver in a motor vehicle crash. His head struck and fractured the windshield. He sustained a left frontal lobe injury. Which symptoms do you expect from this patient?
    A. Hearing and balance impairment
    B. Sensory and memory problems
    C. Personality changes, poor short-term memory
    D. Loss of motor function, hearing problems

54. What does the acronym RIND represent?
    A. Recurrent ischemic neurologic default
    B. Reversible intracerebral neurologic deficit
    C. Recurrent intracerebral neurologic default
    D. Reversible ischemic neurologic deficit

55. What differentiates a transient ischemic attack (TIA) from a reversible ischemic neurologic deficit (RIND)?
    A. A TIA lasts less than 24 hours, a RIND lasts more than 24 hours.
    B. A TIA lasts less than 6 hours, a RIND lasts more than 48 hours.
    C. A TIA lasts more than 24 hours, a RIND lasts less than 24 hours.
    D. A TIA lasts less than 24 hours, a RIND lasts less than 6 hours.

56. Your patient has had a major left sided stroke. What is the most common cause of stroke in the United States?
    A. Uncontrolled diabetes mellitus
    B. Cocaine abuse
    C. Uncontrolled hypertension
    D. Tobacco addiction

57. You are educating your patient and her family about stroke. Part of your talk involves modifiable risk factors for stroke. Which of the following are modifiable risk factors for stroke?
    A. Alcohol use, obesity, family history
    B. Alcohol use, smoking, obesity
    C. Alcohol use, family history, smoking
    D. Alcohol use, family history, hypertension

58. What are the two major types of stroke?
    A. Ischemic and lacunar
    B. Ischemic and hemorrhagic
    C. Hemorrhagic and transient ischemic attack
    D. Hemorrhagic and reversible ischemic neurologic deficit

59. Why does diabetes mellitus increase the risk of stroke?
    A. Increased risk of hypertension
    B. Decreased neuroreceptor response in cerebral circulation
    C. Accelerated arthrosclerosis of the large arteries
    D. Increased risk of clot formation

60. Your patient with uncontrolled hypertension is most likely to have which type of stroke?
    A. Ischemic
    B. Lacunar
    C. Transient ischemic attack
    D. Reversible neurologic deficit

61. Which hemisphere, cerebral or cerebellar, is likely to be affected by stroke?
    A. Right cerebellar hemisphere
    B. Right cerebral hemisphere
    C. Left cerebral hemisphere
    D. Left cerebellar hemisphere

62. You are caring for a 72-year-old man who has experienced a left-side cerebrovascular accident. What symptoms do you expect to see?
    A. Hearing deficits, left vision problems, left facial droop
    B. Speech deficits, loss of right visual field, right facial droop
    C. Loss of right visual field, receptive aphasia, left facial droop
    D. Speech deficits, left visual field loss, left facial droop

63. Your priority in caring for a patient with a cerebrovascular accident is
    A. Preventing decubitus ulcers.
    B. Preventing aspiration of food or fluid.
    C. Preventing contractures.
    D. Preventing depression.

64. **What area in the cerebrum controls verbal expression?**
    A. Wernicke's area
    B. Broca's area
    C. Limbic area
    D. Pontine area

65. **Fred F., an 80-year-old African American man, has had a left temporal cerebrovascular accident due to uncontrolled hypertension. As the ICU nurse, you know that Fred is likely to have which of the following deficits?**
    A. Motor deficits
    B. Expressive aphasia
    C. Receptive aphasia
    D. Balance deficits

66. **What is the homunculus?**
    A. A strip of the frontal lobe that affects motor skills
    B. A strip of the parietal lobe that affects sensory reception
    C. A strip in the cerebellum that affects balance and fine motor coordination
    D. A strip of cerebral cortex that involves the sensory and motor functioning

67. **Georgia, a 35-year-old woman, has Guillain-Barré syndrome. What is the most important measurement for this patient?**
    A. Blood pressure
    B. Negative inspiratory force (NIF)
    C. Pain level
    D. Cerebrospinal fluid study results

68. **Which results would you expect in the evaluation of the cerebrospinal fluid in a patient with Guillain-Barré syndrome?**
    A. Increased white blood cells
    B. Increased protein levels
    C. Increased glucose levels
    D. Anaerobic bacteria

69. **Which of the following nursing diagnoses would be the most appropriate for a patient with Guillain-Barré syndrome?**
    A. Impaired motor weakness, impaired respiratory function, acute pain
    B. Impaired respiratory function, impaired nutrition, acute pain
    C. Impaired motor weakness, impaired bowel function, acute pain
    D. Impaired respiratory function, impaired bowel function, acute pain

70. **Your patient with Guillain-Barré syndrome is experiencing a great deal of pain. Why is this occurring?**
    A. Parasympathetic function
    B. Sympathetic inactivity
    C. Autonomic dysfunction
    D. Sympathetic function

71. **Nursing management of a patient with Guillain-Barré syndrome includes which of the following?**

A. Monitoring labs and neurologic signs
B. Monitoring respiratory status and neurologic signs
C. Monitoring respiratory status and lab results
D. Monitoring labs results and urinary output

72. **A nursing diagnosis for a patient with Guillain-Barré syndrome includes**
    A. Impaired nutrition.
    B. Risk for impaired respiratory function.
    C. Impaired fluid balance.
    D. Impaired body image.

73. **What is the vector for West Nile virus?**
    A. Fleas
    B. Field mice
    C. Birds
    D. Cockroaches

74. **What differentiates West Nile virus from other forms of vector-borne encephalitis?**
    A. Extreme fatigue and a diffuse papular rash
    B. Lymphadenopathy and extreme fatigue
    C. Erythematous rash and lymphadenopathy
    D. Bull's-eye rash and lymphadenopathy

75. **Jenny B. has had a transphenodial resection of a pituitary tumor. As the ICU nurse, you know postoperative care for this patient includes**
    A. Monitoring vital signs, I&O monitoring, and neurologic signs.
    B. Monitoring neurologic signs, urinary output, and moustache dressing changes.
    C. Monitoring I&O, moustache dressing changes, and daily weights.
    D. Changing nasal packing daily, monitoring neurologic signs, and daily weights.

76. **Mark H. has three large aneurysms in his Circle of Willis. What methods are used to treat aneurysms?**
    A. Clipping the aneurysms and endovascular coiling
    B. Clipping of the aneurysms and tPA administration
    C. Medical management of blood pressure and Amicar infusion
    D. Amicar infusion and tPa administration

77. **Death from status epilepticus is usually caused by what mechanism?**
    A. Airway blockage, leading to severe cerebral hypoxia
    B. Creation of a hypermetabolic state within the brain
    C. Falls from seizure, causing head trauma
    D. Aspiration pneumonia

78. **Nancy is an ICU patient with new-onset grand mal seizures. While at her bedside, you witness a seizure. What should your first action be?**
    A. Hold the patient down to prevent injury.
    B. Roll Nancy to her right side and protect the airway.
    C. Insert an oral airway and call for help.
    D. Hit the Code Blue button.

79. Jerry has a grand mal seizure lasting 70 seconds. As soon as the seizure has passed, he is fully awake and asking for food. The ICU nurse should
    A. Tell the patient she knows he faked the seizure.
    B. Feed the patient.
    C. Notify the attending physician and anticipate a psychological evaluation.
    D. Give Dilantin 1 gram slowly.

80. John Doe is admitted to the MICU for seizure activity. The nurse should anticipate which of the following laboratory tests?
    A. CBC, lipid panel, toxicology screen
    B. CBC, toxicology screen, LFTs
    C. CBC, CMP, lipid panel
    D. CBC, CMP, sedimentation rate, CRP, RPR, toxicology screen

81. Continuing with the scenario from Question 80, which diagnoses should be considered possible causes of John Doe's seizures?
    A. Alcohol abuse and hypertension
    B. Panic attack and psychological illness
    C. Panic attacks and transient ischemic attack
    D. Cardiac arrhythmias and hypertension

82. Mary, an 85-year-old woman with a recent TIA, has been sent to the intensive care unit after a carotid endarterectomy (CEA). What are important signs to document in this patient?
    A. Vital signs, neurologic signs, carotid artery pulses
    B. Vital signs, neurologic signs, subclavian pulses
    C. Vital signs, temporal artery pulses, neurologic signs
    D. Vital signs, neurologic signs, no pulses are necessary

83. What level of carotid stenosis is necessary for a carotid endarterectomy or endovascular stenting before the patient is considered for treatment?
    A. Greater than 50%
    B. Greater than 65%
    C. Greater than 70%
    D. Greater than 85%

84. What would be an indication for use of Aggrenox?
    A. Post myocardial infarction
    B. Post cerebrovascular accident
    C. Post pulmonary embolism
    D. Post deep vein thrombosis

85. Fran, a 28-year-old female, has been diagnosed with multiple sclerosis (MS). She was admitted to the intensive care unit after an acute exacerbation in which she experienced left-side weakness. You know that multiple sclerosis is which type of disease?

    A. Motor disorder of the spinal cord

    B. Demyelinating disorder of the brain and spinal cord

    C. Motor disorder of the brain and spinal cord

    D. Demyelinating disease of the spinal cord

86. **Continuing with the scenario from Question 85, Fran is very depressed. She states, "I don't want to die like my mother did with MS." Which Kubler-Ross stage of grief is Fran experiencing?**

    A. Denial

    B. Bargaining

    C. Anger

    D. Acceptance

87. **Common symptoms of an exacerbation of multiple sclerosis can include which of the following?**

    A. Hyperthesia, fatigue, hyporeflexia

    B. Paresthesias, urinary incontinence, constipation

    C. Diplopia, ataxia, emotional labiality

    D. Ataxia, dementia, temporal neuralgia

88. **What is the cause of multiple sclerosis?**

    A. Heredity

    B. Unknown

    C. Chemical exposure

    D. Heavy-metal poisoning

89. **Lab studies for multiple sclerosis identification include**

    A. Cerebrospinal fluid evaluation, sedimentation rate, and fluorescent treponomal antibody absorption.

    B. Cerebrospinal fluid evaluation, syphilis testing, and drug screen.

    C. Cerebrospinal fluid evaluation, CBC, and HIV testing.

    D. Cerebrospinal fluid evaluation, lipids, and sedimentation rate.

90. **What are the two major types of multiple sclerosis?**

    A. Progressive and relapsing–resolving

    B. Relapsing–remitting and static

    C. Progressive and relapsing–relapsing

    D. Relapsing–remitting and progressive

91. **What are the four types of Guillain-Barré syndrome?**

    A. Ascending, progressive, relapsing–remitting, pure motor

    B. Ascending, descending, Miller–Fischer Variant, pure motor

    C. Ascending, descending, relapsing, pure sensory

    D. Ascending, relapsing–remitting, pure motor, pure sensory

92. **Myasthenia Gravis is diagnosed using which test?**

    A. Weber test

    B. Rinne test

    C. Tensilon test

    D. Clonus test

93. **What is myasthenia gravis?**
    A. A neuromuscular disorder in which myelin is destroyed at varying rates
    B. A neuromuscular disorder at the neuromuscular junctions
    C. A neuromuscular disorder seen after viral infections
    D. A fatal neuromuscular disorder of upper motor neurons and lower motor neurons causing muscle wasting

94. **What are some common symptoms of myasthenia gravis?**
    A. Ptosis, proximal muscle weakness, spasticity
    B. Dysphonia, sialorrhea, atrophy
    C. Fatigue, proximal muscle weakness, respiratory weakness
    D. Generalized weakness, hyperreflexia, dyspnea

95. **Betty is a 50-year-old female who was admitted to the intensive care unit for Acute coronary syndrome. She also has myasthenia gravis and is allowed to keep her pyridostigmine at her bedside so she does not miss a dose. Suddenly her monitor alarm goes off, signaling a severe bradycardia. You suspect an overdose of pyridostigmine. If that is true, Betty's problem is**
    A. Cholinergic crisis.
    B. Acetylcholine crisis.
    C. Myasthenia gravis crisis.
    D. The bradycardia is related to the acute coronary syndrome, not myasthenia gravis.

    This concludes the Neurology questions.

ANSWERS

1. **Correct Answer: A**
   There are many responses to sympathetic stimuli as the body prepares for "flight, fright, or fight." Other responses include dilated pupils for increased visual acuity, increased heart rate, increased myocardial contractility, increased blood pressure, increased respiratory rate, decreased gastric motility, decreased gastric secretion, decreased urine output, decreased insulin production, and decreased renal blood flow.

2. **Correct Answer: A**
   Spinal shock can occur hours to weeks after an injury to the spinal cord. The patient develops flaccidity, loss of sensation, and loss of bowel and bladder function. Answer B (hyperreflexia and spasticity after spinal cord injury) occurs after spinal shock resolves.

3. **Correct Answer: A**
   Spinal shock occurs hours to weeks after a cord injury causing autonomic loss. The severity of a spinal cord injury cannot be fully assessed until the shock has resolved.

4. **Correct Answer: B**
   Neurogenic shock is a much more severe form of shock that may occur with spinal cord injuries at or above T6. The autonomic dysfunction causes increased vagal tone, which results in severe bradycardia, decreased cardiac output, peripheral dilatation, and decreased SVR.

5. **Correct Answer: B**
   Eighty-five percent of cerebral aneurysms are located at the anterior bifurcations of the Circle of Willis. Fifteen percent occur at the posterior bifurcations.

6. **Correct Answer: D**
   An explosive headache is the most common symptom. It frequently is the last thing patients say before losing consciousness.

7. **Correct Answer: C**
   AVMs lack the normal blood flow from arterial to venous flow without going through a capillary bed. This high pressure flow makes them more likely to bleed. They are not common, they occur slightly more often in men, and AVM's are the most common cause of stroke in children younger than 12 years of age.

8. **Correct Answer: B**
   A Glasgow Coma Scale assessment is imperative in monitoring for vascular spasm, a potentially life-threatening problem for a patient with a cerebral aneurysm. Vascular spasm occurs secondary to meningeal irritation caused by the presence of blood in the subarachnoid space.

9. **Correct Answer: A**
   An altered mental state is the primary symptom of encephalopathy. "Encephalopathy" is an umbrella term for a collection of symptoms produced by other illnesses. It can include liver or renal failure, infection, brain tumors, increasing hydrocephalus, and environmental hazard exposure.

10. **Correct Answer: C**

    Because there are so many potential causes, management of encephalopathy must focus on treating its cause. Examples of treatment include antibiotics, hemodialysis, and electrolyte replacement.

11. **Correct Answer: B**

    Blood tests can include CMP, CBC, and sedimentation rate, tests for specific illness or toxin, and potentially lumbar puncture to rule out neurologic infection. Other tests include electroencephalograms and imaging studies of specific structures (e.g., hepatic or renal imaging).

12. **Correct Answer: C**

    Level of consciousness is the most sensitive indicator of a patient's neurologic status. The brain tissue is extremely sensitive to even minute changes in oxygen and glucose levels. When cerebral edema occurs, as in a closed head injury, changes in these levels very quickly affect the patient's level of consciousness.

13. **Correct Answer: C**

    Battle's sign is seen as ecchymosis over the mastoid bone 12 to 24 hours after the injury. Rhinorrhea, raccoon's eyes, and subconjunctival hemorrhage are signs of an anterior fossa fracture.

14. **Correct Answer: A**

    The halo sign is indicative of a basilar skull fracture. This can be a dangerous sign for the patient, as meningitis can easily develop.

15. **Correct Answer: B**

    Because the catheter is inserted directly into one of the lateral ventricles, intraventriculosotomy is the most direct and accurate method of measuring intracranial pressure. The drain is inserted on the right side of the head. The ventriculostomy allows for not only drainage of excess CSF, but also sampling of CSF to monitor for infection.

16. **Correct Answer: B**

    Normal intracranial pressure is in the range of 4–15 mm Hg.

17. **Correct Answer: C**

    The foramen of Monroe is the junction between the lateral ventricles and the third ventricle. It is located just above the ear.

18. **Correct Answer: A**

    Cushing syndrome is also known as Cushing's triad. This triad of symptoms—increased systolic blood pressure, widening pulse pressure, and bradycardia—is a late indicator of a serious deterioration of neurologic status. This patient is at very high risk for herniation and death.

19. **Correct Answer: D**

    Lumbar punctures in a patient with increased intracranial pressure can lead to herniation of the tentorium or brain stem.

20. **Correct Answer: C**

    Absorption of cerebrospinal fluid at an increased rate decreases intracranial pressure. The other answers contribute to increased intracranial pressure.

21. **Correct Answer: C**
    Changes in level of consciousness are seen before other symptoms develop because the cerebral cortex is extremely sensitive to changes in oxygen pressure.

22. **Correct Answer: C**
    Diabetes insipidus (DI) is characterized by a serious decrease in antidiuretic hormone (ADH). The most common causes of neurogenic DI are closed head injury and posterior pituitary tumor removal. ADH is produced by the posterior pituitary gland. Closed head injury and cerebral edema lead to pressure on the pituitary gland, thereby decreasing ADH production. Other common causes of DI include lung cancer (small-cell or oat-cell carcinoma), leukemia, and lymphoma.

23. **Correct Answer: B**
    Intravenous replacement with $D_5W/\frac{1}{2}NS$ with 20 mEq of potassium is titrated to replace hourly urine output. Other therapies include DDAVP (Desmopressin) nasal spray or Pitressin infusion. Strict I&O and daily weights, monitoring electrolytes, and measurement of serum and urine osmolalities are also done.

24. **Correct Answer: A**
    Triple H therapy reduces the chance of vasospasm of the affected arteries by maintaining full vessels. Cerebral vasospasm after an aneurysm bleed greatly increases the patient's mortality risk.

25. **Correct Answer: C**
    Continued seizures deplete glucose and oxygen levels in the brain. The hypoxia causes cerebral edema and can lead to damage of the neurons.

26. **Correct Answer: B**
    Communicating hydrocephalus is caused when the blood cells from a subarachnoid hemorrhage block the arachnoid villi from reabsorbing the cerebrospinal fluid. This condition may be transient. If it is permanent, a ventriculo-peritoneal (VP) shunt will be placed.

27. **Correct Answer: B**
    Cerebral perfusion pressure equals mean arterial pressure minus intracranial pressure. CPP is a calculated measurement of the pressure gradient that allows blood to flow to the brain. It may also be calculated using the CVP instead of the ICP because it is a measure of vascular resistance.

28. **Correct Answer: A**
    Cerebral perfusion pressure is a calculated measurement of the pressure gradient that allows blood to flow to the brain. The goal is a CPP in the range of 50–80 mm Hg.

29. **Correct Answer: A**
    CN I is the most frequently affected cranial nerve in a basilar skull fracture; damage to this nerve leads to loss of the sense of smell. CN VII and CN VIII are less likely to be affected except in the case of a severe head injury. CN VII (Facial nerve) injury causes ipsilateral (same-side) paralysis. CN VIII (Acoustic nerve) injury can interrupt balance and hearing.

30. **Correct Answer: C**

Nystagmus indicates pressure or damage to Cranial nerve VIII (Acoustic) in the vestibular portion. Shaking is usually stronger on one side and may occur in any of the cardinal eye directions.

31. **Correct Answer: B**

Syndrome of inappropriate antidiuretic hormone is caused by interrupted feedback of the osmotic stimuli and continuous antidiuretic hormone secretion, which lead to fluid intoxication and electrolyte imbalance. Oat-cell carcinoma is a common cause of SIADH due to its high rate of metastasis to the brain.

32. **Correct Answer: A**

SIADH has many causes. The most common include bronchogenic (oat cell) cancer, pneumonia, and head injury. Less common causes include stroke, tuberculosis, Guillain-Barré syndrome, meningitis, encephalitis, multiple sclerosis, subarachnoid hemorrhage, pancreatic cancer, and lymphoma.

33. **Correct Answer: D**

The knee jerk (also known as the patellar reflex or deep tendon reflex) is an example of a functional lower motor neuron. These reflexes are also known as deep tendon reflexes. The nerve impulse makes an arc from the tendon to the sensory portion of the spinal cord to the motor root and back to the patella, causing extension of the lower leg.

34. **Correct Answer: C**

The spinothalamic tract carries impulses from the spine to the thalamus; thus it is a sensory motor tract. The lateral spinothalamic tract senses pain and temperature; the anterior tract senses light touch and pressure.

35. **Correct Answer: C**

Autonomic hyperreflexia, also known as autonomic dysreflexia, is caused by numerous stimuli such as bowel or bladder dysfunction, cool breezes, a clogged urinary catheter, or constipation.

36. **Correct Answer: B**

Autonomic hyperreflexia is a potentially life-threatening response to a minor stimulus; it is seen after spinal cord injury at T6 or higher. It occurs after the initial spinal shock has resolved. Symptoms can include severe hypertension, dysrhythmias, severe headache, and photophobia.

37. **Correct Answer: B**

SIADH causes hemodilution and therefore the treatment is centered on normalizing serum and urine osmolality.

38. **Correct Answer: B**

In a normal doll's eyes (oculocephalic) reflex, the eyes appear to move to the opposite direction from the head turn. For example, if the head is turned quickly to the patient's left, the eyes normally appear to move to the far right side. If the reflex is absent, the eyes appear fixed and do not move. This is a poor neurologic sign. It represents pontine and midbrain damage. It may be utilized in determining brain death.

39. **Correct Answer: B**
The Glasgow Coma Scale measures eye opening, motor response, and verbal response. It rates each parameter so that possible total scores range from 3 to 15, where 15 indicates a fully responsive patient. A score of 6 or 7 is comatose level. The longer the patient remains in the lower score ranges, the worse the projected outcome.

40. **Correct Answer: B**
A score of 6 or 7 is comatose level on the Glasgow Coma Scale. A score of 15 is a patient who is fully awake. A score of 3 means there is no eye, motor, or verbal response from the patient.

41. **Correct Answer: C**
Decerebrate posturing indicates pressure on the midbrain and pons. It is a very poor neurologic sign, especially if it continues for more than 4 hours.

42. **Correct Answer: D**
Brown–Sequard syndrome causes ipsilateral (same-side) motor paralysis and contralateral (opposite-side) loss of pain and temperature sensation. This syndrome occurs because of the way the pyramidal tracts cross in the spinal column.

43. **Correct Answer: B**
Ipsilateral (same-side) pupil dilation is a symptom seen with uncal herniation across the tentorium. The tentorium is a fold of dura mater that supports the temporal and occipital lobes. This herniation puts pressure directly on CN III, causing pupil dilation.

44. **Correct Answer: B**
Neisseria meningitidis is the causative agent for meningococcal meningitis. *Streptococcus pneumoniae* causes pneumococcal meningitis. *Haemophilius influenzae* causes *Haemophilius* meningitis. *Staphylococcus aureus* is not likely to cause meningitis but can cause infection in the brain when the patient has ventriculostomy drains or bolts.

45. **Correct Answer: B**
Petechiae are the hallmark symptom of meningococcal meningitis. The other symptoms can be seen with any form of meningitis.

46. **Correct Answer: A**
Guillain-Barré syndrome is a demyelinating autoimmune process affecting the spinal and cranial nerves. It is seen after viral infections.

47. **Correct Answer: C**
A positive Babinski or Plantar reflex is a sign of an upper motor neuron lesion. This pathologic sign can be seen with spinal cord compression, head injury, or stroke.

48. **Correct Answer: B**
The proper technique is to stroke the lateral sole of the foot from the heel up to and across the ball of the foot. It should be done in one motion with a relatively sharp instrument such as the end of a reflex hammer.

49. **Correct Answer: B**
Cerebrospinal fluid is formed by the choroid plexus of the third ventricle. The arachnoid villi—projections from the subarachnoid space—reabsorb the cerebrospinal fluid.

50. **Correct Answer: C**

The choroid plexus in the third ventricle produce 400 to 800 mL of cerebrospinal fluid each day. Approximately 125 to 150 mL of CSF is circulating in the ventricular system and spinal column at any one time.

51. **Correct Answer: C**

Cerebrospinal fluid should be clear and colorless, with a protein count of 16–45 mg/dL, WBC of 0–5 cells/mm^2, and glucose levels approximately 80% of serum glucose levels.

52. **Correct Answer: B**

The six cardinal eye movements test CN II (Oculomotor), CN IV (Trochlear), and CN VI (Abducens). CN III is assessed by having the patient follow the examiner's finger or light up and out, up and in, down and out, and inward toward the nose. CN IV is assessed by having the patient follow the examiner's finger down and in toward the tip of the nose. CN VI is assessed by having the patient follow the examiner's finger out toward the ear.

53. **Correct Answer: C**

The frontal lobe is responsible for personality, memory, motor function, contains Broca's area, and critical thinking skills.

54. **Correct Answer: D**

A RIND is a reversible ischemic neurologic deficit. It is similar to a TIA, but the symptoms last more than 24 hours. The patient recovers completely from a RIND.

55. **Correct Answer: A**

TIAs typically last a very short time—sometimes less than an hour but no longer than 24 hours—and do not cause any neurologic deficits. With a RIND, the symptoms last more than 24 hours but the patient still has a complete recovery. Both TIAs and RINDs may be precursors of a major stroke within a year.

56. **Correct Answer: C**

Uncontrolled hypertension is the most common cause of stroke in the United States. More than 360,000 strokes occur each year as a result of hypertension. For many patients, stroke is the first symptom of hypertension. Diabetes mellitus can lead to cardiovascular disease and hypertension, but it is less common than hypertension alone.

57. **Correct Answer: B**

Alcohol use, smoking, and obesity are all modifiable risk factors in preventing stroke.

58. **Correct Answer: B**

Hemorrhagic strokes are usually caused by hypertension and may include aneurysm rupture. Ischemic strokes are usually caused by an occlusion of an atherosclerotic cerebral artery secondary to an embolus or occlusion.

59. **Correct Answer: C**

Diabetes mellitus causes accelerated atherosclerosis in the large arteries of the cerebral circulation, thereby narrowing the lumens of the arteries.

60. **Correct Answer: B**

A lacunar infarction is caused by thrombosis of the small arteries that penetrate the cerebrum. It causes facial, arm, and leg deficits.

61. **Correct Answer: C**
    The dominant side of the brain is the most likely site for a cerebrovascular accident. Since more than 90% of the population is right side dominant, the left hemisphere is most likely to suffer a stroke.

62. **Correct Answer: B**
    A left-side cerebrovascular accident causes right-side deficits because of crossing of the cerebrospinal tracts in the brain and spinal cord.

63. **Correct Answer: B**
    Prevention of aspiration should be the priority of the critical care nurse. The other answers are also a part of caring for a patient with a cerebrovascular accident, but the ABCs (airway, breathing, circulation) are always the first priority.

64. **Correct Answer: B**
    Broca's area at the lower edge of the frontal lobe is responsible for verbal expression. A deficit in this area is called expressive aphasia. The patient can comprehend what is said but lacks the ability to form the words due to loss of motor skills.

65. **Correct Answer: C**
    This patient has had a stroke affecting Wernicke's area in the temporal lobe, which affects verbal reception. Damage to Wernicke's area leads to an inability to interpret speech. It can also affect comprehension of written words.

66. **Correct Answer: D**
    The homunculus is the outer strip of the cerebral cortex that involves the motor functioning of the frontal lobe and the sensory functioning of the parietal lobe. It demonstrates how much of the cortex controls each body part. For example, in the parietal lobe, very large sections of the cortex are devoted to the face, hands, and feet due to the complexity of the sensations necessary for the protection of these extremities. In the frontal lobe, a larger portion of the motor cortex is devoted to the face, hands, and tongue.

67. **Correct Answer: B**
    The negative inspiratory force measures the ability of the patient to take a deep breath to minus 28 mm Hg. Once the effort is less than 28 mm Hg, the patient should be evaluated for intubation to prevent respiratory arrest.

68. **Correct Answer: B**
    Protein in the CSF is always increased with Guillain-Barré syndrome due to the destruction of the myelin sheath. Because Guillain-Barré syndrome is an autoimmune disorder, WBCs, abnormal glucose levels, and bacteria would not be present in the CSF.

69. **Correct Answer: A**
    Patients with Guillain-Barré syndrome experience motor weakness, impaired respiratory function, and acute pain. These are the most important nursing diagnoses. The pain is caused by an accentuated sympathetic response secondary to the loss of parasympathetic counterbalance.

70. **Correct Answer: C**
    The autonomic dysfunction observed in Guillain-Barré syndrome is caused by a lack of balance in the autonomic nervous system. The sympathetic nervous system is unopposed, causing heightened sensitivity and leading to an over-response to minor stimuli.

71. **Correct Answer: B**
Respiratory status and neurologic signs are the most important nursing management issues, especially in the early onset of the demyelinating process.

72. **Correct Answer: B**
Risk for impaired respiratory function is the most important nursing diagnosis. Other nursing diagnoses include acute pain, risk for impaired verbal communication, and potential for neuromuscular weakness related to demyelination.

73. **Correct Answer: C**
Crows are a well-known vector for the mosquitoes that spread West Nile virus. Fleas are the vector for bubonic plague and field mice are the vector for Hantavirus.

74. **Correct Answer: C**
Erythematous rash and lymphadenopathy are indicative of infection with West Nile virus. Other common signs of any vector-borne viral encephalitis include flu-like symptoms such as fever, chills, malaise, headache, nausea, and vomiting.

75. **Correct Answer: B**
Monitoring neurologic signs, urinary output, and moustache dressing changes are the most important post-operative cares for the patient with a transphenoidal resection of a pituitary tumor. Daily weights are important, as are vital signs. Patients who undergo this surgery are at risk for developing diabetes insipidus due to a lack of ADH.

76. **Correct Answer: A**
Clipping of the aneurysm and endovascular coiling are the two most common methods of managing aneurysms. Tissue plasminogen activator (tPA) is a thrombolytic and would not be given to this patient. Controlling the blood pressure involves maintaining good cerebral perfusion pressure to reduce the risk of vasospasm. Amicar inhibits plasminogen activator, allowing fibrin production.

77. **Correct Answer: B**
Status epilepticus decreases the amount of oxygen and glucose in the brain leading to the release of glutamate. The increased glutamate causes an influx of calcium into the neurons, destabilizing them electronically and leading to cell injury and death.

78. **Correct Answer: B**
The best action is to turn Nancy to her right side and protect her airway. Because the seizure has already started, it would be impossible to safely insert an oral airway. Never try to restrain a patient who is having a seizure. Hitting the Code Blue button is certainly an option but it doesn't help the patient immediately. Precipitating events, aura, onset, duration, nursing actions, and postictal state should be included in the nursing notes.

79. **Correct Answer: C**
This patient should be given a psychological evaluation. If he had a genuine grand mal seizure, the postictal state is expected to last several hours and the patient would not be able to request food.

80. **Correct Answer: D**
CBC, CMP, sedimentation rate, CRP, RPR, and toxicology screen are the tests that need to be performed to establish the cause of John Doe's seizures. Seizures can be caused by

illness, infection, overdose on drugs or alcohol, tertiary syphilis, dehydration, electrolyte imbalance, and cardiac arrhythmia.

81. **Correct Answer: C**
    Panic attacks, transient ischemic attacks, cardiac arrhythmias, and syncope are some causes of seizures.

82. **Correct Answer: C**
    It is important to monitor the temporal artery for blood flow in patients with CEA. A change in the flow can signal bleeding or swelling at the surgical site. Neurologic signs are important to monitor for possible stroke.

83. **Correct answer: C**
    A 70% stenosis has a significant risk–benefit ratio to justify surgery.

84. **Correct Answer: B**
    Aggrenox is a persantine-based medication given twice-daily to patients with stroke or TIA.

85. **Correct Answer: B**
    Multiple sclerosis is a demyelinating disorder of the white matter of the brain and spinal cord. It can be intermittent, progressive, or relapsing. It follows an acute or progressive course. Multiple sclerosis is the major cause of disability in young adults ages 16 to 40, and it affects females more frequently than males.

86. **Correct Answer: C**
    Fran is angry at her diagnosis and afraid she will suffer the same fate as her mother. The five stages of grief identified by Kubler-Ross (1969) are denial, anger, bargaining, depression, and acceptance. The patient can move through the stages in any order and can revisit a stage at any time. The nurse should try to encourage the patient to express her feelings. The physician should also be notified, and the patient should receive counseling. Antidepressants may be considered.

87. **Correct Answer: C**
    Multiple sclerosis produces a wide variety of symptoms depending on the white matter affected by the exacerbation. These symptoms include both motor and sensory problems, include ataxia, Babinski reflex, vision disturbances, clumsiness, emotional lability, fatigue, paresthesias, paralysis, hyperactive deep tendon reflexes, loss of proprioception, loss of vibratory sense, impotence in men, and urinary problems in women.

88. **Correct Answer: B**
    Although the exact cause of multiple sclerosis is unknown, it is thought to be an autoimmune disorder triggered by environmental exposure or viral illness. Clusters have been found in Northern European families, and there is a higher incidence of the disease in people who work with manganese.

89. **Correct Answer: A**
    Cerebrospinal fluid evaluation includes negative syphilis (RPR), abnormal; colloid gold curve, increased IgG, myelin debris, slightly increased protein. Other tests include FTA-ABS, sedimentation rate, and HTLV-1 serology. The patient should also be checked for vasculitic disorders. Neurologic testing includes evoked responses that are highly predicative for MS. An MRI scan will show plaques as white spots in the brain.

90. **Correct Answer: D**
Relapsing–remitting and progressive are the most common forms of multiple sclerosis. The frequency of relapsing–remitting episodes is related to stress and illness. Progressive disease may follow a continuous but slow route, or it may advance quickly to the patient's death. Relapsing–remitting disease may worsen to progressive MS.

91. **Correct Answer: B**
Ascending, descending, Miller–Fischer Variant, and pure motor are the 4 types of Guillain-Barré syndrome. Ascending disease is the classic form of weakness and numbness that starts in the legs and moves up the trunk to involve the cranial nerves in some patients. The weakness is symmetrical. Descending disease affects the cranial nerves first; and the weakness progresses caudally. Respiratory failure is a major problem for patients with the descending form of Guillain-Barré syndrome. Miller–Fisher Variant is a very rare form of Guillain-Barré syndrome that is characterized by a triad of symptoms that includes ophthalmoplegia, areflexia, and pronounced ataxia. The pure motor form of Guillain-Barré syndrome is identical to the ascending form, but there is limited sensory involvement and, therefore, no pain.

92. **Correct Answer: C**
The Tensilon test is often used to diagnose myasthenia gravis because of the ease of administration. The medication, given as 10 mg intravenously, has a quick onset and a short half-life. If there is improvement in a weak muscle, the Tensilon test is considered to be positive. The Weber and Rinne tests assess hearing. Clonus is a reflex used to test spasticity.

93. **Correct Answer: B**
Myasthenia gravis is a pure motor disorder that occurs when an autoimmune response at the neuromuscular junction destroys acetylcholine receptors on the muscle membrane. Answer A is multiple sclerosis, answer C is Guillain-Barré syndrome, and answer D is amyotrophic lateral sclerosis (ALS).

94. **Correct Answer: C**
Most myasthenia gravis symptoms are linked to the weakness caused by the lack of acetylcholine receptors at the neuromuscular junction. These symptoms include ptosis, diplopia, facial weakness, dysphagia, dysarthria, neck weakness, proximal limb weakness, respiratory weakness, and generalized weakness.

95. **Correct Answer: A**
Cholinergic crisis is a life-threatening problem that may occur with any overdose—accidental or otherwise. It causes bradycardia, severe weakness, cardiac arrest, and occasionally respiratory arrest.

BIBLIOGRAPHY

Ahrens, T. (2006). *Critical care nursing certification*. Columbus, OH: McGraw-Hill.

Akopian, G., Gaspard, D. J., & Alexander, M. (2007). Outcomes of blunt head trauma without intracranial pressure monitoring. *American Surgeon, 73*(5), 447–450.

Alspach, J. G. (2006). *American Association of Critical-Care Nurses: Core curriculum for critical care nursing* (6th ed.). Philadelphia: Saunders.

American Association of Critical-Care Nurses. (2006). *Core curriculum for critical care nursing* (6th ed.). Philadelphia: Saunders.

American Association of Critical-Care Nurses. (2007). *AACN certification and core review for high acuity and critical care* (6th ed.). Philadelphia: Saunders.

American Heart Association. (2007). *Guidelines 2005 for cardiopulmonary resuscitation and emergency cardiovascular care*. Retrieved July 24, 2008, from http://circ.ahajournals.org/content/vol112/24_suppl/

Bader, M. K., & Littlejohns, L. R. (2004). *AANN core curriculum for neuroscience nursing* (4th ed.). St. Louis: Saunders.

Ball, C., & Westhorpe, R. N. (2006). Muscle relaxants: Reversal agents. *Anaesthesia and Intensive Care, 34*(4), 415.

Barker, E. (Ed.). (2002). *Neuroscience nursing: A spectrum of care* (2nd ed.). St. Louis, MO: Mosby.

Bickley, L. S., & Szilagyi, P. G. (2003). *Bates' guide to physical examination and history taking* (8th ed.). Philadelphia: Lippincott, Williams & Wilkins.

Brain Injury Association of America. (2006). *Facts about traumatic brain injury*. Retrieved January 15, 2008, from http://www.biausa.org/aboutbi.htm

Braunwald, E., Fauci, A. S., Kasper, D. L., Hauser, S. L., Longo, D. L., & Jameson, J. L. (Eds.). (2001). *Harrison's principles of internal medicine* (15th ed.). New York: McGraw-Hill.

Burns, S. M. (Ed.). (2007). *American Association of Critical-Care Nurses (AACN): AACN protocols for practice: Healing environments* (2nd ed.). Sudbury, MA: Jones and Bartlett.

Centers for Disease Control and Prevention. (2008). *Spinal cord injuries: Acute injury care*. Retrieved March 23, 2008, from http://www.cdc.gov/ncipc/dir/AcuteInjuryCare.htm

Chen, H., Richard, M., Sandler, D. P., Umbach, D. M., & Kamel, F. (2007). Head injury and amyotrophic lateral sclerosis. *American Journal of Epidemiology, 166*(7), 810–816.

Chernecky, C. C., & Berger, B. J. (2001). *Laboratory tests and diagnostic procedures* (3rd ed.). Philadelphia: Saunders.

Chieregato, A., Tanfani, A., Compagnone, C., Turrini, C., Sarpieri, F., Ravaldini, M., et al. (2007). Global cerebral blood flow and CPP after severe head injury: A xenon-CT study. *Intensive Care Medicine, 33*(5), 856–862.

Cho, S. J., Minn, Y. K., & Kwon, K. H. (2007). Stroke after burn. *Cerebrovascular Diseases, 24*(2–3), 261–263.

Conover, M. B. (2003). *Understanding electrocardiography* (8th ed.). St. Louis, MO: Mosby/Elsevier.

Copstead, L., & Banasik, J. L. (2000). *Pathophysiology: Biological and behavioral perspectives* (2nd ed.). Philadelphia: Saunders/Elsevier.

Crawford-Faucher, A. (2008). When is CT indicated after minor head injury? *American Family Physician, 77*(2), 228, 231.

Curley, M. A. Q. (1998). Patient–nurse synergy: Optimizing patients' outcomes. *American Journal of Critical Care, 7,* 64–72.

Delye, H., Verschueren, P., Depreitere, B., Verpoest, I., Berckmans, D., Vander Sloten, J., et al. (2007). Biomechanics of frontal skull fracture. *Journal of Neurotrauma, 24*(10), 1576–1586

Dossey, B. M., Keegan, L., & Guzzetta, C. (2003). *Holistic nursing: A handbook for practice* (3rd ed.). Boston: Jones & Bartlett.

Edwards, D. F. (1999). The Synergy Model: Linking patient needs to nurse competencies. *Critical Care Nurse, 19*(1): 88–98.

Eide, P. K., Bentsen, G., Stanisic, M., & Stubhaug, A. (2007). Association between intracranial pulse pressure levels and brain energy metabolism in a patient with an aneurysmal subarachnoid haemorrhage. *Acta Anaesthesiologica Scandinavica, 51*(9), 1273–1276.

Emergency Nurses Association & Newberry, L. (2003). *Sheehy's emergency nursing: Principles and practice* (5th ed.). St. Louis, MO: Mosby/Elsevier.

Finkelmeier, B. A. (2000). *Cardiothoracic surgical nursing* (2nd ed.). Philadelphia: Lippincott, Williams & Wilkins.

Flachenecker, P. (2007). Autonomic dysfunction in Guillain-Barré syndrome and multiple sclerosis. *Journal of Neurology, 254*(suppl), II96–II101.

Gilman, S., & Newman, S. W. (2003). *Manter and Gatz's essentials of clinical neuroanatomy and neurophysiology* (10th ed.). Philadelphia: F. A. Davis.

Greim, B., Engel, C., Apel, A., & Zettl, U. K. (2007). Fatigue in neuroimmunological diseases. *Journal of Neurology, 254*(suppl), II102–II106.

Hardin, S. R., & Kaplow, R. (Eds.). (2004). *Synergy for clinical excellence: The AACN Synergy Model for Patient Care.* Boston: Jones and Bartlett.

Hickey, J. V. (2002). *The clinical practice of neurological and neurosurgical nursing* (5th ed.). Philadelphia: Lippincott, Williams & Wilkins.

Hoge, C. H., McGurk, D., Thomas, J. L., Cox, A. L., Engel, C. C., & Castro, C. A. (2008). Mild traumatic brain injury in U.S. soldiers returning from Iraq. *New England Journal of Medicine, 358*(5), 453–463.

Hughes, R. A. C., Swan, A. V., Raphaël, J. C., Annane, D., van Koningsveld, R., & van Doorn, P. A. (2007). Immunotherapy for Guillain-Barré syndrome: A systematic review. *Brain, 130*(9), 2245–2257.

Iseki, K., Mezaki, T., Kawamoto, Y., Tomimoto, H., Fukuyama, H., & Shibasaki, H. (2007). Concurrence of non-myasthenic symptoms with myasthenia gravis. *Neurological Sciences, 28*(2), 114–115.

Juurlink, D. N., Stukel, T. A., Kwong, J., Kopp, A., McGeer, A., Upshur, R. E., et al. (2006). Guillain-Barré syndrome after influenza vaccination in adults. *Archives of Internal Medicine, 166*(20), 2217–2221.

Keris, V., Lavendelis, E., & Macane, I. (2007). Association between implementation of clinical practice guidelines and outcome for traumatic brain injury. *World Journal of Surgery, 31*(6), 1352–1355.

Kilpatrick, A. M., LaDeau, S. L., & Marra, P. P. (2007). Ecology of West Nile virus transmission and its impact on birds in the Western hemisphere. *Auk, 124*(4), 1121–1136.

Labuz-Roszak, B., & Pierzchala, K. (2007). Difficulties in the diagnosis of autonomic dysfunction in multiple sclerosis. *Clinical Autonomic Research, 17*(6), 375–377.

Lipson, J. G., Dibble, S. L., & Minarik, P. A. (Eds.). (1996). *Culture and nursing care: A pocket guide.* San Francisco, CA: UCSF Nursing Press.

Logullo, F., Manicone, M., Di Bella, P., & Provinciali, L. (2006). Asymmetric Guillain-Barré syndrome. *Neurological Sciences, 27*(5), 355–359.

McCance, K. L., & Huether, S. E. (2002). *Pathophysiology: The biologic basis for disease in adults and children* (4th ed.). St Louis, MO: Mosby.

McNally, P. (2001). *GI/liver secrets* (2nd ed.). Philadelphia: Hanley & Belfus/Elsevier.

McQuillan, K. A., Von Rueden, K. T., Hartsock, R. L., Flynn, M. B., & Whalen, E. (Eds.). (2002). *Trauma nursing: From resuscitation through rehabilitation* (3rd ed.). Philadelphia: Saunders/Elsevier.

Medina, J., & Puntillo, K. (2006). *AACN protocols for practice: Palliative care and end-of-life issues in critical care.* Sudbury, MA: Jones and Bartlett.

Pagana, K. D., & Pagana, J. (2005). *Mosby's manual of diagnostic and laboratory tests* (3rd ed.). St. Louis, MO: Mosby/Elsevier.

Papadakis, M., Fee, P., Wilhelm, T., Davenport, A., & Connolly, J. (2007). Facial weakness in a haemodialysis patient. *Lancet, 369*(9562), 714.

Parker, T. M., Osternig, L. R., van Donkelaar, P., & Chou, L. S. (2007). Recovery of cognitive and dynamic motor function following concussion. *British Journal of Sports Medicine, 41*(12), 868.

Pascual, J. L., Maloney-Wilensky, E., Reilly, P. M., Sicoutris, C., Keutmann, M. K., Stein, S. C., et al. (2008, March). Resuscitation of hypotensive head-injured patients: Is hypertonic saline the answer? *American Surgeon, 74*(3), 253–259.

Rios, M., Daniel, S., Chancey, C., Hewlett, I. K., & Stramer, S. L. (2007). West Nile virus adheres to human red blood cells in whole blood. *Clinical Infectious Diseases, 45*(2), 181.

Ruts, L., van Koningsveld, R., Jacobs, B. C., & van Doorn, P. A. (2007). Determination of pain and response to methylprednisolone in Guillain-Barré syndrome. *Journal of Neurology, 254*(10), 1318–1323.

Sammarco, C. L. (2007). A case study: Identifying alcohol abuse in multiple sclerosis. *Journal of Neuroscience Nursing, 39*(6), 373–376.

Sejvar, J. J. (2007). The long-term outcomes of human West Nile virus infection. *Clinical Infectious Diseases, 44*(12), 1617.

Seneviratne, J., Mandrekar, J., Wijdicks, E. F. M., & Rabinstein, A. A. (2008). Noninvasive ventilation in myasthenic crisis. *Archives of Neurology, 65*(1), 54.

Shafi, S., Diaz-Arrastia, R., Madden, C., & Gentilello, L. (2008). Intracranial pressure monitoring in brain-injured patients is associated with worsening of survival. *Journal of Trauma, 64*(2), 335–340.

Siedel, H. M., Ball, J. W., Dains, J. E., & Benedict, G. W. (2003). *Mosby's physical examination handbook* (3rd ed.). St. Louis, MO: Mosby.

Siegel, A., & Siegel, H. (2002). *Neuroscience: Pretest self-assessment and review* (5th ed.). New York: McGraw-Hill.

Skidmore-Roth, L. (2004). *Mosby's 2004 nursing drug reference.* St. Louis, MO: Mosby/Elsevier.

Smeltzer, S., & Bare, B. G. (2003). *Brunner and Suddarth's textbook of medical–surgical nursing* (10th ed.). Philadelphia: Lippincott, Williams & Wilkins.

Sole, M. L., Hartshorn, J., & Lamborne, M. L. (2001). *Introduction to critical care nursing* (3rd ed.). Philadelphia: Saunders/Elsevier.

Stewart-Amidei, C., & Kunkel, J. A. (2001). *AANN's neuroscience nursing: Human responses to neurologic dysfunction* (2nd ed.). Philadelphia: Saunders.

Stocchetti, N., Colombo, A., Ortolanoet, F., et al. (2007). Time course of intracranial hypertension after traumatic brain injury. *Journal of Neurotrauma, 24*(8), 1339–1346.

Swinton, F., & Schuster-Bruce, M. (2007). Epidural haematomas. *Anaesthesia, 62*(12), 1299.

Takahashi, M., Tsunemi, T., Miyayosi, T., & Mizusawa, H. (2007). Reversible central neurogenic hyperventilation in an awake patient with multiple sclerosis. *Journal of Neurology, 254*(12), 1763–1764.

Tarek, D., Sharshar, O., Porcher, R., Annane, D., Claude, J., & Clair, B. (2006). Prognosis and risk factors of early onset pneumonia in ventilated patients with Guillain-Barré syndrome. *Intensive Care Medicine, 32*(12), 1962–1969.

Tiemstra, J. D., & Khatkhate, N. (2007). Bell's palsy: Diagnosis and management. *American Family Physician, 76*(7), 997–1002.

Urden, L. D., Stacy, K. M., & Lough, M. E. (2007). *Thelan's critical care nursing: Diagnosis and management* (5th ed.). St. Louis, MO: Mosby.

van de Beek, D., Kremers, W., Daly, R. C., Edwards, B. S., Clavell, A. L., McGregor, C. G., et al. (2008). Effect of neurologic complications on outcome after heart transplant. *Archives of Neurology, 65*(2), 226.

Venes, D. (2001). *Taber's cyclopedic medical dictionary* (19th ed.). Philadelphia: F. A. Davis.

Wiegand, D. J. L., & Carlson, K. K. (Eds.). (2005). *AACN procedure manual for critical care* (5th ed.). Philadelphia: Elsevier.

Woods, S., Sivarajan Froelicher, E. S., & Motzer, S. U. (2000). *Cardiac nursing* (4th ed.). Philadelphia: Lippincott, Williams & Wilkins.

World Health Organization. (2006). Meningococcal vaccine and Guillain-Barré syndrome. *WHO Drug Information, 20*(4), 247–248.

Zhao, X., Rizzo, A., Malek, B., Fakhry, S., & Watson, J. (2008). Basilar skull fracture: A risk factor for transverse/sigmoid venous sinus obstruction. *Journal of Neurotrauma, 25*(2), 104–111.

Gastrointestinal

QUESTIONS

1. A regular diet would be inappropriate for a stroke patient with which of the following cranial nerve(s) directly involved?
   A. Cranial nerve I
   B. Cranial nerves II and III
   C. Cranial nerves V and VII
   D. Cranial nerve VIII

2. Assessment of the abdomen should occur in which order?
   A. Inspection, palpation, auscultation, percussion
   B. Auscultation, inspection, palpation, percussion
   C. Percussion, inspection, palpation, auscultation
   D. Inspection, auscultation, percussion, palpation

3. Your patient has been diagnosed with chronic liver disease. In addition to a venous hum or murmur, which finding might you note during abdominal auscultation?
   A. Aortic bruit
   B. Hepatic bruit
   C. Iliac artery bruit
   D. Renal artery bruit

4. Your patient is suspected to have a biliary obstruction. Which of the following diagnostic procedures would confirm this diagnosis?
   A. Flexible sigmoidoscopy
   B. Colonoscopy
   C. Angiography
   D. Endoscopic retrograde cholangiopancreatography (ERCP)

5. Melena stools indicate bleeding from which area?
   A. Mouth
   B. Upper gastrointestinal area
   C. Descending colon
   D. Melena stools are not caused by bleeding, but from iron ingestion.

6. Normal portal pressures are
   A. 5–10 mm Hg.
   B. 10–20 mm Hg.
   C. 5 mm Hg below the inferior vena cava pressure.
   D. 10 mm Hg above the inferior vena cava pressure.

7. Your patient has acute esophageal and gastric varices. Which esophagogastric tamponade tube is the best choice for differentiating bleeding from the esophagus or the stomach?
   A. Minnesota tube
   B. Sengstaken–Blakemore tube
   C. Linton–Nachlas tube
   D. Standard nasogastric tube

8. Your patient has a history of transphenoidal hypohysectomy. Which of the following procedures is absolutely contraindicated?
   A. Nasal placement with gastric tube
   B. Oral placement with gastric tube
   C. Oral intubation with endotracheal tube
   D. Tracheal intubation

9. You have just assisted with the insertion of an esophageal and gastric balloon. Tamponade therapy duration should be carefully documented because
   A. Prolonged inflation may lead to necrosis or ulceration.
   B. Patient comfort increases 24 hours after balloon placement.
   C. Hgb and Hct should drop after placement.
   D. Enteral feeding may be given via the tube after 36 hours.

10. Your patient with a Minnesota tube has a sudden drop in oral secretions and esophageal balloon pressures. You should
    A. Provide oral care and check the patient again in 2 hours.
    B. Document pressures and check the patient again in 2 hours.
    C. Check for bleeding and notify the physician.
    D. Attempt to reinflate the balloon to 70 mm Hg.

11. Your 18-year-old patient overdosed on Valium and Paxil. Gastric lavage is ordered. This is best accomplished if
    A. It is done within 60 minutes of ingestion.
    B. 0.45% normal saline is used.
    C. Lavage is not recommended for this type of overdose.
    D. The ingestion is liquefied first.

12. The wife of your 55-year-old patient with newly diagnosed acute hepatitis A asks if her husband is getting better. Her husband's AST, ALT, alkaline phosphate, and GGT levels are returning to normal after being severely high. The PT, INR, and bilirubin levels are still rising. You tell her:
    A. "Of course. The important labs are improving."
    B. "I can't talk to you. You don't have power of attorney."
    C. "No, but you have to wait for the doctor to explain more."
    D. "Although some of the labs are stabilizing, the increasing PT, INR, and bilirubin indicate that your husband is still very ill."

13. **Which of the following are late signs of acute liver failure?**
    A. Increased ICP, increased mean arterial pressure, and normal CPP
    B. Decreased ICP, decreased mean arterial pressure, and elevated CPP
    C. Increased ICP, decreased mean arterial pressure, and decreased CPP
    D. Decreased ICP, increased mean arterial pressure, and normal CPP

14. **The daughters of your patient with severe biliary obstruction notice that their father has multiple scratches and excoriations over his skin. They are concerned that their father is being abused. You explain:**
    A. "Do not panic, we are not abusing him."
    B. "I understand you are concerned. Because of the high bilirubin levels, he scratches unconsciously."
    C. "He must have gotten out of the restraints."
    D. "He did it to himself as a result of ICU psychosis."

15. **The most common cause of death related to acute hepatic failure is**
    A. Brain stem herniation.
    B. Anemia.
    C. Pulmonary embolism.
    D. Pulmonary edema.

16. **The family of your 48-year-old patient with chronic liver failure would like to know what they can do to make him more comfortable. You tell them that they can**
    A. Provide deep tissue massage every 2 hours.
    B. Apply a moisturizing lotion when visiting.
    C. Assist with rapid range-of-motion exercises every 4 hours.
    D. Limit visitation to once a day.

17. **Hepatic encephalopathy has _____ grades based on _____ clinical findings.**
    A. 3; 4
    B. 4; 4
    C. 4; 5
    D. 5; 5

18. **Hepatorenal syndrome is a complication of hepatic failure caused by**
    A. Increased circulating plasma.
    B. Vasodilatation.
    C. Increased renal circulation.
    D. Release of mediators.

19. **Your 19-year-old patient was involved in a motor vehicle accident and suffered blunt abdominal trauma related to the seat belt placement. He complains of severe abdominal pain around the epigastric area that is knife-like and twisting. You also note a low-grade fever with diaphoresis, abdominal distention, decreased bowel tones, and rebound tenderness. You suspect**
    A. Pancreatitis.
    B. Acute liver failure.
    C. Gastrointestinal bleeding.
    D. Abdominal bruising.

20. A patient with acute pancreatitis had labs drawn this morning. A result you would expect to see would be:
    A. Elevated serum amylase
    B. Decreased serum lipase
    C. Elevated albumin
    D. Decreased trypsin level

21. Cullen's sign is
    A. A marbled appearance to the abdomen.
    B. Bruising of the scrotum or labia.
    C. A bluish discoloration of the flanks.
    D. A bluish discoloration of the periumbilical area.

22. Mrs. Jones has been in the ICU for 2 weeks and has developed a stress ulcer. Family members ask why the patient had developed an ulcer. You acknowledge their concern and explain
    A. There is a decrease in mucosal blood flow.
    B. There is an increase in mucus production.
    C. Ulcers are caused by fungal infections.
    D. Mrs. Jones had the ulcer before she was admitted to the hospital.

23. Mr. Gonzalez, a non-alcohol-abusing patient, was diagnosed with portal hypertension with direct variceal bleeding. His wedge hepatic venous pressure is less than his portal pressure due to portal vein thrombosis. This may be due to
    A. Chronic active hepatitis.
    B. Umbilical vein catheterization as a neonate.
    C. Metastatic carcinoma.
    D. Congestive heart failure.

24. Mr. Smith, who is 86 years old, is frequently admitted to your unit for alcohol-induced coma. Just prior to his transfer to a step-down unit, he begins projectile vomiting bright blood. You would first
    A. Position the patient flat.
    B. Obtain and insert a Linton–Nachlas tube.
    C. Place the patient on NPO and verify IV access.
    D. Start dopamine at 5 mcg/kg/min.

25. Mr. Naples is a 38-year-old businessman who is in town for an important conference. He was brought to the hospital after collapsing with continuous right upper quadrant pain, nausea, vomiting, and fever. He complains to you about his work schedule and his inability to take time off from work. He asks you which course of treatment will result in less in-hospital time. You tell him:
    A. "I understand your concern. I will ask the physician to speak to you about treatment options."
    B. "Delaying surgery may increase mortality."
    C. "Fifty percent of patients who choose to delay surgery eventually require emergency surgery."
    D. "Laparoscopic surgery requires even less hospital time and has a decreased risk of bile duct injury."

26. Tony, an 18-year-old student, was admitted with an acute appendix 4 days ago. Antibiotics and morphine have controlled his symptoms. As you are transferring him to a medical–surgical unit, he asks if the pain will ever come back. You tell him:
    A. "No. You should never have this problem again."
    B. "Yes, but not for several years."
    C. "Yes, but the pain will not be as severe."
    D. "Possibly. Approximately 33% of patients are readmitted and require surgery within 1 year."

27. Jake, a 21-year-old student, had an appendectomy in another state while on Spring break 1 week ago. He is admitted to the ICU with fever, nausea and vomiting, and abdominal pain with a red, swollen surgical incision. You anticipate
    A. Immediate surgery with IV antibiotics.
    B. Hydration and antibiotics.
    C. Bedside excision of abscess.
    D. Bedside wound debridement.

28. Joan, a 41-year-old housewife, just had surgery for peritonitis related to diverticulitis. During drug reconciliation, which of the following medications should Joan continue?
    A. Advil for headaches
    B. Prednisone for bronchitis
    C. Morphine for surgical pain
    D. Verapamil for atrial fibrillation

29. Jillian, a 20-year-old student, is 6 feet tall and weighs 80 pounds. She was found unconscious by her roommate in the bathroom. She was admitted for severe dehydration and starvation. You would expect to see
    A. Decreased serum lactate.
    B. Normal urinary nitrogen excretion.
    C. Decreased serum catecholamines, glucagon, and cortisol.
    D. Conservation of body fluids with third spacing.

30. Sarah, an 18-year-old model, is a recovering anorexic. You are preparing to transfer her to a medical–surgical unit when you notice that she has not touched her lunch. You would tell her:
    A. "It's okay. I know that hospital food is not gourmet, but the dinners are more appetizing."
    B. "If you don't eat, we will have to put a feeding tube in you."
    C. "You need to eat to regain strength and prevent complications. We will work with you to find foods that you like."
    D. "Food is not your enemy. Eating this is not going to make you fat."

31. Eric, a 45-year-old alcoholic with chronic pancreatitis, develops respiratory distress with dyspnea and pulmonary edema. These symptoms are due to
    A. Pulmonary capillary endothelial damage related to phospholipase A_2.
    B. Bronchospasm related to stress.
    C. Aspiration.
    D. Atelectasis.

32. Bill, a 58-year-old construction worker with cirrhosis, was admitted yesterday after attending a weekend party involving alcohol, drugs, and smoking. His A.M. lab results were as follows:

ALT 250 U/L   AST 150 U/L
Bilirubin 10 mg/dL   PT 23 sec   PLT 76×10^3/mm^3
Hgb 8.2 g/dL   Hct 32%

These results would indicate a high risk for
   A. Peptic ulcer disease.
   B. Variceal bleeding.
   C. Gastritis.
   D. Boerhaave's syndrome.

33. Nicolae, a 62-year-old Russian immigrant, is admitted to the ICU with vague epigastric discomfort, vomiting times one week, inability to eat more than a few bites of solid foods, weight loss, weakness, and postprandial fullness. Labs showed a Hgb level of 10.8 g/dL and a positive stool guiac. Based on these findings, you would expect to see which result after the upper gastrointestinal studies?
   A. "Unitis plastia"—leather bottle stomach
   B. Localized ulcer
   C. Esophageal varices
   D. Pyloric stenosis

34. Jerry, a 76-year-old retired teacher, is being admitted for dehydration and malnutrition after collapsing in his apartment. His daughter reports that he has been eating very bland, soft foods for 3 weeks due to reflux and difficulty swallowing. You suspect
   A. Partial tongue paralysis.
   B. Gastric cancer.
   C. Tracheal neoplasm.
   D. Esophageal neoplasm.

35. Joan's grandmother was diagnosed with colorectal cancer. Joan asks you how the location of the cancer is determined. You tell her:
   A. "All locations present in the same way."
   B. "Only with an MRI test do we know the location for certain."
   C. "We will be able to tell only by interpreting the lab results."
   D. "The symptoms present differently. A lower gastrointestinal series allows direct internal visualization of the location."

36. Robert is visiting his mother after she has undergone surgery for colorectal cancer. There is a familial history of polyposis and inflammatory bowel disease, and Robert is worried about his own risk of developing cancer. Which of the following statements is true regarding colorectal cancers?
   A. Adenocarcinomas are the least common cancer.
   B. Right colon lesions are rare.
   C. Left colon tumors spread, ulcerate, and erode blood vessels.
   D. Rectal tumors are associated with localized metastasis.

37. **Which form of hepatitis is caused by a DNA virus?**
    A. Hepatitis A
    B. Hepatitis B
    C. Hepatitis C
    D. Hepatitis D

38. **Which form of hepatitis is often misdiagnosed as gastroenteritis?**
    A. Hepatitis A
    B. Hepatitis B
    C. Hepatitis C
    D. Hepatitis E

39. **Rosie, a 22-year-old tattoo artist, complains of flu-like symptoms after a needle stick at work. She has increasing lethargy and decreased appetite with a weight loss of 10 pounds. Generally a cheerful and active person, she reports overwhelming malaise with a sense of foreboding. Nursing interventions include**
    A. Weight-bearing physical therapy every 6 hours.
    B. Extended teaching sessions regarding her disease process.
    C. An order for a low-fat, high-carbohydrate diet.
    D. Allowing 24-hour visitation to cheer up Rosie.

40. **Which of the following statements is true about hepatitis D?**
    A. Hepatitis D is detectable only when it occurs along with HBV infection.
    B. IgM rises late in the course of the hepatitis D infection.
    C. IgG rises slowly, and the increase is limited to only the acute phase of the hepatitis D infection.
    D. Hepatitis D is caused by an RNA virus that is able to self-replicate when it is present concurrently with HBV.

41. **Leena, a 24-year-old exchange student from Hungary, is brought in by her roommate after 9 weeks of flu-like symptoms, increasing bruising, headaches, pounding pulses, and fever. Which diagnosis and cause are mostly likely?**
    A. DIC related to bacterial infection
    B. Acute liver failure related to unintentional overdose of acetaminophen
    C. Vitamin K deficiency related to poor nutritional intake
    D. Anemia related to Gaucher's disease

42. **Which of the following lab tests would support a diagnosis of acute liver failure?**
    A. Decreased creatinine and BUN
    B. Increased serum glucose
    C. Negative hepatitis serology
    D. Factors V and VII levels less than or equal to 20% of normal levels

43. **Which of the following patients with acute liver failure has the best prognosis if liver transplantation does not occur?**
    A. A 51-year-old healthcare worker with hepatitis C
    B. A 32-year-old hippie with *Galerina* poisoning
    C. A 79-year-old patient with an accidental overdose of acetaminophen
    D. A 21-year-old bone marrow transplant recipient with graft-versus-host disease

44. Ascites is a common finding in patients with chronic liver failure. Which of the following statements about ascites is true?
    A. Ascites is a result of an increase in albumin.
    B. Ascites is the result of decreased hydrostatic pressure and increased oncotic pressures in the portal system.
    C. Ascites occurs secondary to aldosteronism.
    D. Ascites is characterized by an increased ventilation/perfusion (V/Q) ratio.

45. Bill's wife is concerned that her husband, who has cirrhosis, is not urinating. You tell her that this is a common complication of the disease process because there is
    A. An increase in the glomerular filtration ratio.
    B. An increase in renal blood flow.
    C. A decrease in the sodium reabsorption rate.
    D. An increase in renin and aldosterone levels.

46. You are admitting an emergency room patient to the MICU post head injury. As you perform your assessment, you note a stoma to the right iliac fossa in the lower abdomen. There are soft, scattered bowel tones. Output is loose, brownish-tinged without form. You would document your findings as a(n)
    A. Sigmoid colostomy.
    B. Ileostomy.
    C. Loop colostomy.
    D. Ascending colostomy.

47. Mrs. Lo, a 42-year-old female with severe Crohn's disease and perforation, returns from surgery with an ileostomy. Mrs. Lo is at greatest risk for which of the following complications?
    A. Prolapsed stoma due to vigorous exercise once discharged
    B. Hypernatremia
    C. Hemorrhage
    D. Dehydration

48. Mr. H. had abdominal surgery for perforation yesterday. Today's abdominal X rays show a double-bubble appearance. He is complaining of nausea with bile-stained emesis, abdominal distention, pain, and fever. The appropriate nursing intervention would be to
    A. Contact the surgeon and prepare for immediate surgery.
    B. Administer morphine and Tylenol, and then call the physician if there is no improvement.
    C. Position the patient flat and give him Tylenol.
    D. Do nothing; this is normal. The physician should be notified only if the abdomen becomes discolored.

49. Which of the following methods for measuring intra-abdominal pressures is most commonly found in the critical care setting?
    A. Intraperitoneal measurement with a peritoneal dialysis catheter
    B. Measurement of the bladder pressures via an indwelling urinary catheter
    C. Intragastric measurement with a nasogastric tube
    D. Rectal measurement with a rectal tube

50. Mr. K. was diagnosed with pancreatic cancer 2 weeks ago. A Whipple procedure is recommended. Which of the following health issues may worsen after the procedure?

    A. Diabetes
    B. Crohn's disease
    C. Hyperbilirubinemia
    D. Obesity

51. During a Whipple procedure, which of the following organs is removed?

    A. Gallbladder
    B. Esophagus
    C. Ascending colon
    D. Jejunum

52. Erin underwent a Whipple procedure 10 days ago for pancreatic cancer. She was started on clear liquids and then advanced to a soft diet. Two hours after lunch, you enter her room and find her sweating profusely, shaking, and confused. On the monitor, you note tachypnea and tachycardia. You suspect she is experiencing

    A. Anxiety or panic attack.
    B. Gastro-esophageal reflux disease (GERD).
    C. Dumping syndrome.
    D. Hypoglycemia.

53. Leah is experiencing dumping syndrome post gastric bypass surgery after eating any meal. Which of the following medications should Leah stop immediately?

    A. Nitroglycerin
    B. Insulin
    C. Pepcid
    D. Reglan

54. Your patient just returned from abdominal surgery. Two hours later you note decreased urine output, increased CVP, increased PAP, increased SVR, and decreased cardiac output. In addition, the ventilator alarm continuously signals low volume despite intact circuits. Based on these findings, you would expect which intra-abdominal pressure value?

    A. 5 mm Hg
    B. 15 mm Hg
    C. 25 mm Hg
    D. 50 mm Hg

55. Helen, a 26-year-old mother of 6 children, is 7 months pregnant and admitted to your unit for severe HELLP syndrome. She is also at risk for which of the following conditions?

    A. Intra-abdominal hypertension (IAH) and abdominal compartment syndrome (ACS)
    B. Decreased intracranial pressure (ICP)
    C. Hypocarbia
    D. Increased platelets

56. You just completed intra-abdominal pressure measurements via the bladder measurement method. When documenting the procedure in your notes, you should
    A. Only write "per policy and procedure"; no other documentation is required.
    B. Identify the number of stopcocks used in the setup.
    C. Include the patient position during the procedure.
    D. Identify when the bladder clamp was released.

57. You are preparing William for a paracentesis. Which of the following actions is the first step in assisting with a paracentesis?
    A. Have the patient void or insert a Foley catheter.
    B. Examine the abdomen for dullness.
    C. Order an upright X ray of the abdomen.
    D. Position the patient with the affected side up.

58. Which of the following lab results would contraindicate peritoneal lavage?
    A. RBC 5.2 million/mm^3
    B. PT 12.5 sec & PTT 75 sec
    C. PLT 70 mm^3/mL
    D. Hgb 14.7 g/dL, Hct 46%

59. Which of the following types of bowel obstruction leads to infarction or strangulation?
    A. Acute
    B. Subacute
    C. Chronic
    D. Intermittent

60. Joab, a 40-year-old Orthodox Jew, presents with an unintentional weight loss of 20 pounds, fatigue, anorexia, and chronic, watery diarrhea with bloody mucus. He is tachycardic, tachypneic, and hyperthermic, with a Hgb of 7 g/dL and Hct of 21%. You suspect
    A. Colonic diverticulitis.
    B. Ulcerative colitis.
    C. Pancreatitis.
    D. Cholecystitis.

61. Sam, a 60-year-old computer programmer, was hospitalized for a myocardial infarction and underwent emergency cardiopulmonary artery bypass graft surgery yesterday. He has been having recurrent uncontrolled atrial fibrillation intermittently for the last 10 hours. This evening he complains of abdominal pain with distention and has intolerance for a soft diet with nausea, vomiting, and fever. The physician orders a plain film of the abdomen. Which of the following results would you expect to see?
    A. Air in the biliary tree, with signs of small bowel obstruction and calculus in the pelvis
    B. Dilated small bowel loops and air–fluid levels
    C. Dilation of the entire bowel including the stomach, "thumb printing," and pneumatosis intestinalis
    D. Air under the diaphragm on the right upper chest or over the right lobe of the liver

62. Janet is being treated in the ICU for burns sustained to 60% of her body after being trapped in her house during a fire. She is at high risk for developing which of the following conditions?
    A. Peptic ulcer
    B. Pancreatitis
    C. Cholecystitis
    D. SRES

63. When checking nasogastric tube placement in your burn patient, you note frank blood returning from the tube. Which of the following therapies would be most effective in managing gastric bleeding in this patient?
    A. Vasopressin infusion
    B. Endoscopic thermal therapy
    C. Endoscopic injection therapy
    D. Variceal ligation

64. The physician orders a gastric lavage to aid in controlling gastric bleeding in your burn patient. The best fluid choice for gastric lavage is
    A. Hot tap water.
    B. Iced 3% saline.
    C. Iced sterile water.
    D. Room-temperature normal saline.

65. During gastric lavage for gastric bleeding related to stress-related erosion syndrome (SRES), your patient becomes hyperthermic, tachycardic, and complains of sudden abdominal pain and abdominal rigidity. You should
    A. Continue with the lavage; these symptoms are normal.
    B. Slow the infusion and change the fluid.
    C. Stop the infusion and rewarm the fluid.
    D. Stop the infusion and contact the physician.

66. Fernando has recurrent gallstones and has been treated medically at home for the last 6 months. He was brought into the ICU for severe dehydration, vomiting, and fever. On admission, your assessment reveals abdominal distention, guarding, tympany, absent bowel tones, jaundice, Grey–Turner's sign, and Cullen's sign. The patient's blood pressure is 75/50, his heart rate is 140, and his respiratory rate is 40 and shallow. You suspect
    A. Cholecystitis.
    B. Pancreatitis.
    C. Cirrhosis.
    D. Gastritis.

67. Your patient with severe acute pancreatitis now has a blood pressure of 70/40, a heart rate of 146, and a respiratory rate of 42. You suspect hypovolemic shock. Hypovolemic shock is caused by
    A. Blood loss with a ruptured gallbladder.
    B. Third spacing related to capillary leaking.
    C. Insufficient volume intake related to vomiting.
    D. Excessive fluid loss due to diarrhea.

68. Your patient was diagnosed with Barrett's esophagus. Which of the following conditions is your patient at greatest risk for?
    A. Esophageal varices
    B. Gastritis
    C. Esophageal cancer
    D. GERD

69. Luis has been medically treated for GERD for the past 3 years. He has been admitted to your unit for aspiration pneumonia due to increasing difficulty swallowing and vomiting. He admits to noncompliance with his GERD medication regimen and was diagnosed with Barrett's esophagus 6 months ago. During his stay in the ICU he is diagnosed with esophageal cancer. Which surgical procedure would Luis likely have to remove his cancer?
    A. Whipple
    B. Modified Whipple
    C. Esophagectomy
    D. Esophagastrectomy

70. Patients considering gastric bypass for weight management control should begin bariatric education
    A. Prior to the decision being made.
    B. When the decision to have surgery is made.
    C. Just prior to surgery.
    D. After surgery.

71. Which of the following assessments is the most important when caring for a patient considering bariatric surgery?
    A. Nutritional assessment
    B. Activity or muscular/skeletal assessment
    C. Psychological evaluation
    D. Physiological assessment

72. You are preparing a patient for gastric bypass surgery when she states, "After surgery, I will be able to eat whatever I want and never be fat again." Your response to her should be:
    A. "That's right, you are so lucky."
    B. "You may not be able to eat high-carbohydrate foods, but you won't ever be fat again."
    C. "You will need to modify your diet to avoid high-carbohydrate and sugary foods. You will still need to increase your activity level and control portions to avoid future weight gain."
    D. "You will need to eat fewer, larger meals of whatever you want."

73. Which of the following bariatric surgical methods does not result in the suturing or removal of gastrointestinal tissue or organs?
    A. Vertical banding
    B. Gastric banding
    C. Biliopancreatic diversion
    D. Roux-en-Y proximal gastric bypass

74. Which of the following complications of gastric banding is the most common?
    A. Stoma obstruction
    B. GERD
    C. Band slippage
    D. Stomach erosion

75. Your patient underwent the Roux-en-Y gastric bypass procedure 3 days ago. Which nutritional complication is this patient most at risk for?
    A. Hypercalcemia
    B. Vitamin C deficiency
    C. Vitamin B_{12} deficiency
    D. Hyperalbuminism

76. Which bariatric surgery method allows for a larger usable stomach pouch?
    A. Vertical banding
    B. Gastric banding
    C. Biliopancreatic diversion
    D. Roux-en-Y proximal gastric bypass

77. Anastomotic leaks are common with bariatric surgeries. Symptoms can be subtle and may include hyperthermia, tachycardia, tachypnea, abdominal pain, and anxiety. If undiagnosed, all of the following complications may result *except*
    A. Hyperoxia.
    B. Sepsis.
    C. MODS.
    D. Death.

78. Management of pain may be challenging in the patient who has undergo bariatric surgery. Management with opioids via a patient-controlled analgesia (PCA) pump is necessary to do all of the following *except*
    A. Prevent pulmonary emboli.
    B. Provide for early mobility.
    C. Prevent atelectasis.
    D. Make an early transition to oral pain medications.

79. The transjugular intrahepatic portosystemic shunt (TIPS) is used in which of the following patients?
    A. Patients with portal hypertension once bleeding has stopped
    B. Patients with a portal pressure gradient of less than 10 mm Hg
    C. Transplant patients
    D. Patients with HITS

80. Sandostatin is ordered for your patient with portal hypertension. Which of the following nursing actions is most important to perform when first starting this drug?
    A. Carefully monitoring input and output
    B. Check nerve stimulation
    C. Blood glucose checks
    D. Check blood pressure every 5 minutes

81. Sarah is admitted to the intensive care unit for abdominal pain. She recently had knee surgery for which she received Tylenol #3 for pain control. She has no bowel sounds, her abdomen is firmly distended, and she is diffusely tender across the abdomen. What is probably wrong with Sarah?
    A. Appendicitis from the pain medications
    B. Pancreatitis from lack of exercise
    C. Gastroenteritis after eating undercooked chicken
    D. Paralytic ileus from the codeine

This concludes the GI questions.

ANSWERS

1. **Correct Answer: C**
   Cranial nerves V and VII control the trigeminal and facial nerves, which are needed for skeletal control during chewing. Cranial nerve I controls the olfactory nerve. Cranial nerves II and III control optic and oculomotor movements. Cranial nerve VIII corresponds with the Vestibulocochlear nerve for auditory control.

2. **Correct Answer: D**
   Inspection to determine landmarks and appearance, auscultation to establish location and quality of bowel tones, percussion notes or tones are different for various internal organs, and palpation to establish wall tone, tenderness, and size of organs. Percussion and palpation prior to inspection or auscultation could affect the assessment findings.

3. **Correct Answer: B**
   Hepatic bruits are heard over the liver and may indicate primary liver cancer, alcoholic hepatitis, or vascular liver metastases. An aortic bruit over the epigastric area indicates a partial aortic occlusion. Iliac artery bruits are heard over the left/right inguinal areas. Renal artery bruits indicate renal artery stenosis.

4. **Correct Answer: D**
   Endoscopic retrograde cholangiopancreatography (ERCP) visualizes the biliary and/or pancreatic ducts via a flexible endoscope. Flexible sigmoidoscopy visualizes the rectum, sigmoid colon, and descending colon via 65 cm of flexible scope. Colonoscopy views the colon from the rectum to the ileocecal valve. Angiography is selective catheterization of the arterial system and venous portal system for blood flow analysis.

5. **Correct Answer: B**
   Melena is black, tarry stool containing 100 to 200 mL of blood from the upper gastrointestinal area or ascending colon. Oral bleeding may result in hematemesis. Descending colon bleeding may lead to bright red stools. Stools with high levels of iron or bismuth and stools resulting from consumption of some other foods may be mistaken for melena, but an occult blood test of the stool will rule out these possibilities.

6. **Correct Answer: A**
   Normal portal pressures are 5 to 10 mm Hg (7 to 14 cm H_2O). A higher pressure would indicate portal hypertension. Portal pressures should be 4 to 5 mm Hg higher than the inferior vena cava pressures. Pressures this high above the inferior vena cava pressures indicate severe portal hypertension.

7. **Correct Answer: A**
   The Minnesota tube has separate suction and balloons that can function independently. The Sengstaken–Blakemore tube has three lumens with only one suction port. The Linton–Nachlas tube is used for gastric varices only. The standard nasogastric tube has no balloon function to tamponade bleeding.

8. **Correct Answer: A**
   Transphenoidal hypohysectomy allows for easier access into the cranial vault. Oral gastric tube placement is safe. Oral intubation does not increase the risk of complications. Tracheal intubations do not increase the risk of complications related to this history.

9. **Correct Answer: A**

Maximum therapy time is 24 to 36 hours for esophageal balloons and 48 to 72 hours for gastric balloons. More time relates to increased risk for necrosis, ulceration, erosion of skin around the nares, airway obstruction, and aspiration of gastric or oropharyngeal contents. Patient comfort decreases over time, and risk of erosion to mucosal lining increases. Hgb and Hct levels should increase or stabilize with cessation of bleeding and blood replacement. The gastrointestinal lining may be inflamed related to the presence of blood in the system, and feedings should be held until bleeding stops.

10. **Correct Answer: C**

A sudden drop in the balloon pressure and the patient's ability to swallow may indicate balloon or esophageal rupture, as evidenced by bleeding, and should be reported to the physician immediately. The patient should not be able to swallow when the balloon is inflated properly. A drop in balloon pressure may indicate a ruptured balloon or esophagus. An inflation pressure of 70 mm Hg is too high.

11. **Correct Answer: A**

Unless taken enterically or in sustained-release form, materials are best lavaged within 60 minutes of ingestion. Normal saline or tap water should be used. Lavage is contraindicated only if the overdose involved corrosive or hydrocarbon materials. Liquid ingestion would have a faster absorption rate than would ingestion of pills, thus requiring faster treatment.

12. **Correct Answer: D**

The lab changes indicate near-complete hepatocellular necrosis. This answer indicates a still-critical condition without diagnosing a condition. Answer A ignores the serious indicators of impending complete hepatocellular necrosis and gives rise to false hope. Answer B is incorrect because the wife of the patient has privilege to the information as next of kin. Answer C does answer the question, but fails to provide appropriate information.

13. **Correct Answer: C**

In late acute hepatic failure, late signs include increased ICP, normal or decreased mean arterial pressures, and decreased CPP. Increased ICP, increased mean arterial pressures, and normal CPP are early indicators of acute hepatic failure.

14. **Correct Answer: B**

This answer acknowledges the daughters' concerns and provides education. Elevated bilirubin levels deposited in the skin result in unconscious scratching and excoriations. With the presence of increased PT, PTT, and INR levels, hematomas may also be present. Answer A provides no explanation for the scratches and decreases communication with the family. Restraints are inappropriate for this patient. ICU psychosis can lead to abnormal behavior, but it is not the reason for this patient's behavior.

15. **Correct Answer: A**

Brain stem herniation is the most common cause of death related to increased coagulation times, intracranial hemorrhaging, and hypoxia leading to cerebral edema. Anemia is a complication of prolonged bleeding times, but is not the primary cause of death. Pulmonary impairment is the result of hemorrhage, not embolism or edema.

16. **Correct Answer: B**

In chronic liver failure, skin becomes very dry, so gentle application of a moisturizer may relieve the patient's discomfort. Deep tissue massage is contraindicated due to the patient's decreased platelet count and increased risk of bruising. Development of orthostatic hypertension prohibits any rapid movement due to dizziness and risks of fall. Patients and family members are at risk for depression; visits may decrease this risk and will provide staff with an opportunity to assess for this issue and intervene if depression is observed.

17. **Correct Answer: C**
There are 4 grades of hepatic encephalopathy based on 5 clinical findings: These are level of consciousness, orientation, intellectual functions, behavior, and neuromuscular function.

18. **Correct Answer: D**
The release of mediators results in vasoconstriction that diverts blood flow to the kidneys. Circulating plasma decreases as the patient develops ascites. Vasoconstriction, not vasodilatation, occurs in end-stage liver failure. There is a decrease in renal circulation due to plasma shifting and vasoconstriction.

19. **Correct Answer: A**
Acute pancreatitis may occur as a result of seat belt trauma to the pancreatic duct or abdominal ischemia. Acute liver failure is characterized by flu-like symptoms, jaundice, confusion, and an enlarged liver. Gastrointestinal bleeding has a history of ulcers and/or esophageal varices with hemodynamic changes, narrowing pulse pressures, hematemesis, and hyperactive bowel tones. Abdominal trauma does not produce the knife-like and twisting pain, and tenderness and a marbled appearance would be noted.

20 **Correct Answer: A**
Serum amylase would be elevated. Serum lipase would be elevated, not decreased. Albumin levels would drop, not increase. Trypsin levels would also increase (not decrease) with the buildup of pancreatic enzymes.

21. **Correct Answer: D**
Cullen's sign is a bluish discoloration of the periumbilical area seen in pancreatitis and abdominal trauma. A marbled appearance is common with abdominal trauma. Coopernail's sign consists of bruising of the scrotum or labia. Turner's sign consists of bruising of the flanks.

22. **Correct Answer: A**
Severe illnesses result in blood shunting to protect cardiac, respiratory, and neurological function. Any mucosal ischemia may lead to a loss of protective functions within the gastrointestinal system. Mucus acts to protect function within the gastrointestinal system, so a decrease in its production would be harmful. Fungal infections involving the gastrointestinal system are rare; instead, bacteria are more common causes of gastric ulcers. Although it is possible to have ulcers on admission to the ICU, the diagnosis here is a new-onset ulcer.

23. **Correct Answer: B**
Pre-hepatic (pre-sinusoidal) factors lead to hepatic venous pressures less than portal pressures. Umbilical vein catheterizations as a neonate (within the first month of life) due to neonatal illness or prematurity may cause damage to the vessel. Chronic active hepatitis is an intrahepatic (sinusoidal) factor. Wedge hepatic venous pressures are either increased or equal to portal pressures. Metastatic carcinoma and cardiac diseases such as CHF can cause portal hypertension and may indirectly cause variceal bleeding.

24. **Correct Answer: C**

This patient has likely ruptured a varice. Priorities are to maintain the airway, stop the bleeding, and verify venous access for blood replacement, fluid management, and homeostasis. Placing the patient NPO and obtaining IV access is the first correct answer listed. You would want to position the patient upright to prevent aspiration, not flat. You would also anticipate the placement of a Minnesota tube, not a Linton–Nachlas tube. Dopamine at 5 mcg/kg/min would better support renal function, rather than blood pressure as needed in this patient.

25. **Correct Answer: A**

Early surgery (within 7 days of signs and symptoms of onset) usually leads to a shorter hospital stay. It is more appropriate for the nurse to refer the patient to the physician to discuss treatment options. A delay in surgery may lead to increased severity of symptoms although there is no change in mortality or complications. Only 25% of delayed surgeries may become urgent. Laparoscopic surgery is associated with a shorter hospital stay compared to open surgery, but there is an increased risk of bile duct injuries. Ultimately, 25% of such surgeries may require open surgical interventions related to complications.

26. **Correct Answer: D**

This situation requires honest communication with the patient regarding possible reoccurrence of symptoms. Approximately 33% of patients with appendicitis who are treated with antibiotics and pain management are readmitted and require appendectomies within 1 year. The remaining answers are stated as absolutes and are inappropriate responses from a practitioner. As the appendix was not removed, the patient may have a reoccurrence of symptoms at a later date. There is no way to predict whether and when an appendix may become infected or diseased. There is also no way to predict the pain of appendicitis, as pain is perceived differently for each patient.

27. **Correct Answer: A**

This patient is exhibiting signs and symptoms of an abscess post surgical intervention for appendicitis; such an abscess occurs in 5% to 33% of these patients. Surgical debridement of the incision and IV antibiotics are appropriate immediate treatment to prevent sepsis. Hydration and antibiotics alone will not treat the abscess. Bedside excision of the abscess alone may reduce the amount of infected fluid and tissue at the site, but will not prevent further infection. Bedside wound debridement is associated with a high risk of further contamination of the site. In approximately 2% of cases, the abscess may be intra-abdominal and may require surgical intervention under anesthesia as well as continued antibiotic treatment.

28. **Correct Answer: D**

This patient may safely continue taking Verapamil for atrial fibrillation. Calcium-channel blockers have been found to provide some protection against complications of diverticulae. Nonsteroidal anti-inflammatory agents, corticosteroids, and opiate analgesics have been noted to increase the risk of perforation of diverticulae.

29. **Correct Answer: D**

Prolonged starvation and protein loss result in fluid shifting and third spacing. Muscle wasting results in an increase in serum lactate levels, not a decrease. Initially there is an increased urinary nitrogen excretion followed by a decrease. There is an increase in serum catecholamine, glucagons, and cortisol as the body releases elements to maintain the amount of energy and glucose available.

30. Correct Answer: C

The goal when working with bulimic and anorexic patients is to support positive nutritional changes while acknowledging and supporting the psychological changes in body and food perception. By acknowledging the difficulties the patient has with food perception and willingness to provide support and counseling with a nutritionist, dietician, and psychologist, the nurse encourages the patient to find foods that are appealing and provide needed nutrition. The remaining answers are abrasive or do not address the patient's physiological or psychological struggle with eating.

31. Correct Answer: A

Chronic pancreatitis results in the release of digestive enzymes into the body. Phospholipase A_2 breaks down the cellular structure of the capillary beds, resulting in tissue injury throughout the body. In the lungs, capillary damage is manifested as pulmonary edema and dyspnea, leading to respiratory distress. Although stress may lead to bronchospasm in patients with existing respiratory diseases such as asthma, that finding is not indicated within the information given. Aspiration and atelectasis are common complications in patients admitted to the ICU, but they do not explain both symptoms as related to the ongoing disease process.

32. Correct Answer: B

Fifty percent of all deaths of patients with cirrhosis are from variceal bleeding. The lab tests cited in this question are used to differentiate causes of bleeding. The patient's history and lab values lean toward varices as a diagnosis. Although Hgb and Hct levels would be decreased in peptic ulcer disease and gastritis, the other lab changes would not be occurring. Boerhaave's syndrome is a full-thickness rupture or perforation of the esophageal wall due to prolonged and frequent vomiting related to eating disorders.

33. Correct Answer: A

This patient is exhibiting subjective and objective signs and symptoms of stomach cancer. There is a higher incidence of stomach cancer in males 50 to 70 years of age from cultures farthest from the equator. Upper gastrointestinal series would show a "leather bottle" stomach. The patient's symptoms do not support a diagnosis of an ulcer. Radiological studies would show ulceration or free air with perforation. Radiological studies for varices would not show any distinct changes. Pyloric stenosis is typically seen in infants and would be manifested as a distended abdomen, and nonbilious, projectile vomiting.

34. Correct Answer: D

This patient is exhibiting classic progression of a developing esophageal neoplasm. Complications that coincide with this disease process are related to changes in nutritional intake. Narrowing of the esophageal lumen results in increasing difficulties and pain when swallowing, prompting the individual to consume a softer diet; eventually, the patient can swallow only liquids. Partial tongue paralysis would be supported if the patient also had difficulty speaking, but that is not a symptom given in the question. Gastric cancer is indicated with indigestion and fullness, not difficulty swallowing. Tracheal neoplasm would be accompanied by more respiratory distress.

35. Correct Answer: D

Colorectal neoplasms present differently depending on their location. A lower gastrointestinal series, such as a sigmoidoscopy, allows for direct visualization of the cancer if it occurs within the lumen. A biopsy provides the definitive diagnosis.

36. **Correct Answer: C**
Left (descending) colon lesions tend to spread, ulcerate, and erode blood vessels within the colon. Obstruction is a very common complication with this type of lesion. Adenocarcinomas are the most common kinds of these neoplasms. Right (ascending) colon lesions are typically polypoid lesions and are associated with a familial history of polyps. Rectal lesions may spread to the vagina or the prostate, but are often associated with systemic metastasis.

37. **Correct Answer: B**
Hepatitis B virus is the only DNA virus listed. The other forms of hepatitis are RNA viruses.

38. **Correct Answer: A**
Hepatitis A is often misdiagnosed initially as gastroenteritis because its symptoms are usually self-limiting. Fecal–oral transmission of this infection may also be mistaken for food poisoning.

39. **Correct Answer: C**
This patient's history and symptomology are consistent with new-onset hepatitis C. Hepatitis C results in a hypermetabolic state. Nursing interventions should focus on minimizing symptoms and reducing stress on the body. A low-fat, high-carbohydrate diet supports an increase in caloric demand and prevent weight loss. The greater the liver compromise related to infection, the lower the patient's fat and protein intake, because the liver may not be able to assist with effective digestion.

This patient should remain on strict bed rest to allow for energy conservation in the acute phase of the disease. Light ambulation is permitted as long as the patient does not become fatigued with the activity. Although teaching is vital for this patient, extended teaching sessions may tax her ability to concentrate. Teaching should be available in multiple forms that can be referred to at the patient's leisure. Family may be supportive, but planned rest periods should be maintained and supported as patient tolerance allows.

40. **Correct Answer: A**
Hepatitis D virus (HDV) can replicate only when hepatitis B virus (HBV) is present. When HDV is present, as either a co-infection or a super-infection, progression of liver disease is more rapid and severe. The IgM level rises early in infection and may remain chronically high. The IgG level rises slowing during infection, but will continue for life. HDV replication occurs only when HBV is present.

41. **Correct Answer: B**
Acute liver failure related to acetaminophen overdose would be consistent with this patient's presentation. Individuals without full command of the English language are at risk for overdose when self-medicating if the medication label is not read and understood correctly. The patient's symptomology is inconsistent with the DIC presentation and vitamin K deficiency. Gaucher's disease is a genetic enzyme-deficiency disease that is typically diagnosed in childhood; its symptoms continue to progress as the glucocerebroside is collected in the spleen and liver. This patient would also present with skeletal weakness, neurological complications, swollen lymph nodes, and pain not restricted to just the last 9 weeks.

42. **Correct Answer: D**
As the liver becomes compromised, symptoms reflect inefficient liver functioning, with clotting Factors V and VII levels less than or equal to 20% of normal levels. In acute

liver failure, creatinine and BUN values will be increased, while serum glucose levels will be decreased. Any patient with new-onset, acute hepatic failure should be tested for all forms of hepatitis. Hepatitis is one of the leading factors for acute liver failures and may be first diagnosed when liver failure presents.

43. **Correct Answer: C**
The patient who has experienced an acetaminophen overdose has the best prognosis, even in the absence of a liver transplant. The patients with viral hepatitis, *Galerina* (poisonous mushrooms), and bone marrow transplant all have very poor prognoses if liver transplants are not available to them. Management goals include stabilizing hemodynamics, preventing infection, maintaining stable glucose levels, protecting the airway, and supporting adequate tissue perfusion.

44. **Correct Answer: C**
Aldosteronism initiates sodium retention, thereby increasing portal hypertension. Low albumin levels accompanied by increased hydrostatic pressure and decreased oncotic pressures result in ascites. Due to fluid shifting, the patient's ventilation/perfusion (V/Q) ratio would decrease.

45. **Correct Answer: D**
Due to the cirrhosis, renal function may be impaired, resulting in poor urine output. Common complications that lead to poor urine output include increased secretion of renin and aldosterone, leading to sodium retention. There is a decrease in both the glomerular filtration rate and renal blood flow.

46. **Correct Answer: B**
An ileostomy is located at the right ileac fossa just prior to the colon. Because the majority of water absorption occurs in the colon, stool from the small intestines is loose and unformed. Sigmoid colostomy stools more closely resemble normal stools, because most of the water has been absorbed. Loop, transverse, and ascending colostomies will yield loose stools with more formation.

47. **Correct Answer: D**
Dehydration is a severe complication with ileostomies as water reabsorption is accomplished by the colon. In this patient, a large portion or all of the large intestine may have been removed related to the Crohn's disease process. Fluids should be encouraged and IV support maintained to prevent hypovolemic shock. Postoperative teaching should include signs and symptoms of shock and preventive home management. Although a stoma prolapse may occur after discharge home, the stoma can be reopened without major complications. Hyponatremia, not hypernatremia, is a serious complication because sodium uptake also occurs in the colon. Hemorrhage is not a concern unless the stoma is scratched or damaged during care. Light pressure should be applied until bleeding stops, but it is not a life-threatening complication.

48. **Correct Answer: A**
This patient is exhibiting signs and symptoms of malrotation and duodenal obstruction related to a volvulus. The nurse should contact the physician immediately and prepare for surgery before necrosis of the bowel occurs. Tylenol and morphine will mask these serious symptoms. The patient's pain is related to ischemia experienced by the intestines as blood supply is prevented by the malrotation. The fever may indicate perforation or necrosis of the intestines impacted by the volvulus. The patient will need to sit

upright to prevent aspiration post vomiting. These symptoms are not normal, and discoloration of the abdomen indicates greater ischemia and a higher risk of perforation.

49. **Correct Answer: B**

The measurement method most commonly used to obtain the intra-abdominal pressure is via the bladder. A specialized catheter with a transducer allows for direct measurement of pressures; such equipment is usually found in the critical care unit.

50. **Correct Answer: A**

If a patient has been diagnosed with diabetes or has uncontrolled blood glucose levels, then removal of the pancreatic head may result in diabetes or worsening symptoms. It is imperative that the patient's blood glucose levels be monitored closely. With removal of part of the pancreas, the pancreas may not produce and release insulin at previous levels. Insulin injections may be required. The Whipple procedure removes part of the bile duct, which may improve bilirubin levels. With removal of part of the stomach and pancreas, patients are at risk of long-term malnutrition and weight loss.

51. **Correct Answer: A**

The Whipple procedure removes the tip or head of the pancreas, the gallbladder, the duodenum, and part of the bile duct. Occasionally, part of the stomach may also be removed. The extent of the cancerous pancreatic tumor will dictate the extent of removal.

52. **Correct Answer: C**

Erin's symptoms are consistent with late dumping syndrome related to the partial gastrectomy during the Whipple procedure. With late dumping syndrome, symptoms occur 1 to 3 hours after meals. Additional symptoms include weakness, fatigue, dizziness, anxiety, palpitations, and fainting. Patients may also exhibit early signs of dumping syndrome approximately 15 to 30 minutes after a meal with nausea, vomiting, cramps or abdominal pain, diarrhea, bloating, tachycardia, dysrhythmias, and dizziness. Although anxiety may be exhibited with dumping syndrome, an alteration in mental status with relation to food consumption and the patient's history support a diagnosis of dumping syndrome. Hypoglycemia is a greater risk for patients who undergo just gastrectomy or bypass. GERD presents with heartburn and epigastric pain.

53. **Correct Answer: D**

Reglan increases gastric emptying by increasing peristalsis, thereby increasing the effects of dumping syndrome. Reglan may be used post gastrectomy when gastroparesis is present. Once peristalsis has resumed, it should be stopped.

54. **Correct Answer: C**

Intra-abdominal pressures of 5 to 15 mm Hg indicate a low to moderate pressure problem. When respiratory function is impaired, these pressures will be approximately 25 mm Hg. You would expect to see increased respiratory distress and compromise. Severe compromise is seen with intra-abdominal pressures of more than 40 mm Hg. Thoracic pressures increase as intra-abdominal pressures increase, inhibiting lung expansion and diaphragm movement and resulting in hypoventilation and hypoxia.

55. **Correct Answer: A**

Due to the patient's pregnancy and resulting HELLP syndrome, there is an increased risk for fluid to collect in the abdominal cavity and tissue edema may occur. Signs and symptoms of IAH and ACS include increased ICP, hypercarbia and decreased platelet values, decreased cardiac output, poor or absent urinary output, and abdominal wall rigidity.

56. **Correct Answer: C**
Documentation for IAP should include vital signs prior to the procedure, patient position and abdominal values, vital signs during and after the procedure, changes in patient assessment, amount of fluid input into the bladder, output amount subtracted from input, any outcomes, interventions, reportable conditions, and any education provided.

57. **Correct Answer: A**
The correct order for these interventions when assisting with paracentesis is (1) have the patient void or insert a Foley catheter, (2) order an upright X ray of the abdomen, (3) position the patient with the affected side up, and (4) exam the abdomen for dullness.

58. **Correct Answer: C**
A patient with a platelet count of 70 mm^3/mL is thrombocytopenic and at risk for coagulation complications. Heparin is normally added to the solution to prevent clotting, but it can lead to further complications—namely, bleeding. The other lab values are within the normal range for either males or females.

59. **Correct Answer: A**
Acute bowel obstruction is the only type of obstruction that leads to infarction or strangulation. Obstruction occurs rapidly and may inhibit blood flow to a portion of the bowel. The other types of obstructions permit limited or intermittent blood flow that sustains but compromises tissue function.

60. **Correct Answer: B**
Based on his presenting symptoms and ethnicity, Joab has ulcerative colitis. He may also have leukocytosis and cachexia. Colonic diverticulitis presents with left upper quadrant pain, hyperthermia, vomiting, chills, diarrhea, and tenderness over the descending colon. Pancreatitis presents with left upper quadrant pain that radiates to the back or chest, hyperthermia, rigidity, rebound abdominal tenderness, nausea and vomiting, jaundice, Cullen's sign, Grey–Turner's sign, abdominal distention, and diminished bowel sounds. Cholecystitis presents with right upper quadrant or epigastric pain, pain that lasts up to 6 hours after a fatty meal, vomiting, and increased white blood cell counts.

61. **Correct Answer: B**
This patient is exhibiting signs of early ischemic bowel. At this time, there will be some dilation of the bowel with loops behind the ischemic bowel because the ischemic bowel is not performing peristaltic actions. Late signs, which may occur if the condition is not diagnosed and treated early, include dilation of the entire bowel including the stomach. "Thumb printing" is when edema of the bowel wall shows the convex indentations of the lumen. In pneumatosis intestinalis, a mottled gas pattern is observed in the bowel wall. Air in the biliary tree is indicative of a gallbladder emergency, and air under the diaphragm is characteristic of pneumoperitoneum.

62. **Correct Answer: D**
The term "stress-related erosive syndrome" (SRES) was once used to explain gastric complications related to critical care illnesses. The stress response within the patient may lead to rapid erosion of the mucosal lining and result in ulcerations. Patients

suffering from severe physiological illnesses are at high risk of SRES and, if left untreated, gastric bleeding.

63. **Correct Answer: A**

This patient is likely having gastric bleeding related to stress-related erosion syndrome. Due to the generalized bleeding associated with this condition, endoscopic therapies are not as effective as arginine vasopressin infusion into the gastric artery to cause splanchnic vasoconstriction. There is no indication that this patient has varices that would require ligation.

64. **Correct Answer: D**

In the past, iced solutions were used to control gastric bleeding. Current research shows that iced solutions may cause additional bleeding by irritating both healthy and compromised portions of the mucosal lining. The lowering of the temperature may also lead to core hypothermia and a shift in the oxyhemoglobin dissociation curve, resulting in decreased oxygen delivery to the tissues. A 3% saline solution would cause a fluid shift. Tap water should be avoided as a lavage measure because it may increase the risk of systemic infection if the water is contaminated.

65. **Correct Answer: D**

The patient is exhibiting signs and symptoms of gastric perforation—a surgical emergency. The lavage should be stopped, fluid aspirated, and the physician notified immediately. Additional actions should include the placement of at least two large-bore IVs, preparation to administer IV fluid replacement if hypovolemic shock occurs, and preparation of the patient for immediate surgery.

66. **Correct Answer: B**

Although the patient's initial symptoms and history may indicate cholecystitis, his current symptoms are classic hallmarks of pancreatitis. Abdominal rigidity, Grey–Turner's sign, and Cullen's sign are late indicators of pancreatitis. In addition, the patient's presentation is one of severe hypovolemic shock. Fluid resuscitation should be initiated immediately to support his cardiovascular function.

67. **Correct Answer: B**

Patients with pancreatitis undergo massive fluid shifting in response to the inflammatory response to pancreatic self-digestion. Mediators released during the inflammatory response leads to vasodilation and increased capillary permeability. Fluid may shift into the bowel, mucosal lining, and within the lungs, leading to acute lung injury (AJI). The drop in blood pressure may lead to acute kidney injury (AKI) and renal failure. Immediate fluid replacement with crystalloids and colloids is required to maintain intravascular volume. A history of poor volume intake only worsens the hypovolemia, but is not the primary and most severe cause of the hypovolemic shock.

68. **Correct Answer: C**

Barrett's esophagus is a result of mucosal changes in the esophagus after repeated and prolonged exposure to gastric secretions seen in untreated gastroesophageal reflux disease (GERD). As a result of cellular changes in the esophageal lining, the patient is at increased risk for esophageal cancer.

69. **Correct Answer: C**

The correct name for the procedure is esophagectomy. It involves removal of the damaged esophagus to the proximal portion of the stomach. The stomach is then resectioned to form a new esophagus. If the stomach is also cancerous, the stomach is removed and the small bowel is resectioned to create a new esophagus.

70. **Correct Answer: A**

Gastric bypass surgery can lead to permanent gastric changes and places the obese patient at risk for both surgical and anesthesia-related complications. For many bariatric patients, the initial gastric bypass surgery is not the only surgery required. Often cosmetic surgery to remove loose skin around the stomach, back, thighs, arms, and chest is required to improve self-image. Each surgery has additional risk. Therefore, complete bariatric education should be provided to any patient who is considering bariatric surgery. Education should include preoperative changes in diet, nutritional consultation, psychological evaluation, and full medical evaluation including lab work and cardiovascular testing. Education and support for the bariatric surgery patient should continue throughout the surgical process, with ongoing education, nutritional support, and physiological support for years after the surgery.

71. **Correct Answer: C**

Although each of these assessments is vital prior to bariatric surgery, psychological evaluation assesses the patient's psychological health regarding weight management, food, diet, nutrition, activity, exercise, health, surgery, coping mechanisms, self-image, and self-esteem and may estimate the long-term success of surgery. Obesity has many different causes, and assessing the patient's psychological health may reveal dangerous beliefs and behaviors related to food and nutrition that should be addressed prior to surgery.

72. **Correct Answer: C**

Regardless of the type of bariatric surgery performed, the stomach size is always altered or restricted. Some forms of bypass also alter the normal pathway of food through digestion or malabsorption. Either method results in poor tolerance for large volumes of food and fluid requiring patients to eat more frequently, but smaller meals. Foods that are high in carbohydrates and sugar are also harder to digest when malabsorptive surgical methods are used. When such foods are consumed, the patient may experience "dumping syndrome," which can be extremely painful. This physical reaction provides a level of behavior modification meant to deter patients from consuming carbohydrates or sugary foods.

Patients must understand the mandatory changes in diet that come with bariatric surgery. The leading cause of failure with restrictive surgical techniques is that patients consume foods in ever-increasing amounts, which eventually leads to stretching of the pouch (stomach). Over time, the stomach can be restretched to almost its original size.

73. **Correct Answer: B**

In gastric banding, an adjustable band is placed around the upper portion of the stomach to create a small, 1- to 2-ounce area to act as the stomach. Because the size is restricted without suturing off stomach or removal of any tissue, this procedure may be reversed for medical reasons such as pregnancy. Vertical banding, biliopancreatic diversion, and Roux-en-Y proximal gastric bypass all include some permanent change to the normal gastric pathway.

74. **Correct Answer: B**

Gastroesophageal reflux disease (GERD) is a common complication of gastric banding. Due to the smaller gastric size and the close proximity of the band to the sphincter, the patient may experience reflux, and possibly nausea and vomiting, after eating. Deflation of the band with slower reinflation adjustments every 2 weeks will ease symptoms. Stoma obstruction may occur if the patient fails to chew food properly and thoroughly. Band slippage may lead to erosion and perforation of the stomach or a folding of the larger portion of the stomach over the smaller portion.

75. **Correct Answer: C**
Because the gastric size is greatly reduced, less intrinsic factor is available to assist in vitamin B_{12} absorption, which is essential to prevent pernicious anemia. Oral supplements are not recommended, because they may not be absorbed quickly enough. Sublingual or injected vitamin B_{12} may be required. Iron, thiamin, and calcium are all absorbed in the duodenum. In gastric bypass, the duodenum is bypassed as well, which greatly limits the absorption of these vitamins and minerals. Careful supplementation is mandatory to prevent malnutrition. Protein deficiencies are also common following Roux-en-Y gastric bypass, and supplementation is necessary, especially in early postoperative recovery, to prevent muscle wasting during the rapid-weight-loss period.

76. **Correct Answer: C**
Biliopancreatic diversion uses a 5-ounce stomach pouch and wide anastomosis. The biliary branch or limb connects a portion of the small bowel to the biliary tract to allow for normal biliary excretion. To prevent further preoperative or postoperative complications associated with cholecystitis, the gallbladder may be removed during the procedure.

77. **Correct Answer: A**
Hyperoxia is not a complication of bariatric surgery and anastomosis leakage. Symptoms may present as an acute abdomen. If they are subtle, however, sepsis may lead to multiple-organ dysfunction or failure, and ultimately death.

78. **Correct Answer: D**
Pain management via a PCA pump should only allow transition to oral pain medications after anastamoses have healed. Effective pain management allows for early ambulation to improve lung expansion and blood circulation to prevent atelectasis, pneumonia, and pulmonary embolism. Due to the high fat ratio, pain medications may need to be adjusted to ensure their greatest effectiveness.

79. **Correct Answer: C**
TIPS is used in transplant patients to bridge between the two livers in a hemodynamically unstable patient, thereby increasing the patient's stability. TIPS can be used during active bleeding via varices. Patients must have a directly measured portal pressure gradient of more than 10 mm Hg. This procedure should be postponed if bleeding is due to heparin-induced thrombocytopenia (HITS) until the patient is stabilized.

80. **Correct Answer: C**
Glycemic emergencies may occur with administration of Sandostatin, especially in the diabetic patient. It is important to monitor blood glucose to prevent hyperglycemia and/or hypoglycemia. Blood pressure and urinary function may also be affected, but these changes are not as quickly life-threatening as the changes in glucose levels.

81. **Correct Answer: D**
Codeine slows gastric motility throughout the GI tract. This patient needs a nasogastric tube and motility medications such as metoclopramide.

BIBLIOGRAPHY

Ahmed, I., & Beckingham, I. J. (2007). Liver trauma. *Trauma, 9*(3), 171–180.

Ahrens, T. (2006). *Critical care nursing certification.* Columbus, OH: McGraw-Hill.

American Association of Critical-Care Nurses. (2006). *Core curriculum for critical care nursing* (6th ed.). Philadelphia: Saunders.

American Association of Critical-Care Nurses. (2007). *AACN certification and core review for high acuity and critical care* (6th ed.). Philadelphia: Saunders.

American Heart Association. (2007). *Guidelines 2005 for cardiopulmonary resuscitation and emergency cardiovascular care.* Retrieved July 24, 2008, from http://circ.ahajournals.org/content/vol112/24_suppl

Barry, M., Cahill, R. A., & O'Connor, J. (2006). Duodenal hematoma secondary to blunt abdominal trauma. *European Journal of Trauma, 32*(6), 576–577.

Betz, T. G., Lee, P., & Victor, J. C. (2008). Hepatitis A vaccine versus immune globulin for postexposure prophylaxis. *New England Journal of Medicine, 358*(5), 531–532.

Britt, R. C., Gannon, T., Collins, J. N., Cole, F. J., Weireter, L. J., & Britt, L. D. (2005). Secondary abdominal compartment syndrome: Risk factors and outcomes. *American Surgeon, 71*(11), 982–985.

Brolin, R. E., & Cody, R. P. (2007). Adding malabsorption for weight loss failure after gastric bypass. *Surgical Endoscopy, 21*(11), 1924–1926.

Burns, S. M. (Ed.). (2007). *American Association of Critical-Care Nurses (AACN): AACN protocols for practice: Healing environments* (2nd ed.). Sudbury, MA: Jones and Bartlett.

Cho, Y. P., Kwon, Y. M., Kwon, T. W., & Kim, G. E. (2003). Mesenteric Buerger's disease. *Annals of Vascular Surgery, 17*(2), 221–223.

Conover, M. B. (2003). *Understanding electrocardiography* (8th ed.). St. Louis, MO: Mosby/Elsevier.

Copstead, L., & Banasik, J. L. (2000). *Pathophysiology: Biological and behavioral perspectives* (2nd ed.). Philadelphia: Saunders/Elsevier.

Curley, M. A. Q. (1998). Patient–nurse synergy: Optimizing patients' outcomes. *American Journal of Critical Care, 7,* 64–72.

Delaet, I., Hoste, E., Verholen, E., & De Waele, J. J. (2007). The effect of neuromuscular blockers in patients with intra-abdominal hypertension. *Intensive Care Medicine, 33*(10), 1811–1814.

Dossey, B. M., Keegan, L., & Guzzetta, C. (2003). *Holistic nursing: A handbook for practice* (3rd ed.). Sudbury, MA: Jones and Bartlett.

Edwards, D. F. (1999). The Synergy Model: Linking patient needs to nurse competencies. *Critical Care Nurse, 19*(1), 88–98.

Emergency Nurses Association, & Newberry, L. (2003). *Sheehy's emergency nursing: Principles and practice* (5th ed.). St. Louis, MO: Mosby/Elsevier.

Finkelmeier, B. A. (2000). *Cardiothoracic surgical nursing* (2nd ed.). Philadelphia: Lippincott, Williams & Wilkins.

Hamza, S. M., & Kaufman, S. (2007). Effect of mesenteric vascular congestion on reflex control of renal blood flow. *American Journal of Physiology: Regulatory, Integrative and Comparative Physiology, 293*(5), R1917.

Hanchanale, V. S., Rao, A. R., & Gilbert, J. M. (2007). What caused this massive GI hemorrhage? *Contemporary Surgery, 63*(11), 566–568.

Hardin, S. R., & Kaplow, R. (Eds.). (2004). *Synergy for clinical excellence: The AACN Synergy Model for Patient Care.* Sudbury, MA: Jones and Bartlett.

Hickey, J. V. (2002). *The clinical practice of neurological and neurosurgical nursing* (5th ed.). Philadelphia: Lippincott, Williams & Wilkins.

Hiraga, N., Aikata, H., Takaki, S., Kodama, H., Shirakawa, H., Imamura, M., et al. (2007). The long-term outcome of patients with bleeding gastric varices after balloon-occluded retrograde transvenous obliteration. *Journal of Gastroenterology, 42*(8), 663–672.

Horng, M. S. (2006). Beta blockers failed in primary prevention of gastroesophageal varices. *Journal of Clinical Outcomes Management, 13*(1), 15–16.

Jain, P., & Nijhawan, S. (2007). Acute viral hepatitis with pancreatitis: Is it due to the viruses or sludge? *Pancreatology, 7*(5–6), 544–545.

Khan, F., & Morad, N. (2006). Cytomegalovirus enteritis in a mechanically ventilated patient with chronic obstructive pulmonary disease. *Indian Journal of Critical Care Medicine, 10*(1), 40–43.

Knaapen, H. K. A., & Barrera, P. (2007). Therapy for Whipple's disease. *Journal of Antimicrobial Chemotherapy, 60*(3), 457–458.

Köklü, S., Çoban, S., Yüksel, O., & Arhan, M. (2007). Left-sided portal hypertension. *Digestive Diseases and Sciences, 52*(5), 1141–1149.

Lipson, J. G., Dibble, S. L., & Minarik, P. A. (Eds.). (1996). *Culture and nursing care: A pocket guide.* San Francisco, CA: UCSF Nursing Press.

Lisman, T., & Leebeek, F. W. G. (2007). Hemostatic alterations in liver disease: A review on pathophysiology, clinical consequences, and treatment. *Digestive Surgery, 24*(4), 250–258.

Maharaj, D., Perry, A., Ramdass, M., & Naraynsingh, V. (2003). Late small bowel obstruction after blunt abdominal trauma. *Postgraduate Medical Journal, 79*(927), 57–58.

Mayo Clinic Staff. (2007). Dumping syndrome. *Mayo Foundation for Medical Education and Research.* Retrieved March 11, 2008, from http://www.mayoclinic.com/health/dumping-syndrome/DS00715

McNally, P. (2001). *GI/liver secrets* (2nd ed.). Philadelphia: Hanley & Belfus/Elsevier.

McQuillan, K. A., Von Rueden, K. T., Hartsock, R. L., Flynn, M. B., & Whalen, E. (Eds.). (2002). *Trauma nursing: From resuscitation through rehabilitation* (3rd ed.). Philadelphia: Saunders/Elsevier.

Medina, J., & Puntillo, K. (2006). *AACN protocols for practice: Palliative care and end-of-life issues in critical care.* Sudbury, MA: Jones and Bartlett.

Morales, C. H., Villegas, M. I., Villavicencio, R., González, G., Pérez, L. F., Peña, A. M., et al. (2004). Intra-abdominal infection in patients with abdominal trauma. *Archives of Surgery, 139*(12), 1278–1285, discussion 1285.

Morgan, M. Y. (2007). The treatment of hepatic encephalopathy. *Metabolic Brain Disease, 22*(3–4), 389–405.

Okuse, C., Yotsuyanagi, H., & Koike, K. (2007). Hepatitis C as a systemic disease: Virus and host immunologic responses underlie hepatic and extrahepatic manifestations. *Journal of Gastroenterology, 42*(11), 857–865.

Olson, M. M., Ilada, P. B., & Apelgren, K. N. (2003). Portal vein thrombosis. *Surgical Endoscopy, 17*(8), 1322.

Oncel, D., Malinoski, D., Brown, C., Demetriades, D., & Salim, A. (2007). Blunt gastric injuries. *American Surgeon, 73*(9), 880–883.

Pagana, K. D., & Pagana, J. (2005). *Mosby's manual of diagnostic and laboratory tests* (3rd ed.). St. Louis, MO: Mosby/Elsevier.

Reesink, H. W., Engelfriet, C. P., Henn, G., Mayr, W. R., Delage, G., Bernier, F., et al. (2008). Occult hepatitis B infection in blood donors. *Vox Sanguinis, 94*(2), 153–166.

Rogula, T., Yenumula, P. R., & Schauer, P. R. (2007). A complication of Roux-en-Y gastric bypass: Intestinal obstruction. *Surgical Endoscopy, 21*(11), 1914–1918.

Schaefer, P. J., Schaefer, F .K. W., Mueller-Huelsbeck, S., & Jahnke, T. (2007). Chronic mesenteric ischemia: Stenting of mesenteric arteries. *Abdominal Imaging, 32*(3), 304–309.

Shah, V. H., & Kamath, P. (2006). Management of portal hypertension. *Postgraduate Medicine, 119*(3), 14–18.

Shawcross, D., & Jalan, R. (2005). Dispelling myths in the treatment of hepatic encephalopathy. *Lancet, 365*(9457), 431–433.

Shawcross, D. L., Wright, G., Olde Damink, S. W. M., & Jalan, R. (2007). Role of ammonia and inflammation in minimal hepatic encephalopathy. *Metabolic Brain Disease, 22*(1), 125–138.

Shebrain, S., Zelada, J., Lipsky, A. M., & Putnam, B. (2006). Mesenteric injuries after blunt abdominal trauma: Delay in diagnosis and increased morbidity. *American Surgeon, 72*(10), 955–961.

Skidmore-Roth, L. (2004). *Mosby's 2004 nursing drug reference.* St. Louis, MO: Mosby/Elsevier.

Smeltzer, S., & Bare, B. G. (2003). *Brunner and Suddarth's textbook of medical–surgical nursing* (10th ed.). Philadelphia: Lippincott, Williams & Wilkins.

Sole, M. L., Hartshorn, J., & Lamborne, M. L. (2001). *Introduction to critical care nursing* (3rd ed.). Philadelphia: Saunders/Elsevier.

Sonfield, J., Robison, J., & Leon, S. M. (2007). Occult aortic injury after penetrating abdominal trauma. *American Surgeon, 73*(3), 239–242.

Stewart, C. A., & Cerhan, J. (2005). Hepatic encephalopathy: A dynamic or static condition. *Metabolic Brain Disease, 20*(3), 193–204.

Sun, D., & Fang, J. (2007). Two common reasons of malabsorption syndromes: Celiac disease and Whipple's disease. *Digestion, 74*(3–4), 174–183.

Tseng, Y., Wu, M., Lin, M., & Lai, W. (2004). Massive upper gastrointestinal bleeding after acid-corrosive injury. *World Journal of Surgery, 28*(1), 50–54.

University of Southern California, Department of Surgery. (2005). Whipple operation. USC Center for Pancreatic and Biliary Disease. Retrieved February 20, 2005, from http://www.surgery. usc.edu/divisions/tumor/PancreasDiseases

Urden, L. D., Stacy, K. M., & Lough, M. E. (2007). *Thelan's critical care nursing: Diagnosis and management* (5th ed.). St. Louis, MO: Mosby.

Warwick, M., Goonewardene, K., Burton, P. R., Usatoff, V., & Evans, P. M. (2007). HP38P Management of traumative pancreatic injury. *ANZ Journal of Surgery, 77*(s1), A48.

Wiegand, D. J. L., & Carlson, K. K. (Eds.). (2005). *AACN procedure manual for critical care* (5th ed.). Philadelphia: Elsevier.

Williams, O. M., Nightingale, A. K., Hartley, J., Bramkamp, M., Ruggieri, F., Schneemann, M., et al. (2007). Whipple's disease. *New England Journal of Medicine, 356*(14), 1479–1481.

Woods, S., Sivarajan Froelicher, E. S., & Motzer, S. U. (2000). *Cardiac nursing* (4th ed.). Philadelphia: Lippincott, Williams & Wilkins.

Wright, B. E., Reinke, T., & Aye, R. A. (2005). Chronic traumatic diaphragmatic hernia with pericardial rupture and associated gastroesophageal reflux. *Hernia, 9*(4), 392–396.

Zeller, J. L. (2007). Risk of gastric cancer after Roux-en-Y gastric bypass. *Journal of the American Medical Association, 298*(22), 2600.

Zeller, J. L. (2007). Spectrum and risk factors of complications after gastric bypass. *Journal of the American Medical Association, 298*(21), 2461.

QUESTIONS

1. **The definition of acute renal failure would be**
   A. Trauma to one or both kidneys.
   B. A decrease in renal perfusion from shock or anaphylaxis.
   C. A sudden or rapid decline in renal filtration function.
   D. An obstruction to passage of urine.

2. **Intrinsic AKI is most commonly caused by**
   A. Arteriolar vasoconstriction.
   B. Acute ischemic or cytotoxic injury.
   C. Amphotericin.
   D. Hypercalcemia.

3. **Sudden anuria may be due to**
   A. An embolic event.
   B. Congestive heart failure.
   C. Prostate enlargement.
   D. Azotemia.

4. **Postrenal AKI may be caused by**
   A. Malignant hypertension.
   B. Transplant rejection.
   C. Neurogenic bladder.
   D. DIC, preeclampsia.

5. **BUN may be elevated in patients taking**
   A. Steroid treatments.
   B. Streptomycin.
   C. Chloramphenicol.
   D. Low protein intake.

6. **A renal transplant that results from humoral rejection or acute cellular rejection may be definitively diagnosed only via**
   A. Ultrasound.
   B. Nuclear scan.
   C. Doppler scan.
   D. Renal biopsy.

7. In the polyuric phase of AKI, it is important for the nurse to carefully monitor
   A. Nitrogen balance.
   B. Potassium and phosphorus.
   C. Dopamine and mannitol levels.
   D. Desmopressin levels.

8. Anuria is defined as a urine output of
   A. Less than 30 mL/h.
   B. 200 mL/day.
   C. 300 mL/day.
   D. Less than 100 mL/day.

9. Oliguria is a urine output of 100–400 mL/day and is usually the result of
   A. Pyelonephritis.
   B. Rhabdomyolitis.
   C. Prerenal syndrome.
   D. Acute glomerular nephritis.

10. Mrs. F. was admitted to the hospital directly from her physician's office. She had been complaining of fatigue and generalized pain. Her lab work indicated a rapidly rising BUN level, and she was admitted for further tests. While assessing Mrs. F., you note that she has severe acne around the face and neck. You suspect that the rise in BUN may be due to
    A. Tetracycline.
    B. HCTZ.
    C. Bumetanide.
    D. Mannitol.

11. Mannitol and loop diuretics may be used in the treatment of AKI. Mannitol is nontoxic but must be used with caution because
    A. Mannitol may damage the eighth cranial nerve.
    B. Mannitol may cause vestibular impairment.
    C. Mannitol may produce a hyperosmolar state.
    D. Mannitol may bind with proteins in the renal tubule.

12. Nephrotoxity may result from use of
    A. Furosemide.
    B. Aspirin.
    C. Thioguanine.
    D. Acyclovir.

13. NSAIDs may cause
    A. Prerenal AKI.
    B. Intrinsic AKI.
    C. Postrenal AKI.
    D. Increased urine osmolality.

14. **Medications that can decrease BUN levels include**
    A. Neomycin and rifampin.
    B. Chloral hydrate and furosemide.
    C. Bacitracin and gentamycin.
    D. Chloramphenicol and streptomycin.

15. **Which of the following statements about creatinine is true?**
    A. A normal range for creatinine would be 0.8 to 1.4 mg/dL.
    B. Creatinine levels are higher in females than in males.
    C. Lower-than-normal levels of creatinine may indicate pyelonephritis.
    D. Low levels of creatinine are a precursor to eclampsia.

16. **Allergic nephritis may be caused by**
    A. Inadequate protein consumption.
    B. Weight loss.
    C. Cimetidine.
    D. Water intoxication.

17. **The primary site for urea synthesis is in the**
    A. Kidneys.
    B. Liver.
    C. Lungs.
    D. Pancreas.

18. **Increased production of urea may be due to**
    A. GI bleeding.
    B. Consumption of a low-protein diet.
    C. Congenital kidney disease.
    D. Hypothermia.

19. **Your patient was involved in a head-on collision and had to be freed from under the steering column. The patient has been diagnosed with a ruptured bladder. It is important to assess her for signs of**
    A. Bowel perforation.
    B. A ruptured spleen.
    C. A shearing injury.
    D. Rectal injury.

20. **You notice your patient's hand spasming when the automatic blood pressure cuff inflates. When you attempt a manual blood pressure measurement, the same thing happens when you inflate the cuff just past the systolic pressure. This carpopedal spasm is indicative of**
    A. Hypokalemia.
    B. Hyperphosphatemia.
    C. Hypocalcemia.
    D. Hypernatremia.

21. Your patient is becoming confused, is lethargic, and has muscle weakness. A review of her lab reports shows a calcium level of 11.7. A common way to treat this condition would be to use
    A. D_5W and a Kayexalate enema.
    B. Normal saline and a loop diuretic.
    C. Glucose followed by insulin.
    D. Nothing; this is a normal value.

22. While assessing your patient, you notice significant pretibial and pedal edema. When the patient is weighed, you note that the patient has gained 1 kg of weight in 24 hours. This would be equal to at least _____ of excess fluid.
    A. 2,000 mL
    B. 1,000 mL
    C. 2,200 mL
    D. 500 mL

23. Your patient has a calcium level of 7.8. You would expect which of the following EKG changes?
    A. Tall, peaked T waves
    B. A prominent U wave
    C. A first-degree AV block
    D. A prolonged QT interval

24. One way to check for low calcium is to tap over a branch of the facial nerve. If the patient is hypocalcemic, the upper lip on the same side (ipsilateral) will twitch. This is known as
    A. Trousseau's sign.
    B. Chvostek's sign.
    C. Grey–Turner's sign.
    D. Homan's sign.

25. What is the primary acid–base disturbance exhibited by patients with AKI?
    A. Metabolic acidosis
    B. Respiratory acidosis
    C. Metabolic alkalosis
    D. Respiratory alkalosis

26. Peter, a 63-year-old man, is admitted to the intensive care unit for cocaine intoxication. He begins to complain of severe epigastric pain. Labs are WBC 17.3 with 77% neutrophils, hematocrit 40%, LDH 341, platelets 226, BUN 7, and creatinine 1.0. Urine analysis shows trace of proteins, few RBCs, and positive urine toxicology for cocaine. What could cause Peter's pain?
    A. Peptic ulcer disease
    B. Renal infarction
    C. Gastroenteritis
    D. Infarcted mesenteric artery

27. Aldosterone is secreted when the extracellular sodium level is _____ and/or when extracellular potassium is _____.
    A. low, low
    B. low, high
    C. high, low
    D. high, high

28. Marcus is a 24-year-old man with cystic fibrosis. He is at a high risk for
    A. Hypernatremia.
    B. Hypocalcemia.
    C. Hyponatremia.
    D. Hypercalcemia.

29. Hector has a J-tube inserted post peritonitis. For which electrolyte deficit is he at risk?
    A. Sodium
    B. Magnesium
    C. Manganese
    D. Phosphorus

30. Beatrice is a 60-year-old woman with diabetes and congestive heart failure. After 4 days of no contact, her daughter found her in bed, unresponsive. She has a red, dry swollen tongue, a temperature of 102°F, and flushed dry skin. She is tachycardic, hypotensive, and with decreased reflexes. Her urine specific gravity is 1.050. You suspect
    A. Hypernatremia.
    B. Hypocalcemia.
    C. Hypermagnesemia.
    D. Hypokalemia.

31. _____ is the major extracellular cation, and _____ is the major intracellular cation.
    A. Calcium, magnesium
    B. Sodium, calcium
    C. Potassium, sodium
    D. Sodium, potassium

32. What percentage of the body's potassium may be found in the extracellular fluid?
    A. 2%
    B. 5%
    C. 10%
    D. 98%

33. Potassium is reabsorbed in the
    A. Proximal tubules.
    B. Distal tubules.
    C. Ascending colon.
    D. Descending colon.

34. **Aldosterone secretions**
    A. Decrease potassium excretion.
    B. Increase potassium excretion.
    C. Cause potassium excretion to remain the same.
    D. Initially raise, then lower potassium excretion.

35. **Your patient is an alcoholic. What will happen to his potassium level?**
    A. Potassium moves from the vascular circulation into the interstitium.
    B. Potassium moves out of the cell into vascular circulation.
    C. Potassium moves out of the cell into the interstitium.
    D. Potassium from the vascular circulation moves into the cell.

36. **Hypokalemia may cause**
    A. Respiratory alkalosis only.
    B. Metabolic alkalosis only.
    C. Both respiratory and metabolic alkalosis.
    D. Metabolic acidosis only.

37. **Hypokalemia due to excessive urinary excretion can be caused by all of the following *except***
    A. Oliguria.
    B. Renal disease.
    C. Lasix.
    D. Increased production of adrenal cortical hormones.

38. **Jo is hypokalemic. Which of the following would you expect to see on an EKG?**
    A. Peaked T waves
    B. U wave
    C. Shortened QT
    D. Absent P wave

39. **Derek suffered a crush injury when a beam dropped on him. Which of the following results would you expect to see on his electrolyte panels?**
    A. Hyperphosphatemia
    B. Hypomagnesemia
    C. Hypocalcemia
    D. Hyperkalemia

40. **It is recommended that adults consume _____ of potassium daily.**
    A. 500 mg
    B. 1,000 mg
    C. 2,000 mg
    D. 3,500 mg

41. **All of the following foods are high in potassium *except***
    A. Avocadoes.
    B. Raisins.
    C. Potatoes.
    D. Carrots.

42. You are discussing cooking methods for vegetables with your patient's wife. Which of the following cooking techniques leaches the most potassium from vegetables?
    A. Boiling
    B. Baking
    C. Steaming
    D. Microwaving

43. Your patient is receiving potassium in his IV fluid, and the physician has ordered a potassium rider. What is the maximum rate of infusion for potassium solutions?
    A. 2 mEq/h
    B. 4 mEq/h
    C. 10 mEq/h
    D. 15 mEq/h

44. In Addison's disease, what happens to the potassium level?
    A. Hyperkalemia related to the decrease in aldosterone secretion
    B. Hyperkalemia related to the increase in aldosterone secretion
    C. Hypokalemia related to the decrease in aldosterone secretion
    D. Hypocalemia related to the increase in aldosterone secretion

45. All of the following are treatments for hyperkalemia *except*
    A. Glucose and insulin.
    B. Kaon.
    C. Calcium glucanate.
    D. Bicarbonate administration.

46. Jackie has congestive heart failure and was given Lasix for water retention. Her feet and legs continued to swell, so she took extra Lasix this morning. Now Jackie has profound muscle weakness and flat T waves. You would expect her potassium level this morning to be
    A. 1.8.
    B. 3.8.
    C. 4.2.
    D. 6.1.

47. Normal magnesium levels for an adult are in the range
    A. 0.5–1.5 mg/dL.
    B. 1.5–2 mg/dL.
    C. 2–3 mg/dL.
    D. 4–5 mg/dL.

48. Magnesium is required for all of the following *except*
    A. To always act as an antagonist with calcium.
    B. For enzyme activation.
    C. Synthesis of nucleic acid and proteins.
    D. Functioning of the sodium/potassium pump.

49. Magnesium alters intracellular calcium by affecting production of which hormone?
    A. Parathyroid
    B. Aldosterone
    C. Cortisol
    D. Glycosol

50. Where is magnesium most prevalent in the body?
    A. Extra cellular space
    B. In the liver
    C. In the bone
    D. In the spleen

51. As part of his discharge teaching, you are helping Joe determine which foods are rich in magnesium. He asks you what the recommended daily intake of magnesium is for adults. Your answer should be
    A. 50–100 mg per day.
    B. 100–200 mg per day.
    C. 200–350 mg per day.
    D. 350–420 mg per day.

52. Your patient was admitted and treated for torsades de pointes. You are teaching her about adding foods that are rich in magnesium to her diet. Your patient asks about each of the following foods. Which of the following is a poor source of magnesium?
    A. Honey
    B. Broccoli
    C. Almonds
    D. Chocolate

53. Kim had gastric bypass surgery 2 days ago. For which of the following electrolytes is she at most risk for an imbalance?
    A. Potassium
    B. Magnesium
    C. Calcium
    D. Sodium

54. Edna eats a diet high in calcium because her family has a history of osteoporosis. She was admitted status post fractured pelvis and pulmonary embolism—injuries that occurred when she fell down the stairs at her home. Edna has been experiencing increasing weakness and muscle tremors. She has noted an increase of "skipping" beats. She stated that she was very dizzy and disoriented just before she fell. Based on the symptoms, which of the following labs should you assess immediately?
    A. Calcium level
    B. Sodium level
    C. Hemoglobin and hematocrit
    D. Magnesium level

55. Sonia had major abdominal surgery status post motor vehicle accident. She is exhibiting signs and symptoms of hypomagnesemia related to excessive urinary loss. How long will this loss persist?
    A. 12 hours
    B. 24 hours
    C. 36 hours
    D. 48 hours

56. Your patient was admitted for ketoacidosis. Her magnesium level is 0.5 mEq/L. Which symptoms would you expect to see?
    A. Convulsions
    B. Lethargy
    C. Negative Babinski sign
    D. Decreased reflexes

57. Ali was diagnosed with breast cancer 8 years ago. The cancer has now metastasized to the bone. Which changes in her electrolytes would you expect to see?
    A. Decreased magnesium level and increased calcium level
    B. Decreased magnesium and calcium levels
    C. Increased magnesium and calcium levels
    D. Increased magnesium level and decreased calcium level

58. Your patient is status post cardiac arrest. Magnesium replacement is ordered. What is the fastest rate of infusion recommended for magnesium replacement?
    A. 15 mg/min
    B. 30 mg/min
    C. 45 mg/min
    D. 60 mg/min

59. Magnesium is ordered for your patient. You note that the patient exhibits flaccidity, absent patellar reflexes, shallow respirations, and a flushed face. You should
    A. Give the magnesium as ordered; the patient is just sleeping.
    B. Hold the dose for 1 hour.
    C. Give the dose over 3 hours.
    D. Hold the dose, contact the physician, and obtain a magnesium level.

60. The most common cause of hypermagnesemia is
    A. Gastrointestinal bypass.
    B. Gastrointestinal fistulas.
    C. Renal failure.
    D. Overdose.

61. The family of your patient with hypermagnesemia asks why his face is flushed. You reply:
    A. "He has a fever."
    B. "His magnesium level is a little high and causes his faced to look flushed."
    C. "He is embarrassed because the hospital gown does not provide enough coverage."
    D. "He just completed his physical therapy."

62. What percentage of the body's calcium is stored in the bone?
    A. 99%
    B. 85%
    C. 80%
    D. 75%

63. Which of the following statements is true regarding calcium?
    A. Calcium is approximately 40% ionized in the serum.
    B. Calcium levels cannot be correlated with albumin levels.
    C. Calcium that is bonded to protein cannot pass through capillary walls.
    D. Calcium is not necessary for coagulation.

64. Serum calcium is decreased by all of the following *except*
    A. An increase in vitamin D.
    B. Renal tubular excretion.
    C. Gastrointestinal excretion.
    D. Bone demineralization.

65. As calcium levels _____, the parathyroid _____ secretions.
    A. increase, decreases
    B. increase, increases
    C. decrease, decreases
    D. decrease, remains consistent

66. You are testing for hypocalcemia using Trousseau's sign. You would do this by
    A. Tapping the patient's cheek.
    B. Lifting the left leg up and looking for head lifting to the chest.
    C. Inflating a BP cuff to greater than the systolic pressure for 3 minutes and waiting for a carpal spasm.
    D. Taking a sharp object up from the patient's heel to the toes and watching for the toes to spread.

67. Maria is scheduled to undergo continuous renal replacement therapy (CRRT) this week. Which of the following drugs should be stopped 2 to 3 days prior to therapy?
    A. Beta blockers
    B. ACE inhibitors
    C. Heparin
    D. Calcium-channel blockers

68. For non-pumped continuous renal replacement therapy (CRRT) to function correctly, the minimal mean arterial blood pressure must be
    A. 40 mm Hg.
    B. 50 mm Hg.
    C. 60 mm Hg.
    D. 80 mm Hg.

69. Alice has renal failure and is preparing to have continuous renal replacement therapy (CRRT). She asks if she can have visitors during the procedure. You tell her:

A. "Of course. There are no restrictions."

B. "No. They would be in the way of the equipment."

C. "No. They will increase your risk of infection."

D. "Yes, but if they are sensitive to the sight of blood, they may want to wait until after the procedure to see you."

70. **Which of the following continuous renal replacement therapies (CRRT) require only venous access and pumping function?**
    A. CVVHDF, SCUF
    B. CVVH, CVVHD
    C. CAVH, CAVHD
    D. CVVH, CAVH

71. **Trace is a patient in renal failure post multiple cardiac arrests and cardiogenic shock. He has continued cardiovascular instability. The best method for removal of fluid is by**
    A. Hemodialysis.
    B. Peritoneal dialysis.
    C. Continuous renal replacement therapy (CRRT).
    D. Plasmapheresis.

72. **Adam is undergoing hemodialysis for renal failure as a result of uncontrolled Type II diabetes. His wife asks how you know the hemodialysis is effective. Adequacy of dialysis is measured by**
    A. Urine creatinine clearance.
    B. Sodium, chloride, and potassium levels.
    C. Blood pressure.
    D. Urea clearance.

73. **You are assessing your patient's vascular access prior to hemodialysis. You note that there is no thrill or bruit. Your next nursing action would be to**
    A. Call the surgeon to do a new graft.
    B. Use a Doppler to determine graft patency.
    C. Administer a bolus of heparin.
    D. Continue with the hemodialysis, there is nothing wrong.

74. **Hemodialysis is used to treat many metabolic abnormalities as well as renal failure. One possible treatment is**
    A. Vitamin C and calcium carbonate to treat osteoporosis.
    B. Erythropoietin to counteract excessive iron.
    C. Phosphate binders to treat hyperphosphatemia.
    D. Glucose to treat hyperglycemia.

75. **Communication between all staff members who are treating a patient is vital. When transferring your patient with a graft, which of the following is a priority to communicate to all personnel who may come in contact with this patient?**
    A. Last dialysis date
    B. Location of the graft
    C. Type of dialysis machine used
    D. Total fluid removed with last dialysis

76. **The usual amount of dialysate used in peritoneal dialysis is**
    A. 0.5–1 L.
    B. 1–2 L.
    C. 2–3 L.
    D. 3–4 L.

77. **Which of the following is the correct fluid exchange sequence in peritoneal dialysis?**
    A. Dump, dwell, drain
    B. Instillation, dwell, drain
    C. Drain, instillation, dwell
    D. Instillation, drain, dwell

78. **Peritoneal dialysis functions by using which two principles?**
    A. Diffusion and ultrafiltration
    B. Osmotic pressure and osmosis
    C. Ultrafiltration and oncotic pressure
    D. Diffusion and osmosis

79. **You are preparing Leena for her first peritoneal dialysis session. It is important to tell her which of the findings is normal?**
    A. During the instillation phase, the insertion site may leak.
    B. During the dwell phase, you may feel abdominal fullness and shortness of breath.
    C. During the dwell phase, subcutaneous fluid may be seen in the groin.
    D. During the drain phase, you may feel dizzy and have palpitations.

80. **During the drain phase of peritoneal dialysis, you note only 50% return in the collection bag. What is your first action?**
    A. Position the patient prone.
    B. Check for kinks, bends, or cracks in the tubing.
    C. Double-check the amount installed.
    D. Assess for subcutaneous fluid.

81. **You are providing discharge teaching to the family and a patient who is receiving peritoneal dialysis. As part of the discharge instructions, your patient will receive a home glucometer. The daughter questions the need for the glucometer because her mother is not a diabetic. You would tell her:**
    A. "Peritoneal dialysis can cause diabetes."
    B. "She didn't tell you? Your mother was just diagnosed with diabetes."
    C. "The dialysate contains glucose and can lead to hyperglycemia."
    D. "Peritoneal dialysis may lead to pancreatitis."

82. **For which of the following disease processes is immunoadsorption used as a treatment?**
    A. Paraneoplastic neurologic syndromes
    B. Multiple sclerosis
    C. Cutaneous T-cell lymphomas
    D. Heart transplant rejection

83. **Aphaeresis is best defined as**
    A. The removal of plasma and/or proteins from the blood.
    B. The selective removal of cells, plasma, and substances from the blood.
    C. The selective removal of cellular components from the blood.
    D. The removal of an antigen in the blood.

84. **The exchange plasma volume used in aphaeresis is usually delivered at a ratio of**
    A. 1.5:1.
    B. 2:1.
    C. 2.5:1.
    D. 3:1.

85. **Kathy, a 26-year-old teacher, is undergoing lymphocytopheresis and plasma exchange for progressive multiple sclerosis, with citrate as the anticoagulant. She begins to feel tingling. Which of the following lab results should you check first?**
    A. ABGs, ionized calcium, PT/PTT levels
    B. Potassium, magnesium, PT/PTT levels
    C. INR, potassium, sodium, chloride levels
    D. ACT, ionized calcium level, ABGs

86. **Jeff has been diagnosed with hypertension. He states that in order to control his blood pressure, he "will never eat another thing with salt." You would tell him:**
    A. "That is not easy. Most fresh vegetables and fruit have tons of sodium."
    B. "Great. Sodium plays only a minor part in water balance and cellular activity, so your body won't know the difference."
    C. "You cannot completely eliminate sodium from your diet. Your body has an intricate system of safety measures to protect the level of sodium in your body."
    D. "Okay. Sodium is controlled by aldosterone that is released by the pituitary gland."

87. **The recommended sodium daily intake for someone limiting sodium from their diet should range between**
    A. 100 mg and 900 mg.
    B. 1,000 mg and 2,000 mg.
    C. 3,000 mg and 5,000 mg.
    D. 4,000 mg and 6,000 mg.

88. **Liam was put on a limited-sodium diet and has been working with a nutritionist. He was admitted to your unit for chest pain (angina) and pulmonary edema. He reports that he has stopped all additional sodium intake, has been following his diet regimen closely, stopped eating out, is drinking 8 to 10 eight-ounce glasses of tap water every day, and is voiding well. His sodium level is 155 mEq/L. What is the likely cause of his hypernatremia?**
    A. Renal failure
    B. Hypotonic fluids
    C. Diabetes mellitus
    D. Water softener system

89. Which of the following fruits has the lowest sodium content per 3.5-ounce serving?
    A. Cantaloupe
    B. Grapes
    C. Peaches
    D. Blackberries

90. Henry is trying to limit his salt intake. Which of the following meat products would you recommend for Henry to eat?
    A. Chicken without the skin
    B. Canned beef hash
    C. Fresh pike
    D. Canned crab

91. Andrew loves cheese, but must limit his sodium intake. Which of the following cheeses has the highest sodium content per 3.5-ounce serving?
    A. Swiss cheese
    B. Mozzarella cheese
    C. Cheddar cheese
    D. Parmesan cheese

92. You are receiving report on Alec, who was injured when he seized while working on his roof. His sodium level on admission was 120 mEq/L. Which symptom of hyponatremia would you expect to see?
    A. Twitching
    B. Tachypnea
    C. Lethargy
    D. Flattened T waves

93. A common cause of hyponatremia is
    A. Salt water drowning.
    B. Over-hydration.
    C. Administration of hypertonic solutions.
    D. Hyperoxia.

This concludes the Renal questions.

ANSWERS

1. **Correct Answer: C**
   Acute renal failure is now known as acute renal injury (AKI) and can be classified as either prerenal, intrinsic, or postrenal. Because material covered on the CCRN exam reflects practice up to 2 years ago, we thought that the new terminology should be added here. Some item writers may use this new terminology on the exam.

2. **Correct Answer: B**
   Other causes include cell detachment, dilatation of the lumen, and injury to the distal nephron. Answers A, C, and D are causes of prerenal AKI.

3. **Correct Answer: A**
   Anuria is usually due to postrenal AKI. Mechanical obstruction of the urinary collection system is involved. The collection system is comprised of the renal pelvis, the ureters, the bladder, and the urethra.

4. **Correct Answer: C**
   Other causes include tumor, tricyclic antidepressants, fibrosis, BPH, prostate cancer, urethral obstruction, stone disease, and ligation during surgery. Answers A, B, and D are causes of intrinsic failure/injury.

5. **Correct Answer: A**
   The BUN may also be elevated in cases of GI or mucosal bleeding or excessive protein intake.

6. **Correct Answer: D**
   Ultrasound may be difficult to obtain or interpret due to ascites, obesity, or fluid in the retroperitoneal area. Doppler scans measure blood flow and the flow may be diminished due to prerenal and intrinsic AKI. Nuclear scans are of limited value because the excretion rates may be slowed by disease. The renal biopsy is the gold standard for diagnosing rejection.

7. **Correct Answer: B**
   Potassium and phosphorus levels must be diligently monitored because of the potential for dysrhythmias.

8. **Correct Answer: D**
   Anuria is defined as urinary output of less than 100 mL/day.

9. **Correct Answer: C**
   Answers A, B, and D are causes of non-oliguria (urine output of more than 400 mL/day). Hepatorenal syndrome is another cause of oliguria.

10. **Correct Answer: A**
    Tetracycline decreases anabolism, which in turn increases BUN.

11. **Correct Answer: C**
    Answers A, B, and D are characteristics of loop diuretics such as furosemide, bumetadine, and torsemide.

12. **Correct Answer: D**

    Acyclovir can crystallize in the kidney and cause AKI. It is important for the nurse to carefully monitor the infusion time and the amount of fluid used to dilute intravenous drugs. Additional drugs that can crystallize in the kidney include sulfonamides, idinivir, and triamterine.

13. **Correct Answer: A**

    NSAIDs block prostaglandin production, which in turn alters glomerular arteriolar perfusion.

14. **Correct Answer: D**

    Answers A, B, and C are medications that increase BUN levels.

15. **Correct Answer: A**

    Females have less muscle mass than males, so they have lower levels of creatinine. Higher-than-normal levels of creatinine may indicate pyelonephritis or eclampsia.

16. **Correct Answer: C**

    Cimetidine interferes with creatinine excretion in the renal tubules. Renal function does not decrease, but the creatinine level does rise. If diminished renal function exists, the patient may develop an allergic nephritis.

17. **Correct Answer: B**

    More than 99% of urea synthesis occurs in the liver. Dietary protein is converted into amino acids and peptides. Approximately 90% of these molecules are absorbed and transferred to the liver. Any excess nitrogen is converted into urea.

18. **Correct Answer: A**

    Approximately 500 mL of whole blood equals 100 g of protein. The extra protein must be converted into urea.

19. **Correct Answer: D**

    Individuals who are trapped under a steering column as the result of a motor vehicle accident often have rectal injures, pelvic fractures, and injured iliac vessels.

20. **Correct Answer: C**

    This procedure elicits Trousseau's sign, which is an indication of hypocalcemia. You can also elicit this response by having the patient hyperventilate. When the patient becomes alkalotic, the serum calcium level decreases and a carpopedal spasm occurs.

21. **Correct Answer: B**

    The patient has hypercalcemia. A loop diuretic prevents reabsorption of calcium, and normal saline is used to increase the patient's glomerular filtration rate. Administration of a thiazide diuretic would actually decrease calcium excretion. Administration of glucose, insulin, and Kayexalate is not indicated because these agents are treatments for hyperkalemia.

22. **Correct Answer: B**

    1 kilogram = 2.2 pounds= 1,000 milliliters. Although you may think this is too basic a piece of information for a CCRN review, little pieces of information like this often trip people up on the exam.

23. **Correct Answer: D**
    This patient is hypocalcemic. Lack of calcium slows cardiac contractility (the prolonged QT), and the patient might develop torsades de pointes (polymorphic ventricular tachycardia). The torsades is also caused by hyperkalemia.

24. **Correct Answer: B**
    Trousseau's sign utilizes a BP cuff to elicit a carpopedal spasm indicative of hypocalcemia. Grey–Turner's sign is ecchymosis around the umbilicus, indicating abdominal issues. Homan's sign may indicate DVT.

25. **Correct Answer: A**
    The patient with AKI cannot excrete ammonium or acid ions in quantities that are necessary to aid in the excretion of hydrogen. The buildup of the hydrogen causes the acidosis.

26. **Correct Answer: B**
    Renal infarction can occur with cocaine intoxication. Cocaine abuse can lead to any infarction, including MI. The proteinuria and RBCs in the urine are indicative of renal infarction.

27. **Correct Answer: B**
    Aldosterone is a hormone secreted by the adrenal glands. Aldosterone will also be secreted if an individual's blood pressure is too low and when a person is under extreme physical stress.

28. **Correct Answer: C**
    Because of a defect in chromosome 7, patients with cystic fibrosis lose sodium through their skin and mucous membranes. This results in a thickening of the mucous layers, leading to infection and hyponatremia.

29. **Correct Answer: A**
    Large amounts of extracellular fluids are present in the peritoneal cavity. If sodium is lost in this area, then it is no longer available to be absorbed into the vasculature.

30. **Correct Answer: A**
    Due to her medical condition, Beatrice was unable to drink; the lack of fluids led to dehydration and hemoconcentration. As a result of her diabetes, she may have additional renal injury. Coupled with the decreased blood flow through her kidneys from the CHF, this injury meant that Beatrice's kidneys were unable to filter the excess sodium from her body.

31. **Correct Answer: D**
    Sodium is the major extracellular cation, and potassium is the major intracellular cation.

32. **Correct Answer: A**
    Approximately 2% of potassium is extracellular; the remaining 98% is intracellular. Intracellular electrolytes cannot be directly measured, but extracellular levels can be measured. Normal values are 3.5 to 5.0 mEq/L.

33. **Correct Answer: B**
    Regulated excretion of potassium occurs in the distal tubules.

34. **Correct Answer: B**

As aldosterone is secreted, potassium excretion increases. The reverse is also true: If aldosterone secretion is inhibited, potassium excretion decreases and more potassium is retained.

35. **Correct Answer: D**

Consumption of alcohol leads to an alkalotic state. Because potassium ions have a positive charge, hydrogen ions move in the opposite direction. As potassium moves into the cell, hydrogen moves out to correct the alkalosis.

36. **Correct Answer: C**

Potassium ions and hydrogen ions move in opposition to each other. With hypokalemia, hydrogen moves into the extracellular fluid, leading to both respiratory and metabolic alkalosis.

37. **Correct Answer: A**

Oliguria is the result of hyperkalemia. Renal disease, administration of Lasix, and increased production of adrenal cortical hormones lead to hypokalemia.

38. **Correct Answer: B**

A U wave is seen in hypokalemia. A peaked T wave, a shortened QT segment, and an absent P wave are seen in hyperkalemia.

39. **Correct Answer: D**

The patient will become hyperkalemic as the potassium from the cells is released into the vasculature as a result of the crush injury.

40. **Correct Answer: C**

Some people may take in 800 to 11,000 mg of potassium per day through their diet.

41. **Correct Answer: D**

Carrots have the lowest amount of potassium per serving (233 mg), as compared to avocadoes (1,484 mg), raisins (751 mg), and potatoes (610 mg).

42. **Correct Answer: A**

Boiling leaches out most of the nutrients into the water. Baking is the best method allowing the vegetables to retain most of their potassium and other nutrients.

43. **Correct Answer: C**

Potassium should not be infused at any rate greater than 10 mEq/h to prevent extravasation, pain, or spasms related to rapid electrolyte changes.

44. **Correct Answer: A**

Addison's disease results in a decrease in aldosterone secretion. The lower level of aldosterone leads to both hyperkalemia and hyponatremia, because sodium cannot be retained and potassium cannot be removed.

45. **Correct Answer: B**

Kaon is another name for potassium glucanate, a common potassium replacement medication. The glucose/insulin combination, calcium glucanate, and bicarbonate all bind or push the potassium back into the cell from the intravascular, thereby leading to lower extracellular potassium levels.

46. Correct Answer: A

Jackie is exhibiting signs and symptoms of hypokalemia. Hypokalemia is defined as any potassium level less than 3.5 mEq/L. When patients are given new medications, it is important to educate them about how those drugs will affect their electrolyte levels.

47. Correct Answer: C

The current recommended serum magnesium level is 2–3 mg/dL. This level may be higher for patients with cardiac disease or for patients in their third trimester of pregnancy to treat pregnancy-induced hypertension and to control premature contractions.

48. Correct Answer: A

Magnesium usually acts synergistically with calcium to control neuromuscular function within all muscle groups.

49. Correct Answer: A

The parathyroid controls the calcium level within the body. Magnesium has been found to influence the secretion rate of the parathyroid and, therefore, calcium levels.

50. Correct Answer: C

Approximately 50% of the body's magnesium is within the bone marrow. The measured serum magnesium reflects only approximately 1% of the body's magnesium; the remaining 49% is found intracellularly.

51. Correct Answer: D

Currently, the recommended adult intake of magnesium is 350 to 420 mg per day. For pregnant women, the recommended intake is at the higher end of this range. Children's intake should be less and should be based on age.

52. Correct Answer: A

Honey contains the smallest amount of magnesium. It is better to recommend foods such as leafy vegetables that have a deep, green color, whole grains, nuts, legumes, seafood, cocoa, and chocolate.

53. Correct Answer: B

Because magnesium is absorbed in the small intestines, surgical procedures that remove or alter the small intestines (such as gastric bypass) place the patient at risk for hypomagnesemia. Gastric surgeries also affect water reabsorption, time processing in the intestines, calcium level, and amount of lactose in the diet.

54. Correct Answer: D

Edna is exhibiting signs and symptoms of hypomagnesemia related to her high calcium intake. Calcium and magnesium are absorbed in the small intestines. Calcium, when consumed in extremely high doses (either through supplements or as part of dietary intake), competes with magnesium for absorption. Edna will need nutritional teaching so that she can learn to balance her diet.

55. Correct Answer: B

Abdominal surgery and trauma lead to increased stress on the body and increased aldosterone secretion. This increase in aldosterone secretion leads to an increase in magnesium excretion, which contributes to hypomagnesemia. This condition lasts for approximately 24 hours. There is an additional risk with any abdominal injury or surgery that impairs small bowel absorption of magnesium.

56. **Correct Answer: A**

    Ketoacidosis leads to excessive urinary secretion of magnesium as a result of osmotic diuresis caused by the elevated glucose concentration. In addition, the insulin therapy used to treat the hyperglycemia forces magnesium into the cells, which further decreases the extracellular concentration of magnesium. As magnesium levels drop, cellular irritability increases and the risk of convulsions increases. The patient would demonstrate increased overall irritability, a positive Babinski sign, and increased reflexes.

57. **Correct Answer: A**

    As cancer spreads through bone, calcium is released into the serum. In a hypercalcemic state, magnesium secretion increases, leading to hypomagnesemia.

58. **Correct Answer: B**

    Only if a patient is in cardiopulmonary arrest would you infuse magnesium at a rate of 1–2 g over 5 to 10 minutes. IV infusion should be no faster than 30 mg per minute. Careful monitoring should be performed, along with venous access and monitoring of EKG changes. If using stock magnesium or ampules, be aware of the concentrations available. Solutions are available in 10%, 20%, and 50% concentrations. To prevent medication errors, orders should specify the milliliters of a concentration in an amount of dilute solution to be given over a specific time frame. For example, the order might state that the patient is to be given 2 mL of 50% magnesium sulfate (do not use the abbreviation $MgSO_4$, which may be confused with MS or morphine) to be diluted in 100 mL of normal saline (or 9% sodium chloride) over 2 hours.

59. **Correct Answer: D**

    The patient is exhibiting the signs and symptoms of hypermagnesemia. The dose should be held, the physician contacted, and the magnesium level evaluated.

60. **Correct Answer: C**

    Renal failure is one of the most common causes of hypermagnesemia. The patient is unable to excrete excess magnesium via the urine. Gastrointestinal bypass and fistulas will lead to hypomagnesemia.

61. **Correct Answer: B**

    Magnesium levels greater than 5 mEq/L lead to vasodilation of the facial vessels.

62. **Correct Answer: A**

    Approximately 99% of the body's calcium is stored in the bone.

63. **Correct Answer: C**

    If calcium is bonded with protein, the resulting molecule is too large to pass from the extracellular fluid into intracellular space due to restrictive capillary permeability. Approximately 50% to 70% of serum calcium is ionized in the serum. Because of the protein-binding ability of calcium, albumin and calcium levels can be directly correlated. Calcium plays a role in coagulation.

64. **Correct Answer: A**

    Vitamin D increases serum calcium.

65. **Correct Answer: A**

    Parathyroid hormone is the hormone most closely related to serum calcium management. In response to rising calcium levels, the parathyroid decreases its secretion to decrease or stabilize calcium levels.

66. **Correct Answer: C**

The technique for eliciting Trousseau's sign is to inflate a blood pressure cuff to greater than the systolic blood pressure for 3 minutes. A positive sign is noted when the carpal nerve spasms, causing the hand to curve inward with all fingers touching.

67. **Correct Answer: B**

Beta-blockers may cause an anaphylactic reaction with the membranes or the filter in the CRRT. Bradykins are released as a result, which leads to systemic anaphylaxis.

68. **Correct Answer: C**

The patient's blood pressure provides the gradient on which the system functions. If the blood pressure is too low, the system will not filter appropriately.

69. **Correct Answer: D**

Some individuals cannot tolerate the sight of blood. Because CRRT occurs outside the body, blood is in full sight. To improve communication between both patient and visitors, it is best for the patient to let visitors know when procedures are occurring so that they may visit at a time when CRRT is not occurring. There are some restrictions to how many people may fit in one room with the equipment, but this number will vary by facility. The more people in a room, the higher the risk that the equipment could be touched and/or disconnected. Visitors should be informed not to touch equipment while in the room. Simple hand washing will prevent many infections. Other infection control measures should be implemented based on the patient's specific disease process.

70. **Correct Answer: B**

The "C" in the acronym stands for "continuous." The second and third letters refer to the access and return sites, respectively. CVV types of dilution require a pump function, because the blood must be pumped through the system. CAV types of filtration use arterial pressures to drive the flow and the filtration. H, HD, and HDF refer to the type of filtration: hemofiltration, hemodialysis, or hemodiafiltration respectively. SCUF, or slow continuous ultrafiltration, is used to remove fluid from the patient and no replacement is given.

71. **Correct Answer: C**

Continuous renal replacement therapy (CRRT) results in slower volume regulation in an effort to avoid rapid shifts in volume. This method results in continuous removal and/or regulation of solutes and volume.

72. **Correct Answer: D**

The rate of urea clearance in the blood is the best method of monitoring dialysis effectiveness. Electrolytes may be altered due to fluid shifting and the distillate used. Blood pressure may fluctuate with fluid removal, so it is not the best measurement method. The urine creatinine clearance rate indicates residual renal function.

73. **Correct Answer: B**

Lack of thrill and/or bruit may indicate that the graft is occluded and dialysis is not possible. It is best to use a Doppler to determine graft patency prior to making any calls or administering any medication. Although you may not hear or feel the thrill and bruit, the graft may still be patent. The surgeon should be notified if the Doppler study is negative. Heparin will not break an existing clot.

74. **Correct Answer: C**

Hemodialysis is used to administer phosphate binders to patients with hyperphosphatemia. In addition, it may be used to provide vitamin D and calcium carbonate for osteoporosis, erythropoietin for iron deficiencies (anemia), and glucose for hypoglycemia.

75. **Correct Answer: B**

It is imperative that all staff members be made aware of the graft site location, including lab personnel, nursing assistants, student nurses, medical staff, physical therapy personnel, and respiratory therapy providers. All personnel should avoid any lab or blood draws, blood pressures, or occlusions in the grafted limb.

76. **Correct Answer: C**

Approximately 2–3 L of dialysate is used in peritoneal dialysis.

77. **Correct Answer: B**

The correct sequence for fluid exchange in peritoneal dialysis is (1) install the dialysate, (2) allow the fluid to dwell within the abdomen for a predetermined time, and (3) drain the fluid. The number of exchanges is determined by the physician and the desired outcome.

78. **Correct Answer: D**

Peritoneal dialysis functions by the principles of diffusion and osmosis. Diffusion is the passive movement of solutes across a membrane. The direction of diffusion is based on concentration (solutes move from areas of higher concentration to areas of lower concentration), heat, and pressure. The speed at which diffusion occurs is based on the grade or steepness of the differences in concentrations on each side of the membrane and the molecule moving across the membrane (size, polarity).

Osmosis is the passive movement of solvents (i.e., water) over a permeable membrane. Movement of the solvent depends on the permeability of the membrane. The more permeable the membrane, the more passive movement of solutes and solvents occurs. Permeability may determine which types of solutes are able to unintentionally cross the membrane.

79. **Correct Answer: B**

It is common for patients to have a feeling of abdominal fullness related to the 2–3 L of dialysate installed in the abdomen and allowed to dwell there. Leaking at the insertion site must be reported to the physician because the patient may develop peritonitis and the patient should be monitored closely. Dialysis cannot continue until the insertion site is repaired. If fluid is felt or seen in the groin, it indicates a hernia. A hernia may lead to strangulation of any bowel that enters the groin during the dwell phase and is trapped there when the dialysate is drained.

If a patient feels dizzy or has palpitations during the drain phase, this reaction indicates a too-rapid fluid shift or triggering of the vagal nerve. The drain time may need to be lengthened.

80. **Correct Answer: B**

Kinking, bends, and cracks in the tubing are the most likely causes of decreased dialysate return. If eliminating these problems does not correct the fluid flow, then reposition the patient, assess for any subcutaneous fluid, fluid within the groin, double-check the amount of fluid installed, and complete an assessment prior to reporting the situation to the physician.

81. **Correct Answer: C**
The dialysate often contains an amount of glucose. During diffusion, glucose may cross the membranes and lead to hyperglycemia. It is important for the patient to monitor this complication at home. Careful education will assist the family in managing any complications and knowing when to notify the physician.

82. **Correct Answer: A**
Each of the answers is a condition often treated with aphaeresis, but paraneoplastic neurologic syndromes are treated with immunoadsorption. Multiple sclerosis is treated with plasma lymphocytes. Cutaneous T-cell lymphoma is treated using a combination of photopheresis and leukopheresis. Heart transplant rejections are treated with a combination of photopheresis and plasmapheresis.

83. **Correct Answer: B**
Aphaeresis is the general term used for all pheresis techniques and encompasses any selective removal of cells, plasma, and substances from blood with the return of remaining components and volume to the patient. Plasmapheresis is the removal of plasma and/or proteins from the blood or as a plasma exchange. Cytopheresis is the selective removal of cellular components from the blood (i.e., WBCs). Leukocytopheresis is the specific removal of WBCs. Erythroctytopheresis is the removal of RBCs. Plateletpheresis is the removal of platelets. Plasma-adsorption/perfusion is the filtering and treatment of plasma via adsorptive fiber filters. Immunoadsorption is the removal of an antigen via an antibody filter. Photopheresis is the removal and return of blood after exposure to ultraviolet light to destroy specific cells (in solid-organ transplant rejection).

84. **Correct Answer: A**
Replacement of plasma volume in plasmapheresis is usually at a 1:1 or 1.5:1 ratio. Replacement fluids include FFP, thawed plasma, albumin, and electrolytes and other fluids based on the patient's condition.

85. **Correct Answer: D**
Citrate binds with calcium in the blood and metabolizes into sodium bicarbonate, thereby increasing sodium and phosphate alkaline levels. ACT, ionized calcium levels, and ABGs will show the extent of this binding. The tingling results from a decrease in the amount of calcium available to the tissues.

86. **Correct Answer: C**
Sodium cannot be completely eliminated from the diet. Sodium is a major cation in the extracellular fluid within the body. Sodium plays a key part in the sodium/potassium pump and in stabilizing the polarization of cells and water balance. The body will protect sodium levels by titrating aldosterone and antidiuretic hormone (ADH), and by changing the filtration rate within the kidneys.

Fresh fruits and vegetables contain minimal amounts of salt. Canned vegetables typically use sodium to preserve flavor and will contain the highest sodium levels.

87. **Correct Answer: B**
The daily recommended sodium intake for someone limiting sodium in their diet should be between 1,000 and 2,000 mg per day. This challenges the body to use sodium efficiently without overstressing the body's systems. A low-sodium diet aims to restrict sodium intake to less than 1,000 mg per day.

88. **Correct Answer: D**

Many water softening systems filter out calcium and magnesium (these minerals make water "hard") and replace them with sodium. The longer the filter has been in place, the greater the sodium content of the water. Not all water softeners use sodium, so recommend that patients check their systems first before abandoning these devices. Possibly, instead of drinking tap water, the patient should drink—and food should be prepared with—distilled or bottled water. He may also consider replacing the water filter with a reverse-osmosis system.

Liam is following his diet as prescribed and does not exhibit any signs of renal failure. Hypertonic fluids would lead to higher sodium levels. Diabetes insipidus would lead to elevated sodium levels due to the lack of ADH.

89. **Correct Answer: D**

Blackberries have 1 mg of sodium per 3.5-ounce serving, which is less than the amount of sodium found in same-size servings of peaches (2 mg), grapes (3 mg), and cantaloupe (12 mg).

90. **Correct Answer: C**

Most fresh fish is low in sodium. Pike has only 51 mg of sodium per 3.5-ounce serving—much less than chicken (60–80 mg), canned beef hash (540 mg), and canned crab (1,000 mg). Any canned or processed meat will contain some kind of preservative. If it is not marked as being "low sodium," the patient should check the sugar content—it could be too high. For most people, eating fresh or fresh frozen meats, vegetables, and fruits will aid in limiting sodium, fat, and sugar intake.

91. **Correct Answer: D**

Parmesan cheese contains 1,862 mg of sodium per serving, compared to 260 mg in Swiss cheese, 620 mg in cheddar cheese, and 373 mg in mozzarella.

92. **Correct Answer: A**

With hyponatremia, sodium levels drop below 135 mEq/L. Twitching and seizures are common, as are apnea (not tachypnea), irritability (lethargy is seen with hypernatremia), and generalized muscle weakness (a late sign). Flattened T waves are seen with hypokalemia.

93. **Correct Answer: B**

Over-hydration is a common cause of hyponatremia. It is not a real hyponatremia, in that the level falls below normal because of dilution rather than a disease process or injury. Intake, orally or intravenously, has caused an artificial drop in sodium. The imbalance can be corrected through fluid restriction or a decrease in the IV rate. Other potential causes of hyponatremia include loss of sodium through sweating or vomiting, shock, bleeding, SIADH, renal failure (inability to save sodium), hypoxia, fresh water drowning, and administration of excessive hypotonic fluids.

BIBLIOGRAPHY

Ahrens, T. (2006). *Critical care nursing certification*. Columbus, OH: McGraw-Hill.

American Association of Critical-Care Nurses. (2006). *Core curriculum for critical care nursing* (6th ed.). Philadelphia: Saunders.

American Association of Critical-Care Nurses. (2007). *AACN certification and core review for high acuity and critical care* (6th ed.). Philadelphia: Saunders.

American Heart Association. (2007). *Guidelines 2005 for cardiopulmonary resuscitation and emergency cardiovascular care*. Retrieved July 24, 2008, from http://circ.ahajournals.org/content/vol112/24_suppl

Bossola, M., Giungi, S., Tazza, L., & Luciani, G. (2007). Long-term oral sodium bicarbonate supplementation does not improve serum albumin levels in hemodialysis patients. *Nephron, 106*(1), c51–c56.

Brindley, P. G., Butler, M. S., Cembrowski, G., & Brindley, D. N. (2007). Case report: Falsely elevated point-of-care lactate measurement after ingestion of ethylene glycol. *Canadian Medical Association Journal, 176*(8), 1097–1099.

Burns, S. M. (Ed.). (2007). *American Association of Critical-Care Nurses (AACN): AACN protocols for practice: Healing environments* (2nd ed.). Sudbury, MA: Jones and Bartlett.

Conover, M. B. (2003). *Understanding electrocardiography* (8th ed.). St. Louis, MO: Mosby/Elsevier.

Copstead, L., & Banasik, J. L. (2000). *Pathophysiology: Biological and behavioral perspectives* (2nd ed.). Philadelphia: Saunders/Elsevier.

Curley, M. A. Q. (1998). Patient–nurse synergy: Optimizing patients' outcomes. *American Journal of Critical Care, 7*, 64–72.

Dessap, A. M., Lellouche, N., Audard, V., Roudot-Thoraval, F., Champagne, S., Lim, P., et al. (2008). Effect of renal failure on peak troponin Ic level in patients with acute myocardial infarction. *Cardiology, 109*(4), 217–221.

Dossey, B. M., Keegan, L., & Guzzetta, C. (2003). *Holistic nursing: A handbook for practice* (3rd ed.). Sudbury, MA: Jones and Bartlett.

Eastwood, G., Gardner, A., & O'Connell, B. (2007). Low-flow oxygen therapy: Selecting the right device. *Australian Nursing Journal, 15*(4), 27–30.

Edwards, D. F. (1999). The Synergy Model: Linking patient needs to nurse competencies. *Critical Care Nurse, 19*(1), 88–98.

Emergency Nurses Association, & Newberry, L. (2003). *Sheehy's emergency nursing: Principles and practice* (5th ed.). St. Louis, MO: Mosby/Elsevier.

Eslamifar, A., Hamkar, R., Ramezani, A., Ahmadi, F., Gachkar, L., Jalilvand, S., et al. (2007). Hepatitis G virus exposure in dialysis patients. *International Urology and Nephrology, 39*(4), 1257–1263.

Finkelmeier, B. A. (2000). *Cardiothoracic surgical nursing* (2nd ed.). Philadelphia: Lippincott, Williams & Wilkins.

Hardin, S. R., & Kaplow, R. (Eds.). (2004). *Synergy for clinical excellence: The AACN Synergy Model for Patient Care*. Sudbury, MA: Jones and Bartlett.

Herzog, H. A. (2008). Kidney disease in cardiology. *Nephrology, Dialysis, Transplantation, 23*(1), 42–46.

Hickey, J. V. (2002). *The clinical practice of neurological and neurosurgical nursing* (5th ed.). Philadelphia: Lippincott, Williams & Wilkins.

Hodgman, M. J., Horn, J. F., Stork, C. M., Marraffa, J. M., Holland, M. G., Cantor, R., et al. (2007). Profound metabolic acidosis and oxoprolinuria in an adult. *Journal of Medical Toxicology, 3*(3), 119–124.

Kawada, T., Yamazaki, T., Akiyama, T., Li, M., Zheng, C., Shishido, T., et al. (2007). Angiotensin II attenuates myocardial interstitial acetylcholine release in response to vagal stimulation. *American Journal of Physiology: Heart and Circulatory Physiology, 293*(4), H2516.

Komaba, H., Igaki, N., Goto, S., Yokota, K., Takemoto, T., Hirosue, K., et al. (2007). Adiponectin is associated with brain natriuretic peptide and left ventricular hypertrophy in hemodialysis patients with Type 2 diabetes mellitus. *Nephron, 107*(3), c103–c108.

Laine, J., Jalanko, H., Alakulppi, N., & Holmberg, C. (2005). A new tubular disorder with hypokalaemic metabolic alkalosis, severe hypermagnesuric hypomagnesaemia, hypercalciuria and cardiomyopathy. *Nephrology, Dialysis, Transplantation, 20*(6), 1241–1245.

Lankisch, P. G., Weber-Dany, B., Maisonneuve, P., & Lowenfels, A. B. (2008). Frequency and severity of acute pancreatitis in chronic dialysis patients. *Nephrology, Dialysis, Transplantation, 23*(4), 1401–1405.

Lin, S. H., & Halperin, M. L. (2007). Hypokalemia: A practical approach to diagnosis and its genetic basis. *Current Medicinal Chemistry, 14*(14), 1551–1565.

Lipson, J. G., Dibble, S. L., & Minarik, P. A. (Eds.). (1996). *Culture and nursing care: A pocket guide.* San Francisco, CA: UCSF Nursing Press.

Livingston, E. H., & Langert, J. (2006). The impact of age and Medicare status on bariatric surgical outcomes. *Archives of Surgery, 141*(11), 1115–1120, discussion 1121.

Madias, J. E. (2007). Loss of QRS voltage in renal failure. *Journal of Electrocardiology, 40*(5), 400.

McNally, P. (2001). *GI/liver secrets* (2nd ed.). Philadelphia: Hanley & Belfus/Elsevier.

McPhatter, L., & Lockridge, R. S. (2004). Daily dialysis: Nutritional implications and advantages for a state-of-the-art treatment option. *Nephrology Nursing Journal, 31*(2), 223–224.

McQuillan, K. A., Von Rueden, K. T., Hartsock, R. L., Flynn, M. B., & Whalen, E. (Eds.). (2002). *Trauma nursing: From resuscitation through rehabilitation* (3rd ed.). Philadelphia: Saunders/Elsevier.

Medina, J., & Puntillo, K. (2006). *AACN protocols for practice: Palliative care and end-of-life issues in critical care.* Sudbury, MA: Jones and Bartlett.

Mocini, D., Leone, T., Tubaro, M., Santini, M., & Penco, M. (2007). Structure, production and function of erythropoietin: Implications for therapeutic use in cardiovascular disease. *Current Medicinal Chemistry, 14*(21), 2278–2287.

Morgera, S., Haase, M., Ruckert, M., Krieg, H., Kastrup, M., Krausch, D., et al. (2005). Regional citrate anticoagulation in continuous hemodialysis: Acid–base and electrolyte balance at an increased dose of dialysis. *Nephron, 101*(4), c211–c219.

Morris, C. G., & Low, J. (2008). Metabolic acidosis in the critically ill: Part 1. Classification and pathophysiology. *Anaesthesia, 63*(3), 294–301.

Pace, R. C. (2007). Fluid management in patients on hemodialysis. *Nephrology Nursing Journal, 34*(5), 557–559.

Pagana, K. D., & Pagana, J. (2005). *Mosby's manual of diagnostic and laboratory tests* (3rd ed.). St. Louis, MO: Mosby/Elsevier.

Palomar, R., González-Martín, V., Martín, L., Morales, P., de Francisco, A. L. M., & Arias, M. (2007). Is abdominal surgery still a contraindication for peritoneal dialysis? *Nephrology, Dialysis, Transplantation, 22*(8), 2360–2361.

Rosival, V. (2006). Treating metabolic acidosis. *QJM, 99*(12), 881; author reply 881–882.

Sinert, R., Zehtabchi, S., Bloem, S., & Lucchesi, M. (2006). Effect of normal saline infusion on the diagnostic utility of base deficit in identifying major injury in trauma patients. *Academic Emergency Medicine, 13*(12), 1269.

Skidmore-Roth, L. (2004). *Mosby's 2004 nursing drug reference.* St. Louis, MO: Mosby/Elsevier.

Smeltzer, S., & Bare, B. G. (2003). *Brunner and Suddarth's textbook of medical–surgical nursing* (10th ed.). Philadelphia: Lippincott, Williams & Wilkins.

Sole, M. L., Hartshorn, J., & Lamborne, M. L. (2001). *Introduction to critical care nursing* (3rd ed.). Philadelphia: Saunders/Elsevier.

Sood, M. M., & Richardson, R. (2007). Negative anion gap and elevated osmolar gap due to lithium overdose. *Canadian Medical Association Journal, 176*(7), 921–923.

Stookey, J. D., Barclay, D., Arieff, A., & Popkin, B. M. (2007). The altered fluid distribution in obesity may reflect plasma hypertonicity. *European Journal of Clinical Nutrition, 61*(2), 190–199.

Upadya, A., Tilluckdharry, L., Muralidharan, V., Amoateng-Adjepong, Y., & Manthous, C. A. (2005). Fluid balance and weaning outcomes. *Intensive Care Medicine, 31*(12), 1643–1647.

Urden, L. D., Stacy, K. M., & Lough, M. E. (2007). *Thelan's critical care nursing: Diagnosis and management* (5th ed.). St. Louis, MO: Mosby.

Webb, S., & Dobb, G. (2007). ARF, ATN or AKI? It's now acute kidney injury. *Anaesthesia and Intensive Care, 35*(6), 843–844.

Westenbrink, B. D., Visser, F. W., Voors, A. A., Smilde, T. D. J., Lipsic, E., Navis, G., et al. (2007). Anaemia in chronic heart failure is not only related to impaired renal perfusion and blunted erythropoietin production, but to fluid retention as well. *European Heart Journal, 28*(2), 166–171.

Wiegand, D. J. L., & Carlson, K. K. (Eds.). (2005). *AACN Procedure manual for critical care* (5th ed.). Philadelphia: Elsevier.

Wiggins, K. J., McDonald, S. P., Brown, F. G., Rosman, J. B., & Johnson, D. W. (2007). High membrane transport status on peritoneal dialysis is not associated with reduced survival following transfer to haemodialysis. *Nephrology, Dialysis, Transplantation, 22*(10), 3005–3012.

Woods, S., Sivarajan Froelicher, E. S., & Motzer, S. U. (2000). *Cardiac nursing* (4th ed.). Philadelphia: Lippincott, Williams & Wilkins.

Multisystem

QUESTIONS

1. Lisa was admitted to the ICU with diffuse abdominal pain and confusion. In the ED, she had generalized seizures and bradycardia. Opioid overdose was suspected, and she was given naloxone with no discernible effect. Lisa is now lethargic, but does tell you that she is a "body packer." Lisa suddenly becomes hypotensive and bradycardic. Appropriate therapy would include
   A. Bowel irrigations, intubation, mechanical ventilation, and anticonvulsants.
   B. Sodium bicarbonate, activated charcoal, and hemodialysis.
   C. Antiemetics, gastric lavage, and bronchodilators.
   D. Activated charcoal, sodium bicarbonate, and vasopressors.

2. Gertrude, age 76, is admitted to your unit with tachycardia (146), RR 34, BP 90/60, T 96.4°F. Her white count is 16,000. Gertrude states she was treated for a "kidney infection" 2 weeks ago. She denies pain at this time. Gertrude probably has
   A. MODS.
   B. A kidney stone.
   C. SIRS.
   D. Appendicitis.

3. Jane S., age 42, was admitted to your unit because of increased respiratory effort and possible pneumonia. The blood culture revealed the presence of *E. coli*. Which of the following antibiotics would have the best effect on the bacteria?
   A. Ganciclovir
   B. Gentamycin
   C. Cytarabine
   D. Cefoxitin

4. Pat M. is a 19-year-old male admitted to your unit after a burn injury. He was barbequing in the back yard when a sudden flame-up burned his chest and right shoulder and caused loss of his facial hair. Which finding would be indicative of smoke inhalation in this patient?
   A. PaO_2 81, met Hgb level of 2%
   B. PaO_2 76, pCO_2 26
   C. Increased CO_2
   D. CoHgb of 18%, singed facial hair

5. Continuing with the scenario from Question 4, which treatment would be most appropriate for Mr. M. at this time?
   A. Fluid resuscitation at a rate of 300 cc/h
   B. Monitor pulse oximetry continuously
   C. Intubation and place on FiO_2 100%
   D. Antibiotic therapy

6. Continuing with the scenario from Questions 4 and 5, you have now intubated Mr. M. and placed him on mechanical ventilation. His urine output drops significantly. This change is probably due to
   A. Third spacing.
   B. Sepsis.
   C. Underresuscitation.
   D. MODS.

7. Hypertonic solutions are used frequently for burn patients. An advantage of using this type of solution is that it
   A. Minimizes wound edema.
   B. Lessens chances for sepsis.
   C. Eliminates need for vitamin replacements.
   D. Has a lower cost.

8. Signs and symptoms of aspirin overdose include
   A. Metabolic acidosis, tachypnea.
   B. Bradycardia, respiratory acidosis.
   C. Bradycardia, metabolic alkalosis.
   D. Tachycardia, metabolic alkalosis.

9. A 36-year-old male was pumping gas when a spark ignited the fumes. He suffered full-thickness burns of the right arm. During your initial assessment, you note that eschar is present and the right radial pulse is not palpable. A Doppler pulse is also not discernible. Which of the following actions would be appropriate at this time?
   A. Moving the patient's arm away from his torso and elevating it on a pillow
   B. Escharotomy
   C. Morphine 4 mg IV
   D. Ice packs to reduce swelling

10. During the immediate post-burn period, which of the following fluids would be most beneficial?
    A. Normal saline
    B. 0.45% Normal saline
    C. Lactated Ringer's
    D. Albumin

11. The type of burn most likely to cause hemorrhage, thrombus formation, or generalized vascular disruption is a(n)
    A. Chemical burn.
    B. Steam burn.
    C. Direct flame burn.
    D. Electrical burn.

12. **Your patient was in full arrest following a root canal. After a successful resuscitation, the patient has developed Ludwig's angina. This type of angina can be defined as**
    A. A type of painful bradycardia in which the Q-T interval is lengthened.
    B. An infectious process.
    C. Dysrhythmia with severe pain secondary to inhalation of noxious gases.
    D. Cardiac ischemic post-code syndrome.

13. **In sepsis, endotoxins stimulate production of tumor necrosis factor (TNF). The TNF, in turn, stimulates**
    A. Neutrophil activation and platelet aggregation.
    B. Parathyroid hormone production.
    C. Increased CO_2 retention.
    D. Increased CPP.

14. **Acetaminophen overdose may cause hypoglycemia and should be treated with**
    A. Continuous IV of D_5W at 100 cc/h.
    B. A bolus of D_{50}, followed by continuous infusion of D_5W.
    C. A bolus of D_{10}, followed by continuous infusion of 0.45% normal saline.
    D. Continuous IV infusion of Lactated Ringer's.

15. **Patients who are undergoing alcohol withdrawal are frequently hypoglycemic. Treatment should include**
    A. A bolus of $D_{10}W$, q 2 hour blood glucose monitoring.
    B. TPN with high concentrations of sugars, q 2 hour blood glucose monitoring.
    C. Maintenance fluids of $D_{25}W$ at 125 mL/h peripherally.
    D. Thiamine, then bolus with D_{50}, then infusion of D_5W.

16. **Patients who have oral amphetamine overdoses should have which of the following as part of their treatment regimen?**
    A. Ammonium chloride
    B. Ipecac
    C. Caffeine
    D. Theophylline

17. **Your patient is undergoing alcohol withdrawal and exhibits diplopia, peripheral neuropathy, confusion, recent memory loss, and hyper-excitability. You suspect that this patient has**
    A. Jorn's syndrome.
    B. Leucine deficiency.
    C. Increased caritine levels.
    D. Wernicke–Kersakoff syndrome.

18. **Gladys suffered severe respiratory depression following ingestion of a large amount of diazepam. She has now developed atrial fibrillation. Anticipated treatment would include**
    A. Amiodarone.
    B. Lidocaine.
    C. Adenosine.
    D. Prostaglandin.

19. A 44-year-old male was burned over the anterior chest, both arms, anterior neck, and the lateral aspect of the right leg. He was smoking in bed and the bedcovers caught fire. The burns on his chest and right arm have a white, leather-like appearance and the patient has no sensation in that area. Which classification of burn is this?
    A. First degree
    B. Second degree partial thickness
    C. Third degree full thickness
    D. Fourth degree full thickness

20. Continuing with the scenario from Question 19, the burn on the patient's right arm is pink and blistered. When it is touched, the patient screams with pain. This classification of burn is known as a
    A. First degree.
    B. Second degree partial thickness.
    C. Third degree full thickness.
    D. Fourth degree full thickness.

21. If muscle is burned, which classification of burn is involved?
    A. First degree
    B. Second degree partial thickness
    C. Third degree full thickness
    D. Fourth degree full thickness

22. Your patient has burns on the right arm that are circumferential (all the way around the arm). What is a potential risk with this type of burn?
    A. Infection into the bone
    B. Difficulty removing dead tissue
    C. Compartment syndrome
    D. Escharotomy

23. Sustained compartment pressures of _____ are usually suggestive of compartment syndrome.
    A. 15 mm Hg
    B. 30 mm Hg
    C. 40 mm Hg
    D. 50 mm Hg

24. Initially, the burned area is estimated by the Rule of Nines or by using the palm as 1% of the body surface area. There are many ways to calculate the body surface area involved. If your patient was burned over 30% of his body and weighs 70 kg, calculate the total fluid requirements during the first 24 hours using the Parkland formula:
    A. 2,100 mL
    B. 6,300 mL
    C. 4,500 mL
    D. 8,400 mL

25. Calculate the fluid requirements (first 24 hours) for a patient who weighs 65 kg and is burned over 45% of his body using the Parkland formula:
    A. 29,250 mL
    B. 11,700 mL
    C. 26,000 mL
    D. 10,300 mL

26. When using the Parkland formula, the preferred fluid for burn resuscitation is
    A. Normal saline.
    B. D_5/Isolyte M.
    C. Lactated Ringer's.
    D. D_5W.

27. To minimize inflammation in burns, which of the following therapies may be used?
    A. Vitamin C
    B. Hyperbaric therapy
    C. Prednisone
    D. Leaving burns open to air

28. Sally was admitted to the ICU with a recurrent *Pneumocystis carinii* infection. She is currently on protease inhibitors and non-nucleoside reverse transcriptase inhibitors. Which of the following herbal supplements may be contributing to her recurrent infection?
    A. St. John's Wort
    B. Ginseng
    C. Ginkgo Biloba
    D. Thyme

29. The brown recluse spider is also known as the
    A. Hobo spider.
    B. Violet spider.
    C. Fiddleback spider.
    D. Huntsman spider.

30. People often believe that they have been bitten by a brown recluse spider. If they are able to capture the spider and bring it with them, which of the following would confirm a recluse identification?
    A. The spider has 6 eyes.
    B. The spider's legs are a darker brown than its body.
    C. The spider's legs have thick spines.
    D. The spider's web is obvious and may be found between two trees or in bushes.

31. Jay, a 68-year-old retiree, was cleaning out an old basement yesterday. He developed a raised area that initially looked like a mosquito bite but is now red, puss filled, and inflamed. He is admitted to the unit with a necrotizing wound. He may also exhibit all of the following signs and symptoms *except*
    A. Nausea and vomiting.
    B. Dyspnea.
    C. DIC.
    D. Hemolysis and thrombocytopenia.

32. The bite of which spider is most often blamed or misdiagnosed as MRSA and *Streptococcus* infections, ulcerations, or insect bites?
   A. Black widow
   B. Huntsman
   C. Brown recluse
   D. Daddy long-legs

33. Jay, a 68-year-old brown recluse spider bite victim, is leaving your unit. As part of his discharge teaching, you include ways to prevent future bites. Recommendations should include all of the following *except*
   A. Shaking out all clothing prior to getting dressed.
   B. Always wearing gloves when touching wood products, rocks, working in basements, or working in attics.
   C. Changing all storage boxes to cardboard.
   D. Installing yellow or sodium vapor light bulbs outdoors.

34. Black widow spider venom is how many times more potent than cobra or coral snake venom?
   A. 2 times
   B. 5 times
   C. 15 times
   D. 20 times

35. All of the following are found in black widow venom *except*
   A. Thiamine.
   B. Adenosine.
   C. Inosine.
   D. Latrotoxins.

36. Tyler is a 30-year-old gardener brought to your unit after collapsing at home this evening with a severe headache, dizziness, tremors, and severe muscle cramping. He is tachycardic, tachypneic, hypertensive, and restless. You note a rash with erythema, edema, piloerection, and two puncture sites on his anterior left ankle. When questioned, Tyler said that he had been bit by something that morning, but didn't know what. You suspect he was bitten by a
   A. Mosquito.
   B. Bee.
   C. Huntsman spider.
   D. Black widow spider.

37. Continuing with the scenario from Question 36, Tyler, a victim of a black widow spider bite, becomes obtunded, bradycardic, apneic, and hypotensive. You should
   A. Administer morphine 2 mg IV.
   B. Administer antivenin.
   C. Tie a tourniquet around his leg.
   D. Prepare to intubate the patient.

38. Continuing with the scenario from Questions 36 and 37, Tyler is preparing to go home after treatment with antivenin for a black widow spider bite. Which of the following discharge instructions is correct?

A. You may experience muscle spasms for only a few days.

B. You may experience tingling and weakness for 5 years or more.

C. It is normal to have a rash or fever in the next 3 days.

D. Contact your physician immediately if you have joint or abdominal pain or begin to have trouble breathing.

39. Logan, 24 years old, was bitten by a rattlesnake 60 minutes ago while hiking with his wife and friends. He was bitten on the left forearm when he reached down in some grass to pick up a hat that had blown loose. Logan's hand and arm are red and swelling. The puncture sites are bleeding, and he complains of pain and blurred vision. Which of the following actions should you take immediately?

A. Contact his insurance company to verify his coverage.

B. Place a tourniquet around his arm.

C. Remove any rings or watches.

D. Lift his arm above the heart and wrap it in ice.

40. Continuing with the scenario from Question 39, Logan's friends bring in the dead snake that bit him to verify the type of snake. You should tell them

A. That they are crazy for hunting down a snake after it has already bitten someone once.

B. To be careful with the head of the snake, because the snake could bite again even when dead.

C. To get the snake out of the unit as soon as possible.

D. You don't need the snake for verification because all snake bites are the same.

41. All of the following are poisonous snakes *except*

A. Rattlesnake.

B. Coral snake.

C. Cottonmouth.

D. Rat snake.

42. Helen was bitten and envenomated by a baby rattlesnake 40 minutes ago. In caring for Helen, you know which of the following facts will influence your treatment?

A. Baby rattlesnakes bite but do not inject venom.

B. Baby rattlesnake venom is mostly hemolytic.

C. Baby rattlesnake venom is mostly neurotoxic.

D. Baby rattlesnake venom is less concentrated than venom from adult snakes.

43. Many people are adding "exotic herbs" and supplements to their diets. Many of these substances may be very harmful and interact with medicines the patient is taking or may result in serious or deadly complications of existing diseases. Aria is a 20-year-old student who was experimenting with flavorings. She made a roast with Scotch Broom on it for her parents to try. After ingesting only a small portion of the meal, her father began to feel light-headed, have palpitations, and weakness. He is being treated in your unit post cardiac arrest in the emergency room. If not already done in the ER, your priority would be to

A. Insert a nasogastric tube and provide gastric lavage with activated charcoal.

B. Insert a Foley catheter.

C. Continue quinidine medications taken at home.

D. Continue the amiodarone infusion.

44. You have been caring for Mary in the ICU and she has terminal breast cancer. She has stopped eating due to nausea and vomiting. Her son asks if he can bring in her favorite dessert to tempt her to eat. After clearing this action with the physician, he brings in "special" brownies meant only for Mary. Within a few hours after her son leaves, Mary is eating, but is noted to be shaking, anxious, and no longer oriented to time and place. You suspect

A. Mary is exhibiting signs of brain metastasis.

B. Mary is having a stroke.

C. Mary has ingested marijuana and is exhibiting side effects.

D. Mary is hypoglycemic and should continue eating.

45. You are discussing herbal remedies at work when you are approached by a family member of your patient with Alzheimer's disease, who also has pneumonia. She asks if her mother would benefit from drinking ginkgo biloba at home once discharged because she had heard that it would decrease symptoms in the early phase of Alzheimer's. You tell her:

A. "There is a lot of research, but nothing really supports its use."

B. "Sure, there are no interactions with other drugs, so she should be fine."

C. "Her doctor doesn't approve of any natural remedies, so don't tell him if you are using it."

D. "There could be very dangerous side effects if gingko biloba is taken without consulting her physician. I will have him speak with you when he comes in."

46. You are treating Sid, a patient with long Q-T syndrome. Which of the following herbs should he avoid?

A. Ginseng

B. Ginkgo Biloba

C. Marijuana

D. Oregano

47. Your patient has been receiving nitroprusside. When giving this medication, it is necessary to monitor for

A. Tachycardia.

B. Cyanide toxicity.

C. Retinal changes.

D. Ataxia.

48. Ted was admitted to your unit after experiencing abdominal cramping, nausea, and severe diarrhea. His EKG shows sinus tachycardia with frequent PVC. He is currently on an amiodarone infusion. The only significant issue in his history was that Ted ate at a seafood restaurant 3 days ago. Ted is probably suffering from

A. Irritable bowel syndrome.

B. Hypokalemia.

C. Shellfish poisoning.

D. Celiac disease.

49. Paula works in the fashion industry and is a cutter in the wool sweater section of her company. This morning, a fire broke out in her section. Paula did not suffer

any burns, but did inhale large quantities of smoke. What would be the most potent toxin she might have inhaled?

A. Carbon monoxide

B. Smoke

C. Nitrates

D. Cyanide

50. Your patient lives in the country and is self-sufficient. As part of his diet, he eats deer and fish. He was admitted for respiratory distress, weight loss, vomiting, and numbness around the mouth. He is also suffering from mouth sores and drools constantly. His probable diagnosis will be

A. Botulism.

B. *Chlamydia* infection.

C. *Clostridium difficile* infection.

D. Mercury poisoning.

51. Your male patient has been prescribed ergotamine. This drug was probably prescribed for

A. Erectile dysfunction.

B. Headache.

C. Pruritis.

D. Nausea.

52. Patients who are stung by bees numerous times are in danger of developing

A. Kidney failure.

B. Anemia.

C. Long Q-T interval.

D. Hydrocephalus.

53. A possible side effect of cocaine is

A. Malignant hyperthermia.

B. Cherry red skin.

C. Paralytic ileus.

D. Constricted pupils.

54. Harold is 62-years-old and has become septic following a TURP 1 week ago. During his course of treatment, he is prescribed naloxone. The purpose of the naloxone is

A. To block prostaglandins.

B. To stabilize the cell membrane.

C. To block endorphins.

D. To block histamine.

55. Harold is also receiving activated protein C. The actions of this drug include

A. Blockade of angiotensin II.

B. Antimicrobial agent.

C. Antiviral agent.

D. Pro-fibrinolytic action.

56. Which of the following drugs may promote anaphylaxis in a patient receiving treatment for status asthmaticus?

   A. Oxygen

   B. Acetylcysteine

   C. Codeine

   D. Guaifenesin

57. Your patient was very anxious prior to a bronchoscopy. He received an IM injection of 0.20 mg/kg of Versed. His blood pressure dropped from 142/80 to 88/56, and he became bradycardic. To counter this reaction, he should be given

   A. Xanax.

   B. Ativan.

   C. Valium.

   D. Romazicon.

58. A nursing consideration with administration of norepinephrine (Levophed) would be

   A. Do not administer it with alkaline solutions.

   B. Do not administer it for low coronary artery perfusion states.

   C. It is not indicated for vasogenic shock.

   D. Do not use it for hypotensive states.

59. Levophed may cause tissue necrosis. You should treat extravasations with

   A. Regitine.

   B. Benadryl.

   C. An antihistamine.

   D. Hydrazazine.

60. Which of the following vasodilators should not be mixed with Ringer's lactate?

   A. Nesiritide

   B. Captopril

   C. Cardene

   D. Epinephrine

61. Patients should be monitored for thiocyanate toxicity when receiving

   A. Levophed.

   B. Nitroprusside.

   C. Thiosulfate.

   D. Sodium-channel blockers.

62. If your patient was in the early stage of septic shock, you would expect which of the following hemodynamic parameters?

   A. SVR elevated, PAOP elevated, CO decreased

   B. CO decreased, RAP elevated, PAOP elevated

   C. RAP elevated, SVR decreased, PAOP increased

   D. CO increased, PAOP decreased, SVR decreased

63. Jonathan was stabbed by a burglar in the right anterior chest. He lost approximately 1,500 to 1,600 mL of blood. Which of the following signs and symptoms would be expected with this volume of blood loss?
    A. BP decreased, pulse pressure normal, RR 20–30/min
    B. BP normal, RR increased, capillary refill normal
    C. RR increased, BP normal, pulse pressure normal
    D. BP decreased, RR increased, CO decreased

64. Douglas is a ranch foreman. Yesterday he complained of a stiff neck and was very lethargic. Last night he was found unconscious and had apparently vomited and possibly aspirated. Douglas probably has
    A. Pneumonia.
    B. West Nile virus.
    C. Western equine encephalitis.
    D. A brain tumor.

65. Nancy is a 40-year-old secretary being treated for MRSA. She has been receiving vancomycin, and this morning the trough level result was > 20 mcg/mL. This level
    A. May cause ototoxicity.
    B. May cause nephrotoxicity.
    C. Is therapeutic.
    D. Indicates the current dosage is too low.

66. Mary is a 28-year-old housewife who gave birth 2 months ago to a healthy baby boy. She has been suffering from postpartum depression. Mary was admitted with hallucinations, agitation, ventricular arrhythmias, and a possible seizure (witnessed by her husband). She has probably been taking a tricyclic antidepressant. Which of the following drugs is classified as a tricyclic antidepressant?
    A. Amitriptyline
    B. Gentamycin
    C. Clonidine
    D. Fluvastatin

67. Continuing with the scenario from Question 66, Mary's husband said the last time she took one of the doses of an antidepressant was last evening. A blood level was drawn and is considered a trough level. Her treatment should include
    A. Hemodialysis.
    B. Syrup of Ipecac.
    C. Sodium bicarbonate.
    D. Trazodone.

68. Which of the following conditions would be contraindicated when scheduling a patient for a transesophageal echocardiogram (TEE)?
    A. Cardiac tumors
    B. Dysphagia
    C. Vegetative endocarditis
    D. Mitral valve regurgitation

69. Your patient was stabbed in the chest 2 weeks ago. The damage done to the heart resulted in the patient undergoing a prosthetic mitral valve replacement. The patient is now experiencing transient chest pain and syncopal episodes. A TEE is ordered. You anticipate which of the following actions prior to the procedure?

    A. Hold all medications 8 hours prior to the procedure.

    B. Allow the patient to keep his dentures in.

    C. Administer prophylactic antibiotics.

    D. Position the patient on right side.

70. Which of the following conditions would present with lab results showing a decreased sedimentation rate?

    A. Anemia

    B. Colon cancer

    C. Infection

    D. Congestive heart failure

71. Contraindications for a pulmonary angiogram would include

    A. Perfusion deficits.

    B. Vascular filling defects.

    C. Pulmonary thromboembolism.

    D. Pregnancy.

72. Acetaminophen overdose may take up to 2 weeks to resolve. From 72 to 96 hours from ingestion, symptoms will include

    A. Pallor, lethargy, metabolic acidosis.

    B. Increased renal function.

    C. Right upper quadrant pain, increased serum hepatic enzymes.

    D. Jaundice, confusion, coagulation disorders.

73. The activated coagulation time (ACT) is more sensitive to _____ and _____ than whole blood clotting time.

    A. oxygenation, hemofiltration

    B. factor VIII, heparin

    C. warfarin, leukemia

    D. liver disease, calcium

74. Your patient has been on an amiodarone drip for atrial fibrillation. Today, the serum level returned a result of 3.3 mcg/mL. This result indicates

    A. A therapeutic level.

    B. A subtherapeutic level.

    C. A panic level.

    D. Amiodarone levels are not measured this way.

75. Pulmonary artery catheter infections may be best prevented by which of the following actions?

    A. Using an antibiotic coated catheter

    B. Remove the catheter within 48 to 72 hours after its insertion.

    C. Use of prophylactic antibiotics

    D. Avoid continuous heparin infusions.

76. **Increased protein may occur in cerebrospinal fluid due to spinal anesthetics, measles, and ethyl alcohol.**
    A. True
    B. False

77. **Which of the following statements about cocaine is false?**
    A. Cocaine use, even on just one occasion, can cause rhabdomyolysis.
    B. Cocaine and tobacco use are associated with spontaneous abortion.
    C. Specimens should be kept on ice.
    D. Cocaine causes the placenta to shrink.

78. **Client and family teaching for digital subtraction angiography includes**
    A. The length of the procedure is approximately 90 minutes.
    B. Women who are breastfeeding should substitute formula for breastmilk for 1 or more days after the procedure.
    C. The patient will be able to change position frequently during the procedure.
    D. The patient will be free to move around during the procedure.

79. **An antidote for ethylene glycol toxicity is**
    A. Digoxin.
    B. Anisindione.
    C. Fomepizole.
    D. Narcan.

80. **GHB (Ecstasy) overdoses can lead to amnesia in what percentage of cases?**
    A. 13%
    B. 21%
    C. 24%
    D. 32%

81. **Poisoning by arsenic may result in the following symptoms:**
    A. Pneumonia, renal dysfunction
    B. Tachycardia, hypertension
    C. Paresthesia, cerebral edema
    D. Convulsions

82. **Cadmium accumulates in the lungs, liver, and kidneys after exposure to**
    A. Cigarette smoke.
    B. Asbestos.
    C. Lead paint.
    D. Fungicide.

83. **Your patient was admitted for severe flank pain and hematuria. He is scheduled for a kidney biopsy. Your patient and family teaching should include**
    A. Report any pain in the flank or abdomen post procedure.
    B. A small kidney stone may be passed after the procedure.
    C. The patient will be on bed rest for 24 hours.
    D. No teaching is necessary.

84. Your patient has a history of cluster migraine headaches and has been treated with lithium. Her lithium level on admission was 1.8 mmol/L. This would correspond with her symptoms of
    A. Somnolence and coma.
    B. Ataxia, diarrhea.
    C. Seizures, flattened T wave.
    D. Manic–depressive behavior.

85. Following a lung scan (V/Q), you should observe your patient for
    A. Sixty minutes following the study for possible reaction to the nucleotides.
    B. Signs and symptoms of pneumonia.
    C. Twenty-four hours to measure urine output and maintain strict I&O.
    D. No observation is necessary.

86. When preparing to obtain a wound culture for MRSA, which of the following tasks should *not* be performed?
    A. Obtain a sterile, cotton-tipped culturette swab.
    B. Transport the sample on ice to the lab.
    C. Culture the site using a rotating motion for 10 seconds.
    D. Place the swab in a sodium chloride medium.

87. Factors that may affect results of urine morphine levels include all the following *except*
    A. Poppy seed ingestion may produce false-positive results.
    B. 10 mg MS IV may be detectable in urine up to 84 hours.
    C. Use of a stealth adulterant will cause negative results in a positive sample.
    D. High levels of lymphocytes will mask morphine in urine.

88. Blood osmolality is decreased in
    A. Uremia and dehydration.
    B. Alcoholism and burns.
    C. Diabetes Insipidus.
    D. Hyponatremia and overhydration.

89. Phenytoin serum levels may be affected by
    A. Holding tube feedings 30 minutes after oral phenytoin administration.
    B. Drawing peak levels 2 hours after oral administration of phenytoin.
    C. After a change of dose, allow 24 hours before drawing a phenytoin peak level.
    D. None of the above.

90. Your patient has been scheduled for a PET scan. Your patient teaching should include
    A. The patient is to remain NPO.
    B. The test will require the patient to change position several times during the test.
    C. Avoidance of large quantities of fluids within 2 hours prior to the PET scan.
    D. Lactating women should not breastfeed for at least 48 hours after the scan.

91. Your patient's prothrombin time has an increased INR. You question the patient and determine the patient had taken one of the following medications, which may have affected the INR level:
    A. Antacids
    B. Herbs and natural remedies
    C. Antihistamines
    D. Diuretics

92. Your patient underwent pulmonary function testing. The respiratory therapist tells you the preliminary result is a low peak expiratory flow rate (PEFR). This might indicate
    A. Asthma.
    B. Pneumothorax.
    C. Pulmonary cysts.
    D. Heart failure.

93. Your patient is undergoing a renal arteriogram. After the dye is injected, the patient complains of a "salty taste" in his mouth. You know that
    A. This is the first sign of an anaphylactic reaction.
    B. This will result in termination of the arteriogram.
    C. This is expected and should pass after about 5 minutes.
    D. This is an emergency.

94. Rocky Mountain spotted fever is caused by
    A. A parasite.
    B. Fleas.
    C. A rotavirus.
    D. Fungi.

95. False-positive results for the sickle cell test may be due to all of the following *except*
    A. Polycythemia.
    B. High blood protein levels.
    C. Anemia.
    D. Multiple myelomas.

96. Your hospital has just received word of a mass-casualty incident. You are called on to report to the ED and assist with triage. The preliminary report is that you will be receiving as many as 60 patients. The first patient you see is a male, about 30 years old, with multiple lacerations. He is awake and alert and complaining of pain in the right chest and right upper quadrant. There is no rebound tenderness. You confirm that ribs 7–9 are fractured. You would suspect which of the following underlying conditions/injuries?
    A. Spleen laceration
    B. Liver laceration
    C. Pneumothorax
    D. Mesenteric infarction

97. The second patient you see is a 20-year-old female who was trapped in her car for almost 2 hours by the steering column. She complains of left shoulder pain, left upper quadrant rebound tenderness, and she presents with an obviously fractured lower leg that was splinted by paramedics. The paramedics had listed her as stable and stated that she had no rebound tenderness or guarding at the accident scene. She is tachycardic at 116 and has fractures of ribs 9–10. You suspect
    A. Ruptured pancreas.
    B. Diaphragm rupture.
    C. Spleen injury.
    D. Lacerated liver.

98. The third patient you encounter is a paramedic who was injured on the way to assist with the mass casualties. He is confused, but complains of back pain at the level of L3. He is hypotensive and has swelling at the level of L1–L3. You would suspect which type of injury?
    A. Splenic rupture
    B. Kidney laceration
    C. Large bowel rupture
    D. Retroperitoneal liver injury

99. Marv was a spectator at a golf tournament when he was struck by lightning. He was thrown about 10 feet into a tree. He suffered a fractured left radius, a concussion, and burns on his left arm, chest, and right leg. He has been somewhat confused since the accident. Which of the following statements about lightning injuries is true?
    A. Internal burns are common.
    B. Barotrauma is rare.
    C. Myoglobinuria is rarely seen.
    D. DC current will most likely cause ventricular fibrillation.

100. Binge eating, mutilation, obesity, drug abuse, and alcoholism are all examples of
    A. Self-destruction.
    B. Psychotic behavior.
    C. Neurosis.
    D. Immaturity.

101. All of the following impact an elderly individual's abilities to counter psychiatric emergencies *except*
    A. Altered or reduced problem-solving and coping mechanisms.
    B. Stable health.
    C. Increased loss of or limited support systems.
    D. Greater financial pressures or limited resources.

102. Timothy, a 56-year-old father of 6, has suffered a heart attack and requires an immediate coronary artery bypass graft. His children and wife are present as well as other family and church members. You overhear his wife and children speaking about complete insurance coverage; they state that Timothy's employer has approved significant sick level time for his recovery and has offered the ability to work from home if additional recuperation time is required. You are determining the level of psychiatric distress in this family. Your first priority is to

A. Administer psychotropic medications.

B. Examine the range and effectiveness of their coping mechanisms.

C. Work with any available family members, friends, or religious support systems.

D. Determine if there is a crisis.

103. Amy is the lone survivor of a car crash that killed her parents and 2 siblings. She is recovering from a pneumothorax, hemothorax, and bilateral broken legs. She has been extremely depressed and withdrawn. You are discussing medications, psychiatric therapy, and the increased risk of suicide and suicidal behavior with Amy's distant relatives. The family makes each of the following statements. Which of them is false?

A. "If Amy is considering suicide, she will make statements or give warnings of suicide."

B. "We should trust our instincts if we feel Amy is in danger."

C. "As she recovers from her depression, she is at greater risk of suicide."

D. "If she talks about suicide or asks about pills, she is just voicing the thought and will not attempt suicide."

104. Amy is the sole survivor of a car crash that killed her immediate family. While recovering from massive injuries, her behavior and moods change rapidly. Which of the following behaviors is most concerning and indicates suicidal behavior?

A. Drug seeking with multiple requests for pain medications and sedatives

B. Withdrawal from conversation and other types of interaction

C. Crying and statements of helplessness

D. Screaming at her distant relatives

105. Brody is a 46-year-old male who was admitted to the ICU following a bar-room brawl during which he suffered multiple stab wounds. He is angry and verbally assaultive with the staff. The goal of anger management for this patient is to do all of the following *except*

A. Confront him directly with whatever made him angry.

B. Discuss what in the situation made him angry.

C. Discuss with Brody alternative and positive ways to express his feelings.

D. Decide on positive ways for Brody to express his feelings when confronted with frustrating situations in the future.

106. Cassandra was admitted to the ICU for severe anxiety. Which of the following medical conditions may present with such symptoms?

A. Narcolepsy

B. Asthma

C. Hyperglycemia and/or hypoglycemia

D. Hypercaffeination

107. Jose is an alcoholic admitted to your unit with cirrhosis. Why is thiamine added to his IV fluids?

A. Thiamine is a sedative and will ease Jose's agitation.

B. Thiamine decreases the symptoms of DTs.

C. Thiamine is used to prevent the damage to the brain as a result of Wernicke's syndrome.

D. Thiamine is used to prevent complications of substance abuse.

108. Leon is experiencing delirium tremens. Nursing interventions include keeping the room well lit and minimizing stimulation. Staff members continuously reorient Leon to time, place, and person. Haldol has been given as ordered, and the patient is in four-point restraints. Which of these nursing interventions should be discontinued?
    A. Reorientation
    B. Medication administration
    C. Restraints
    D. Controlling stimulation

109. You are assisting with triaging of patients after an earthquake. Which of the following is your first priority?
    A. Establishing physical conditions
    B. Addressing the media
    C. Getting social services to assist with patients
    D. Reconnecting family members

110. Your patient had a three-vessel CABG procedure and experienced a small stroke during the procedure. The stroke left some residual numbness in the left arm. The family is quite agitated and does not agree with the patient's advance directives. The family informs you that they want everything done for the patient and to ignore the patient's request for no resuscitative measures. Which of the following nursing interventions would be appropriate at this time?
    A. Inform the family that the physician will meet with them to discuss treatment options.
    B. Tell the patient about the family's concerns.
    C. Notify the physician that all orders are to come from the family.
    D. Inform the family that the patient is fully capable of making decisions.

111. Your patient is scheduled for implantation of a VAD. About 20 minutes prior to the scheduled start of the procedure, she informs you that she has concerns about side effects and the procedure itself. Your best nursing intervention would be to
    A. See if the patient signed the consent form for the procedure.
    B. Notify the physician that the patient does not have a full understanding of the procedure.
    C. Cancel the procedure.
    D. Answer the patient's questions yourself.

112. A car carrying 4 teenagers went off a bridge and killed all but 1 of the teens. Today a second EEG was done and brain death was confirmed for the fourth teen. When the family was approached about organ donation, they requested that the patient remain in the ICU for at least 7 to 8 days until the older sister can return from a war zone. The appropriate nursing response would be
    A. Tell the family that other patients are waiting for the bed.
    B. Notify the physician to tell the family organ donation must be made within 24 hours.
    C. Notify social services and arrange for emergency compassionate leave for the sister.
    D. Wait until the family leaves to procure the organs.

113. A woman who is 8 months pregnant was severely injured in an automobile accident. Her condition has been deteriorating over the past week. The husband has been informed of the probable demise of his wife. In addition, the physician suspects fetal demise and notified the husband. The husband wants to bring their only other child, an 8-year-old boy, into the ICU to visit his mother. The ICU has a policy that children must be 15 years old to visit. What is an appropriate nursing action at this time?
    A. Sneak the child in during the night shift.
    B. Take a picture of the mother for the child.
    C. Arrange a patient care conference the next day to discuss options.
    D. Inform the husband that the visiting policy is strictly enforced.

114. Shawn works sorting mail at the local post office. She finds an envelope that is torn and has white powder falling out of the tear. Shawn is sent to the hospital and admitted to the intensive care unit for possible inhalation anthrax. What is the treatment of choice for Shawn?
    A. Penicillin G 2 million units intravenously every 6 hours
    B. Ciprofloxacin 400 mg intravenously every 12 hours
    C. Doxycycline 500 mg intravenously every 12 hours
    D. Augmentin 875/125 mg intravenously every 12 hours

115. What is the incubation period for inhalation anthrax?
    A. 7–10 days
    B. 5–7 days
    C. 7–60 days
    D. 20–30 days

116. What are the initial symptoms of inhalation anthrax?
    A. Mild, flu-like symptoms
    B. Severe dyspnea and productive cough
    C. High fever, cough, and stridor
    D. Cutaneous lesions, cough, and high fever

117. How long is antibiotic therapy continued for inhalation anthrax?
    A. 10 days of intravenous antibiotics
    B. 14 days of intravenous antibiotics, then oral antibiotics
    C. 30 days of intravenous antibiotics, then oral antibiotics
    D. 60 days of combined intravenous and oral antibiotics

118. Which form of isolation should be used for the patient with inhalation anthrax?
    A. Full isolation with laminar air flow
    B. Droplet precautions
    C. Standard contact precautions
    D. Reverse isolation

119. Kathy is a 58-year-old lady who lives on a farm. She home-cans meat and vegetables every year. Kathy is admitted to the intensive care unit with profound weakness, double vision, slurred speech, and dysphagia. Her initial diagnosis is Guillain-Barré syndrome. While you are interviewing her family, you learn that a few days ago Kathy ingested some home-canned green beans that were several years old. No other family members ate the beans because the color was odd. What do you do with this information?
    A. Do nothing, it is of no consequence.
    B. Notify the physician immediately, Kathy may have botulism.
    C. Tell the physician tomorrow during rounds.
    D. Continue the interview.

120. What is the causative organism in botulism?
    A. *Clostridium difficile*
    B. *Clostridium botulinum*
    C. *Clostridium avium*
    D. *Botulinum botulinum*

121. Your hospital is put on an external disaster notice after a ricin poisoning at a local train station. Your intensive care unit prepares to accept casualties. What makes ricin so toxic to humans?
    A. It causes respiratory failure.
    B. It causes renal failure.
    C. It inhibits protein synthesis, leading to cell death.
    D. It destroys the mitochondria in the cell, causing cell death.

122. As the charge nurse for a busy ICU, you note an increased frequency of patients with underlying mental disorders being admitted. You overhear some negative comments regarding assignment to these patients. You ask the nurses to complete a self-awareness survey regarding their beliefs and understanding of mental health issues. You will use this information to
    A. Determine which nurses should never care for patients with mental health issues.
    B. Change nursing assignments immediately.
    C. Determine which nurses should be written up and counseled.
    D. Create an education program for the nurses that will increase understanding of mental health issues and ways to access resources for these patients.

123. You are discussing post-discharge psychiatric resources with a patient's family. You note that they are using the terms "psychiatric emergency" and "crisis" interchangeably. To clarify this issue, you tell them that
    A. A crisis is an immediate danger to someone else, whereas an emergency is a suicide attempt.
    B. A crisis develops over time as a result of a psychological stressor, whereas an emergency is an immediate situation that, if not corrected, will result in violence.
    C. A crisis occurs when no intervention will be effective, whereas an emergency is when interventions have the greatest impact.
    D. A crisis is sudden and precedes an emergency when lives may be threatened.

124. While passing your terminally ill patient's room you see his wife of 50 years crying at the bedside while she pats his hand. She is unkempt, tired, and unable to focus during conversations. You believe that she is in the middle of a situational crisis. Your best action is to
    A. Call the social worker to speak with her.
    B. Call the appropriate spiritual advisor for this patient.
    C. Call the wife's primary doctor for a prescription for Xanax or Paxil.
    D. Call your charge nurse to cover your other patient while you initiate a conversation with the wife to identify stressors and develop a list of resources.

125. Which of the following individuals is at highest risk for a psychological emergency?
    A. An 80-year-old home-bound male whose wife has just died and has no children or living family
    B. A married 20-year-old female delivering a 35-week gestational infant
    C. A married 56-year-old male who was just laid off from his job of 10 years
    D. A married 36-year-old female who is newly diagnosed with systemic lupus erythematosus

126. Your unit has just completed a code lasting 2 hours for an 18-year-old rape and trauma victim. Due to her overwhelming injuries, the patient does not survive. Chaplin services are called in to assist with a nursing staff debriefing. Staff members experiencing which of the following emotions are at highest risk for psychological stress?
    A. Anger
    B. Fear
    C. Anxiety
    D. Denial

127. You are talking to your 24-year-old patient about his newly diagnosed Type II diabetes. He states that he is fine with the diagnosis and knows that he will need to make some changes. His speech is rapid and pressured, he makes frequent jokes, and he talks about playing football with the guys when he is discharged. You would still be concerned about this patient's psychological health because of his
    A. Rapid, pressured speech.
    B. Frequent jokes.
    C. Talk of social activities.
    D. Failure to identify specific lifestyle changes that he needs to make.

128. Zack, a chronic alcoholic with cirrhosis, has returned again to the ICU after failing rehabilitation, which you assisted him in getting admitted to. Although you previously had a friendly and open relationship, Zack will not look at you and answers questions by giving only minimal responses. You tell him:
    A. "I can't believe you wasted the opportunity to get sober at the rehabilitation center."
    B. "I know you want to stay sober, but maybe you need more time."
    C. "I am proud of how long you stayed sober. Let's try again."
    D. "Why don't we work together to find new resources for you to utilize when you are tempted to drink?"

129. Adam, a 24-year-old football player, suffered a spinal injury in a motor vehicle accident while he was intoxicated. He is now a paraplegic without family and financial resources. During wound care, he states, "You shouldn't bother with that, no one cares if I live or die. My life is over. I can't play football and no one wants a cripple around. If I disappear, no one would even notice." Your best response to his statements is to say:

    A. "Don't talk like that, you are still alive and many paraplegics are active and happy."

    B. "Why would you say that? You had visitors yesterday."

    C. "I understand that your injuries are devastating to you, but I cannot allow you to harm yourself."

    D. "Let's just get through the dressing change, and then I'll have the doctor prescribe something for you."

130. Alicia, the 44-year-old estranged daughter of your patient with a myocardial infarction, is overheard in the waiting room telling another family member, "The nurses aren't doing enough for her. If they let her die, I'll make sure they suffer." When she comes in to visit, you note that she is glaring at the staff, her posture is tense, and her movements quick and forceful. Alicia is pacing the room, will not acknowledge staff members, and uses inappropriate language at the bedside. Your priority is to

    A. Call security to assist in removing Alicia from the unit to a secluded area.

    B. Ignore Alicia's behavior and continue to care for the patient.

    C. Call the police and forbid Alicia from returning.

    D. Make jokes and shame Alicia into behaving.

131. You are caring for a 68-year-old woman who was in a motor vehicle accident in which a child was killed. She is combative and restless, hyperventilating, tachy-cardic, and has an elevated blood pressure. The patient states, "I've got to leave here. They'll arrest me, they'll lock me up. I can't believe this. There is no way out." You should tell her:

    A. "Just relax. They can't arrest you while you are in the hospital."

    B. "Calm down. It wasn't your fault if the child darted into traffic."

    C. "Stop it. You are working yourself up. Look at me and focus on what I am telling you to do."

    D. "They should arrest you, you killed a child."

132. You are caring for Mr. B., a 34-year-old gunshot victim from a gang fight that hap-pened 18 hours ago. He was restrained after he became verbally and physically abusive to the staff. You see him thrashing around in the bed and suddenly awake when you enter the room. Mr. B. is shaking, has vomited, and is tachycardic with an elevated blood pressure. He is talking to people not in the room. You suspect he is

    A. Experiencing delirium tremors.

    B. Experiencing drug withdrawal.

    C. Developing septic shock.

    D. Exhibiting signs of paranoid schizophrenia.

This concludes the Multisystem questions.

ANSWERS

1. **Correct Answer: A**
   "Body packer" is a term used for people who transport narcotics in body cavities. In this case, it is probable that a packet may have ruptured. More doses of naloxone may be necessary, along with supportive treatment for opioid overdose. Be alert for brady-cardia, hypotension, respiratory depression, and hypothermia.

2. **Correct Answer: C**
   MODS is usually the result of a direct injury to an organ. A kidney stone or appendici-tis should present with pain and tenderness. SIRS is a systemic infection that can pres-ent in the elderly with hypothermia and even a WBC of < 4,000 or > 12,000.

3. **Correct Answer: B**
   Gentamycin is an aminoglycoside, as are tobramycin and amikacin. These medica-tions are used for gram-negative bacterial infections; however, they must be used with caution because they can cause nephrotoxicity.

4. **Correct Answer: D**
   When a sudden flame-up comes near the face, the first instinct is to gasp. This inhala-tion of superheated air causes swelling of the tissues in the air passages. This patient was probably very near the flame because his facial hair was burned off. He is a great risk of a compromised airway and may need intubation.

5. **Correct Answer: C**
   Because of the immediate danger of airway closure, intubation should be done as soon as possible. Once the airway begins to close, intubation may become impossible. In some cases, even a tracheostomy is extremely difficult.

6. **Correct Answer: C**
   Underresuscitation.

7. **Correct Answer: A**
   Hypertonic solutions minimize wound edema.

8. **Correct Answer: A**
   Aspirin is an acid and causes a profound acidosis. Tinnitus may also be present.

9. **Correct Answer: B**
   This is an emergency. The pressure must be relieved via escharotomy, an incision through multiple layers of tissue. Any circumferential burn of the body may lead to impaired function and escharotomy.

10. **Correct Answer: C**
    Lactated Ringer's is used for burn patients for a variety of reasons and with many of the formulas for burn resuscitation. It is preferred for large volume resuscitation because LR contains 130 mEq/L of sodium compared to normal saline which contains 154 mEq/L of sodium. LR has a higher pH (6.5) compared to normal saline (5.0), so the pH of LR is close to a normal pH. The patient will be in metabolic acidosis, so the metabolized lactate will buffer the acidosis. LR is also an isotonic crystalloid.

11. **Correct Answer: D**
Electrical burns are insidious and follow the path of least resistance. Muscle tissue breaks down, causing rhabdomyolysis from the myoglobin that was released into the circulation.

12. **Correct Answer: B**
Ludwig's angina is a submaxillary infection. It is a cellulitis of the neck and floor of the mouth that usually occurs with, or after, dental disease.

13. **Correct Answer: A**
TNF also stimulates increased capillary permeability and release of IL-1, IL-6, and IL-8.

14. **Correct Answer: B**
Hypoglycemia occurs because of the hepatotoxic effects of acetaminophen. Infusions must also be based on blood glucose results.

15. **Correct Answer: D**
Administer thiamine, then give a bolus of D_{50}, and then start an infusion of D_5W.

16. **Correct Answer: A**
Ammonium chloride can be converted to ammonia and HCl in the liver. This will indirectly correct metabolic alkalosis, although the ammonia that is generated can produce encephalopathy.

17. **Correct Answer: D**
Wernicke–Kersakoff syndrome is a thiamine deficiency and a metabolic encephalopathy.

18. **Correct Answer: A**
Amiodarone is useful in treatment of atrial fibrillation because the drug decreases the sinus rate, increases the PR and Q-T intervals, and results in the development of U waves.

19. **Correct Answer: C**
Full-thickness burns destroy nerve endings because they extend into subcutaneous tissue. The tissue may have a whitish color and will be somewhat firm with a leather-like appearance. Sometimes you can see clotted vessels through the eschar.

20. **Correct Answer: B**
This type of burn may be superficial or a deep partial-thickness burn. The nerve endings are still intact and this burn is very painful. Sometimes burns can be deceptive. A reddened area can be diagnosed as a first-degree burn but may be overlooked when staff calculate the patient's requirements for fluid and nutrient resuscitation. After a few hours, these areas can develop blisters and only then are recognized as dermal burns. A new way of assessing burn levels involves using a laser Doppler during the first week of treatment.

Assessing a burn depth can be tricky. The first step is to determine the factors that caused the burn (chemical, electrical, or thermal), the length of time during which the causative mechanism was in contact with the area, blood flow in the area, and location of the burn. Another issue to consider is the thickness of the skin at the site. Elderly people and children have thinner skin, so burns in those populations tend to be more severe. Burns on the eyelids and genital area are about 1 mm thick, whereas burns on the palms and soles of the feet are on areas about 5 mm thick. Although the thicker skin offers a bit more thermal protection, the palms and soles of the feet become infected more easily.

21. **Correct Answer: D**
    Not many people are familiar with this classification. This type of burn not only involves muscle, but extends through muscle and bone.

22. **Correct Answer: C**
    Escharotomy is a procedure, not a direct risk. The highest risk at this time is compartment syndrome. As a nurse, you must constantly assess for quality of pulses. Edema may be so great as to completely cut off circulation in a limb and cause myoglobin-related renal failure. Elevating the limb may help drain fluid and mitigate further edema. If the pulse is lost, it does not necessarily mean compartment syndrome is the cause. The lost pulse could result from not replacing lost volume secondary to the burn.

23. **Correct Answer: B**
    This level of sustained pressure requires a release to be performed by a physician. If the compartment pressure reaches 40 mm Hg, it requires immediate escharotomy or fasciotomy. In most burn units, some sort of electrocautery device is available at the bedside or close by. The patient should be sedated and medicated for pain if hemodynamically stable. If the patient experiences a lot of pain, it could be that the elevated pressure arises from a fluid deficit. When assessing a burned patient, if the individual has a weak pulse, it is probably due to underresuscitation.

24. **Correct Answer: D**
    The Parkland formula was developed by Dr. Charles Baxter at Parkland Hospital in Dallas, Texas, in the 1960s and is still utilized today. It is used across the United States as a standard for fluid resuscitation. Many other formulas are in use, but this one is widely known and will probably be on the CCRN examination. The formula is

    4 mL fluid × patient's weight (in kg) × body surface area burned (%)

    In this case,

    4 mL × 70 kg × 30% = 8,400 mL fluid requirement for the first 24 hours

    Half the calculated volume is given in the first 8 hours, then the remaining volume is given over the next 16 hours.

25. **Correct Answer: B**
    The formula is

    4 mL × 65 kg × 45% = 11,700 mL fluid replacement

26. **Correct Answer: C**
    Lactated Ringer's is used for a variety of reasons with many of the formulas for burn resuscitation. It is preferred for large volume resuscitation because LR contains 130 mEq/L of sodium compared to normal saline that has 154 mEq/L of sodium. LR has a higher pH (6.5) compared to normal saline (5.0), so the pH of the LR is close to a normal pH. The patient will be in metabolic acidosis, so the metabolized lactate will buffer the acidosis. LR is also an isotonic crystalloid.

27. **Correct Answer: A**

This question is not currently on the CCRN exam, but it may show up as a question within the next year or so. Vitamin C is an antioxidant that is used to counter oxidant-mediated effects on the inflammatory cascade. Studies with animals have shown that if vitamin C is given within 6 hours of the burn, up to 50% of the fluid needed for resuscitation can be eliminated.

With any burn patient, you should start at least 2 large-bore IVs.

Another new treatment involves the use of subatmospheric pressure dressings. These dressings may aid in removing excess fluid and help save areas that would otherwise have to be grafted or removed.

28. **Correct Answer: A**

St. John's Wort is contraindicated in patients with HIV/AIDS because the herb interferes with the metabolism of protease inhibitors and non-nucleoside reverse transcriptase inhibitors.

29. **Correct Answer: C**

Depending on the geographic region in which the spider is found, the brown recluse spider may be referred to as the violin spider or the fiddleback. Although it is normally found in the South, reports have noted its presence from California to Virginia and as far North as Ohio and Michigan. In the United States, there are 13 varieties of recluse spiders.

30. **Correct Answer: A**

The brown recluse spider generally avoids humans whenever possible. Because of its reclusive nature, its web will be difficult to see or find. These spiders have 6 eyes, rather than the 8 eyes seen on most spiders. A dark, violin-shaped mark appears on the part of the body where the legs are attached, with the neck of the "violin" pointing toward the body of the spider. The legs have fine hairs and no spines. The brown recluse spider is no larger than ½ inch in body length.

31. **Correct Answer: B**

Patients presenting post recluse spider bites may not initially know that they were bitten and so may not seek medical help until 12 to 36 hours after the initial bite. Because treatment is delayed, symptoms may be difficult to treat. The majority of patients will present with flu-like symptoms. DIC, hemolysis, and thrombocytopenia are severe symptoms. Treatment includes applying ice to control inflammation, keeping the area clean and protected, and treating symptoms. No specific treatment has been proven 100% effective. Dapsone has limited support for preventing necrosis. Nitroglycerin patches counter the vasoconstrictive properties of the venom and lead to hemodilution in the bloodstream and increased bleeding at the site to wash the venom out.

32. **Correct Answer: C**

The brown recluse spider is often blamed for necrotic wounds that are more likely caused by MRSA, *Streptococcus*, ulcerations, and other insect bites. This spider is generally an isolative spider and will avoid humans whenever possible. Because the bite is rarely felt at the actual time of the bite, capture and identification of the spider that caused the bite is difficult and extremely rare. If the brown recluse is the cause of a bite, and the bite occurs over fatty or soft tissue, the venom may cause necrosis and take months to heal. Necrosis is thought to be caused by the vasoconstrictive properties of the venom.

33. **Correct Answer: C**

It is recommended that all cardboard be removed from houses and populated areas as soon as possible. Because it is made of wood fibers, when cardboard decays it has properties similar to those of a rotting tree stump, a popular haven for the brown recluse. The spiders may hide or nest in folds and between layers of cardboard. Sealed plastic containers and bags provide some barriers to habitation. Gloves protect hands from exposure when handling woods and rocks or when working in storage areas such as basements and attics. Yellow or sodium light bulbs do not prevent spiders from nesting, but will limit their food supply (lights repel other insects) and make the area less inviting.

34. **Correct Answer: C**

Black widow spider venom is 15 times more potent than cobra or coral snake venom. What is fortunate is that black widow spiders are not large, and the puncture from one's bite is at most 1 mm deep (the length of a female's chelicerae or pincher). Males are smaller than the females with smaller chelicerae and, therefore, inject less venom. The high incidence of world-wide deaths by black widow spider bites is mostly reflective of the large and widely distributed populations of this spider.

35. **Correct Answer: A**

Thiamine (vitamin B_1) is not found in the venom of black widow spiders. Adenosine has two effects in the body: It inhibits the central nervous system and it acts as an anti-inflammatory agent. Adenosine is also broken down into inosine within the bloodstream. Inosine is part of the cascade of events leading to muscle movement. Latrotoxin is the main active neurotoxin most responsible for the symptoms felt by victims of black widow spider bites. Low-molecular-weight components within the venom are thought to facilitate higher-molecular-weight toxins in permeating cell membranes. The neurotoxin causes cell death by causing a rapid influx of calcium into the cell.

36. **Correct Answer: D**

Black widow spider venom causes massive muscle contractions as the venom is circulated throughout the body by blood and the lymphatic system from the bite or wound site. Symptoms are most often seen in the first 24 hours after a bite. The neurotoxins cause an influx of calcium into cells, resulting in cellular death. In addition to muscle cramping, other symptoms include joint pain, anxiety, insomnia, diaphoresis, severe abdominal cramping and pain, and lacrimation. If the patient has a compromised immunity or co-morbidities, the effects of the toxins could be more deadly. Extreme cases and complications include priapism, acute renal failure, myocarditis, rhabdomyolysis, and paralysis. If the bite is left untreated, shock, coma, and death may occur.

37. **Correct Answer: D**

The patient is apneic and bradycardic. The first priority is to maintain the airway to provide ventilation and oxygen therapy. The next step is to administer antivenin as soon as available. Morphine may help with pain, but will worsen the bradycardia and hypotension. It is a myth that tying a tourniquet around the affected limb will stop the venom from reaching the bloodstream or lymphatic system. At this point, the venom is already having systemic effects. In minor cases involving healthy adults, symptoms may be managed with pain control, muscle relaxants, and comfort measures. Symptoms should dissipate during the first 3 days after exposure.

38. **Correct Answer: D**

    Joint and abdominal pain (related to splenomegaly) as well as dyspnea may be signs of anaphylaxis or serum sickness that occurs as long as 2 to 4 weeks after antivenin administration. Patients should be taught to contact their physicians immediately so early treatment can be initiated to prevent complications. Administration of corticosteroids and antihistamines will aid in combating the inflammatory response to the animal proteins in the antivenin. The neurotoxin may cause residual muscle spasms, tingling, weakness, and nervousness for weeks to months after the exposure to the venom. Patients may need to slowly increase their activity during their recovery.

39. **Correct Answer: C**

    As swelling continues in the affected limb, it is important to remove any restrictive jewelry or clothing while you are still able to do so without damage. Do not place a tourniquet or ice on the bite, as this will decrease blood flow to the surrounding tissues. A light bandage on the site will absorb the blood; do not bind the site tightly. Do not raise the bitten site above the heart, because gravity will increase venom flow black toward the heart. It is best to keep the limb dependent and stabilized. Keep the patient calm, prevent unnecessary movement, and treat shock symptoms if present.

40. **Correct Answer: B**

    A snake may strike again within 1 hour after death due to reflexes. A snake should never be captured after a strike unless by experienced personnel. The snake may strike again in fear, leading to a second victim. All bites are not the same. It is helpful if you can identify the snake if dead and present, but blood tests can determine which venom is present in the blood.

41. **Correct Answer: D**

    Rattlesnakes, coral snakes, and cottonmouth snakes are all venomous (poisonous). Immediate medical attention should be sought for any bite victim. The rat snake is found mostly on the East Coast from Canada to Florida and as far West as Texas and Minnesota. Often mistaken for a cottonmouth, it has a narrower body than true cottonmouths.

42. **Correct Answer: C**

    The venom of a baby rattlesnake is more potent than the venom of adult snakes and contains more neurotoxins. Hence, symptoms will be more neurologic in presentation. Careful attention should be given to respiratory effort, blood pressure, and muscular control. Baby snakes can bite and inject venom rapidly if they are threatened or cornered. Their venom may be more neurotoxic to paralyze a predator and allow the baby to escape. By comparison, adult snakes use their more hemolytic venom for hunting and consumption. Generally a snake will not strike an animal that it cannot consume unless it is threatened or cornered.

43. **Correct Answer: A**

    Scotch Broom contains sparteine, which has very powerful cardiovascular effects. Arrhythmias, blood pressure changes (increased or decreased), coagulation changes, and vision changes are possible side effects of this herb. The best action listed would be to lavage the stomach to remove any undigested or partially digested Scotch Broom. You will need to insert a Foley catheter, as this herb does have diuretic properties, but it is not a priority. Quinidine and amiodarone should be stopped immediately, as they will interact with the Scotch Broom to cause further cardiovascular collapse by increasing the toxicity of the herb.

44. **Correct Answer: C**

Based on the history presented, it is suspicious that Mary's behavior toward food and her psychomotor skills would be altered so soon after ingesting home-made foods. The brownies should be tested for marijuana. Additional side effects of marijuana ingestion include paranoia, sleeplessness, short-term memory impairment, nausea, respiratory depression, and headaches. Each state has specific regulations regarding marijuana use for medicinal purposes. In any event, the staff should have a family conference with the patient to determine the best course of treatment in regard to Mary's symptoms. Self- or family-prescribing should not be permitted during hospitalization. If marijuana use for medicinal purposes is illegal within your state, local law officials may need to be contacted.

45. **Correct Answer: D**

Although "natural," herbal supplements and herbal use are not regulated. These substances can have varying strengths and resultant side effects. Regardless of their personal beliefs, it is vital that the treating staff be aware of any herbal supplements taken separately or in drinks or foods. Although some research has favored ginkgo biloba's use in increasing cerebral blood flow, there have also been documented cases of severe bleeding, seizures, glucose instability, and allergic reactions to this herb. Extreme caution should be used with herbal products in patients on anticoagulation therapy, antiplatelet therapy, anti-inflammatory medications, a diabetic regimen, MAO inhibitors, antipsychotic drugs, and antiseizure medications.

46. **Correct Answer: A**

Ginseng has been known to increase the Q-T interval, which puts this patient at greater risk for cardiac rhythm complications. Advise patients to carefully read the labels of any sports or high-energy drink, as some contain various herbs and high levels of caffeine. Ginseng may also cause breast tissue enlargement in men, as well as erectile dysfunction. In women, there may be increased menstrual bleeding, hormone imbalances in those with breast cancer, uterine cancer, and endometriosis. This may be due to ginseng exerting similar effects to estrogen. Ginseng may also cause complications or interactions with anticoagulation therapy, calcium-channel blockers, diabetes management, and it increases the potency of some sedatives.

47. **Correct Answer: B**

Sodium nitroprusside, when used in high doses (10 mcg/kg/min) or over a period of days, can raise blood concentrations of cyanide to toxic levels. Patients who are malnourished or are stressed from surgery may have low thiosulfate reserves. These patients are at increased risk for developing symptoms, even with therapeutic dosing. These individuals may become agitated and combative, causing their symptoms to be mistaken for ICU psychosis. If patients are given hydroxocobalamin or sodium thiosulfate along with sodium nitroprusside, the symptoms may be prevented or at least mitigated.

48. **Correct Answer: C**

Shellfish poisoning can produce symptoms days after ingestion of the contaminated food. The toxin contained in shellfish, clams, and oysters is called saxotoxin and is not affected by steaming or cooking. It inhibits sodium channels of membranes, blocking propagation of nerve and muscle action potentials. If the nerves are involved, the patient may experience paresthesias of the lips, tongue, gums, and face. The paresthesias may spread to the trunk and lead to paralysis and respiratory arrest. There is no definite treatment for shellfish poisoning, so care focuses on treating symptoms and providing psychological support.

49. **Correct Answer: D**
Wool and silk give off cyanide gas. Nitriles, like those found in the gloves we wear, will burn and give off cyanide. Household plastics such as melamine dishes, plastic cups, polyurethane foam in furniture cushions, and many other synthetic compounds may produce lethal concentrations of cyanide when burned under appropriate circumstances. Cyanide inhibits cellular respiration, even when the person has adequate oxygen stores. Cellular metabolism changes from aerobic to anaerobic, and the body produces lactic acid. The organs with the highest oxygen requirements are the most affected by cyanide inhalation.

50. **Correct Answer: D**
Fish can contain large amounts of mercury. The concentration of mercury in fish can be more than 1,000 times greater in a fish than in the surrounding water. People who eat fish as a main component of their diet may be at risk of mercury poisoning.

Organic mercury compounds are very toxic. They may be taken into the body by ingestion, inhalation, skin, and eye contact. The mercury compounds can attack all body systems. They can cause nausea, lack of appetite, abdominal pain, kidney failure, swollen gums, and mouth sores. Numbness and tingling in the lips, mouth, tongue, hands, and feet, tremors, and seizures may also occur. Patients may become very uncoordinated and feel disconnected from their surroundings. They may lose part or all of their vision and hearing. Additional neurological issues may include memory loss, personality changes, and headache.

Organic mercury can pass to a baby via breast milk. Methyl mercury may cause serious birth defects.

51. **Correct Answer: B**
Ergotamine (Ergot) is used quite often for migraine headaches, and in females it can be used to promote uterine contraction in childbirth. Because ergotamine causes smooth muscles to contract, it can be used to control bleeding.

In large doses, ergotamine paralyzes the motor nerve endings of the sympathetic nervous system. Excess amounts can cause disorientation, confusion, convulsions, seizures, severe muscle cramping, and dry gangrene of the extremities. LSD (lysergic acid diethylamide) is chemically related to ergotamine.

52. **Correct Answer: A**
Bee venom contains proteins that act as enzymes. The enzymes lyse the cells, causing cellular debris to accumulate very quickly and actually clog the kidneys. The patient then dies from kidney failure. Any patient who has been stung multiple times needs to be monitored for at least 2 weeks following the incident.

53. **Correct Answer: A**
The antidote is Dantrolene. Malignant hyperthermia is usually seen in patients receiving anesthetics. This patient may also require ice packs and a hypothermia blanket. On occasion, bowel irrigations with cold water and cold NG tube irrigations have been necessary. The cherry red skin is a possible effect with carbon monoxide poisoning.

54. **Correct Answer: C**
Excess endorphins need to be mediated. Prostaglandin is blocked by ibuprofen. Corticosteroids are used to stabilize the cell membrane by modifying mediators.

55. **Correct Answer: D**
Activated protein C (Xigris) inhibits factors Va and VIIIa, inhibits human tumor necrosis factor production by monocytes, and limits thrombin-induced inflammatory responses.

56. **Correct Answer: B**
Mucomyst may actually cause bronchospasm, so it must be used with a bronchodilator. Usually, Mucomyst is contraindicated in status asthmaticus. Codeine is generally not used in status asthmaticus. Guaifenesin is Robitussin—a mild cough syrup.

57. **Correct Answer: D**
Xanax, Valium, and Ativan are also benzodiazepines. Flumazenil (Romazicon) is a benzodiazepine antagonist.

58. **Correct Answer: A**
Alkaline solutions may cause the norepinephrine to precipitate. Also, do not use such a solution if it is discolored. Answers B, C, and D are indications for use.

59. **Correct Answer: A**
Regitine is used to counteract this effect. It should be administered subcutaneously around the area of extravasation.

60. **Correct Answer: C**
Cardene cannot be mixed with Lactated Ringer's or sodium bicarbonate infusions. According to studies, although the combination does not cause a precipitate to form, the LR inactivates 15% to 42% of the drug.

61. **Correct Answer: B**
Signs of thiocyanate toxicity include metabolic acidosis, hyperreflexia, confusion, and seizures. You must treat the patient with a simultaneous infusion of thiosulfate to prevent toxicity. If toxicity occurs, sodium thiocyanate, sodium nitrate, or amyl nitrate may be used to treat the patient.

62. **Correct Answer: D**
The patient may have a mild fever and will be in a hyperdynamic state. The endotoxins that are circulating will have vasodilatory effects, so RAP, PAOP, and SVR are decreased. The increase in CO is compensatory.

63. **Correct Answer: D**
This patient is in hypovolemic shock. The normal blood volume in an adult is approximately 5,000 mL, so a loss of 1,500 mL of blood would be equal to about one-third of the total blood volume. You would expect an increased HR (120–150), a decreased BP, a narrowed pulse pressure, an increased RR (25–40), and delayed capillary refill. The skin would be cool and clammy, and the patient may demonstrate neurological issues such as restlessness, anxiety, and confusion.

64. **Correct Answer: C**
Western equine encephalitis is caused by an arbovirus (togovirus); an arbovirus is carried by arthropods. A horse or small mammal was probably infected, and the virus was then vectored by a mosquito. This type of encephalopathy is not directly transmitted

from human to human. In this case, the patient is at high risk for aspiration pneumonia and ARDS.

65. **Correct Answer: B**

This is actually a panic level and, if not addressed, will cause nephrotoxicity. Ototoxicity usually occurs if levels remain at more than 30 mcg/mL for a prolonged period. Vancomycin may cause hypertension, thrombocytopenia, tubular necrosis, colitis, and deafness. The patient may require hemodialysis, hemofiltration, or peritoneal dialysis. Note that charcoal hemofiltration does not remove vancomycin.

66. **Correct Answer: A**

A tricyclic antidepressant acts by blocking norepinephrine and serotonin uptake in the central nervous system; it also has anticholinergic properties. The really interesting thing about this group of drugs is that they metabolize in the liver to one of the other tricyclics. You must test for levels of all of the tricyclics, because the initial drug may have metabolized and added to the effects.

67. **Correct Answer: C**

You can give hypertonic saline for hypotension. The ABG results should guide the amount to be given. Hemodialysis will not remove amitriptyline from the patient's system.

68. **Correct Answer: B**

In a TEE, the patient is sedated and the gag reflex reduced by application of an oral numbing spray. A gastroscope is advanced, and the patient swallows it. The tube is positioned directly behind the heart and allows for sound waves to be reflected off the heart chambers and valves. The left mainstem bronchus can interfere with this view. Some types of scopes can generate a three-dimensional picture.

There is a risk with this procedure that the patient might experience reflex bradycardia, esophageal perforation, transient hypoxia, drug-initiated tachycardia, or oversedation. Additional contraindications for TEE include stenosis and obstruction of the esophagus, penetrating chest injuries, and central nervous system depression (no sedatives). Patients who cannot lie flat are another contraindication.

69. **Correct Answer: C**

The patient should receive prophylactic antibiotics for endocarditis, which may be the cause of his symptoms at this time.

70. **Correct Answer: D**

The sed rate may also be decreased in patients with poikilocytosis. Other causes of a low sed rate include cortisone, lecithin, and corticotrophin.

71. **Correct Answer: D**

In this test, iodine-based radiographic contrast dye is injected into the antecubital or femoral vein via a catheter to the pulmonary artery. The pulmonary vasculature can then be visualized. The radioactive iodine crosses the blood–placental barrier, which is why its use is contraindicated in pregnancy. Other contraindications include allergy to shellfish, iodine, radiographic dye, and renal insufficiency.

72. **Correct Answer: D**

Renal function may be decreased, and the patient may have increased ALT and AST. After approximately 4 days to 2 weeks, the symptoms abate.

73. **Correct Answer: B**
The ACT, which measures the ability of the blood to clot, is easy to perform and quite reliable. Fresh, whole blood is added to a test tube that contains an activator (glass particles, kayolin, or diatomaceous earth). The result indicates how long it takes for a clot to form.

74. **Correct Answer: D**
Amiodarone is measured in micrograms per milliliter and not milligrams. The therapeutic level should be 0.5 to 2.5 mcg/mL.

75. **Correct Answer: B**
One of the major complications associated with use of pulmonary artery catheters is infection. Studies have shown that the initial source of the infection is from an initial colonization of skin bacteria that migrate down the catheter. Additional studies have shown that coating the catheter with antibiotics is not particularly effective in preventing such infection. The point of insertion (subclavian or jugular) also has been found to have no bearing on the risk of infection. Heparin may keep the catheter from clotting, but does not have any bearing on potential infections. Prophylactic antibiotics will not prevent catheter infections and may lead to more antibiotic-resistant strains colonizing the catheter. If the catheter remains in place more than 72 hours, it carries a significant risk of infection.

76. **Correct Answer: A**
We just thought we'd throw you a curve and put in a true/false question. Protein can show up in the cerebrospinal fluid as a consequence of more than 30 conditions. These conditions include brain abscess, brain tumor, diabetic neuropathy, encephalitis, heavy-metal poisoning, meningitis, mumps, myxedema, and phenytoin, to name just a few.

77. **Correct Answer: D**
Cocaine is a Schedule II central nervous system stimulant. It is used as a local anesthetic, a bronchodilator, and a vasoconstrictor. Cocaine compromises the heart's antioxidant defense system, and an overdose can cause an MI. Cocaine can also cause aortic dissection, stroke, intestinal ischemia, hallucinations, and adverse effects on fetuses.

78. **Correct Answer: B**
This test can be done to diagnose aneurysms, aortic valve stenosis, carotid stenosis, pulmonary emboli, ulcerative plaques, hepatocellular carcinomas, and many other conditions. There are risks to the procedure—allergic reactions to the contrast dye, anaphylaxis, aphasia, hemiplegia, paresthesia, hemorrhage, infection, renal toxicity, and thromboemboli.

79. **Correct Answer: C**
Ethylene glycol is a compound found in antifreeze. After ingestion, it is converted to oxalic acid, which is excreted by the kidneys. This process causes crystals in the urine, acidosis, tetany, and renal failure. Hemodialysis and peritoneal dialysis will remove ethylene glycol from the body.

80. **Correct Answer: A**

Ecstasy use can also cause ataxia, central nervous system depression, coma, brady-cardias, hypothermia, hypotension, hypothermia, respiratory depression, and respiratory acidosis.

81. **Correct Answer: D**

Arsenic is found in all human tissues as a trace element. These levels may become elevated with additional exposure. Sixty percent of ingested arsenic is excreted in the urine. Arsenic may be found in well water, pesticides, paints, cosmetics, treated wood, and coal. Chronic exposure can lead to various types of cancers.

82. **Correct Answer: A**

Cadmium is a heavy metal that has a half-life of 15 to 20 years. A respiratory irritant, it can produce pulmonary edema, interstitial pneumonia, and cardiovascular collapse if inhaled. Cadmium is used in the manufacture of storage batteries, in alloys, and in electroplating. If cadmium is ingested, the individual will develop severe gastrointestinal symptoms within 30 minutes. Most cadmium collects in erythrocytes and kidney tissues; it is not metabolized in the body.

83. **Correct Answer: A**

The biopsy may cause bleeding from highly vascular tissue. Flank pain may be the first sign.

84. **Correct Answer: B**

Lithium is an alkali, metal salt used mostly in the treatment of bipolar disorder and to treat cluster migraine headaches. As a treatment for bipolar disorder and alcohol withdrawal, lithium acts by altering sodium transport in nerves and muscles, which helps stabilize mood.

85. **Correct Answer: A**

When you are discarding urine, you should wear gloves while working for 24 hours after the test. You must also wash the gloves with soap and water before removing the gloves. Then, wash your hands again. Many nurses have needlessly exposed themselves because, in their haste to empty fluids for I&Os at shift change, they forget to wear gloves.

86. **Correct Answer: B**

Wound cultures for MRSA do not have to be placed on ice for transport. They may be kept as long as 8 hours at room temperature.

87. **Correct Answer: D**

The stealth adulterant will mask morphine in the urine. When heroin enters the body, it breaks down into morphine. 10 mg of morphine is detectable in urine for 84 hours; the same amount can be measured in corpses for about a week.

88. **Correct Answer: D**

Answers A, B, and C are all causes of increased blood osmolality.

89. **Correct Answer: D**

Phenytoin, which is used as an anticonvulsant and an antidysrhythmic, is metabolized in the liver and excreted in bile and urine. Tube feedings should be held before the test for 2 hours. Peak levels should be drawn 3 to 9 hours after oral use. As much as 5 days must be allowed before a change in dose will change results.

90. **Correct Answer: C**

Patients may eat prior to undergoing a PET scan. They should not drink large quantities of fluid within 2 hours of the scan unless the patient has, or will have, an indwelling catheter. Caffeinated drinks should be avoided within 2 hours of the test. It is important to inform lactating women that they should not breastfeed for at least 20 hours after the scan.

91. **Correct Answer: B**

Many herbs and natural remedies are oral anticoagulants and will affect the INR. They include dan shen, dang gui, dong quai, gingko biloba, garlic, ginseng, and ginger.

92. **Correct Answer: A**

Because of air trapping, patients with asthma have a low peak flow rate during expiration.

93. **Correct Answer: C**

The salty taste is normal. The patient may be slightly nauseous, feel like he wants to cough, or feel flushed. This sensation will pass in about 5 minutes.

94. **Correct Answer: C**

This disease is spread by ticks. Symptoms include a sudden-onset fever for 2 to 3 weeks and a rash that may cover the entire body. Treatment must include both chloramphenicol and tetracycline.

95. **Correct Answer: C**

False-positive results may be caused by polycythemia. A false negative result may be due to anemia or the fact that less than 7 mL of blood was drawn for the test.

96. **Correct Answer: B**

The liver may be lacerated by either blunt or penetrating trauma. In blunt trauma, there will often be fractures of the 7–9th ribs, which overlie the liver. In this case, no history of the mechanism of injury is provided. Right upper quadrant tenderness will be present with a liver laceration. Rebound sensitivity and guarding will not be present because blood has not been in the abdomen for at least 2 hours (long enough to cause peritoneal irritation).

Suspect liver laceration when penetrating trauma involves the right lower chest or right upper abdomen, or when right upper quadrant tenderness accompanies blunt trauma. The patient needs a CT.

97. **Correct Answer: C**

Splenic injury should be suspected when the 9–10th ribs on the left are fractured, or when left upper quadrant tenderness and tachycardia are present. This patient has not complained of pain in the left shoulder, but it is a common complaint. Peritoneal signs such as rebound sensitivity and guarding are delayed until the blood has had adequate time to cause local irritation of the peritoneum; this patient was trapped in her car for almost 2 hours. Hypotension is a sign of an active bleed.

98. **Correct Answer: B**

The kidneys are in the retroperitoneal space at the level of T12 to L3. Kidneys can be damaged by shearing or compression forces, which may cause laceration or contusions. Renal injuries must be suspected with fractures to the posterior ribs or lumbar vertebrae. Rupture of the renal artery with a deceleration injury (as might occur in a car crash) may cause hypovolemia. There is little collateral circulation to the kidney, and damage to the renal artery may lead to acute tubular necrosis and intrarenal failure. Sometimes, the signs of a kidney injury may be confused with a pancreatic injury. Generally, however, hematuria is not observed with a pancreatic injury. Common signs of kidney laceration include Grey–Turner's sign (flank ecchymosis), Cullen's sign (peri-umbilical bruising), and flank pain. This patient also is exhibiting confusion, which could result from causes ranging from a simple concussion to an acute brain injury. The patient needs immediate evaluation.

99. **Correct Answer: C**
First, AC current usually causes ventricular fibrillation and DC current usually causes asystole. In some cases arrhythmias are delayed for up to 12 hours.

   The mechanism of lightning strikes is quite complex. Lightning can injure a person in 5 ways:
   - A side splash from another object, which is probably the cause of this patient's injuries
   - Lightning hits something like a tree, then bounces off
   - A direct strike
   - A person touches an object that has been struck by lightning
   - Ground current effect occurs when energy spreads out across the surface of the earth

   Lightning has 2 strokes, upward and downward. If these strokes do not meet, energy can be directed outward. Internal burns are rare. Myoglobinuria rarely occurs. Generally, lightning will cause cardiac and respiratory arrest, burns from metals touching the victim (e.g., watches, necklaces, golf shoe cleats), and neurological damage.

100. **Correct Answer: A**
Self-destructive behaviors are behaviors that, over time, will shorten or threaten length and quality of life.

101. **Correct Answer: B**
Elderly individuals often have unstable health, which may contribute to psychiatric crisis and emergency. Some elderly persons have limited support systems as time and circumstances result in the loss of loved ones by death or distance. A limited ability to work, poor health or disabilities, or limited funds may lead to greater emotional and psychiatric distress due to financial pressures.

102. **Correct Answer: D**
In any potential psychiatric emergency or crisis, it is important to first determine if such a situation exists. In this scenario, the patient has an extensive and involved support system, financial stability, and effective coping mechanisms. Thus a psychiatric crisis is not likely to develop. Even so, it is still important to carefully monitor the patient and family for any change in status.

103. **Correct Answer: D**
Careful consideration and observation should be given to any person voicing any thought or plan regarding suicide. Many individuals will provide warning about their suicidal thoughts, giving those in the family or in proximity the opportunity to intervene. Warnings are often cries for help and intervention. Family members should pay close attention to any impression or instinct that the person is considering suicide. As

individuals enter and exit depression, they are at greatest risk for suicide, as they have sufficient mental focus to form a plan and energy or motivation to carry it out.

104. Correct Answer: C

Feelings of helplessness or hopelessness indicate psychotic emergencies. Extreme anxiety or ability to recognize options are warning signs that should alert staff and family to a greater risk of suicide, because the patient may see suicide as the only option. The other answers indicate depression and/or levels of grief and emotional expression.

105. Correct Answer: A

Direct confrontation with the object of anger may further exacerbate the situation and limit the person's ability to deal positively with the situation. Instead, engage the person in a conversation regarding the stressor and assist in identifying feelings and options.

106. Correct Answer: A

Alterations in chemical or electrolytes may lead to anxiety and agitation, which might potentially be misdiagnosed as a psychiatric emergency.

107. Correct Answer: C

Wernicke's syndrome is a result of thiamine deficiency and will result in brain damage if not treated immediately.

108. Correct Answer: C

Restraints should be used only if alternative methods of behavioral correction prove ineffective. There is no indication that the patient is violent or represents any threat to staff or self. Restraints should only be used as a last resort to prevent injury to self and staff. Reorientation, medication, and controlling external stimulation are all effective methods for controlling behavior.

109. Correct Answer: A

Physical needs must come before psychological needs in disaster or crisis. In Maslow's hierarchy of needs, physical needs must be met first. Only after physical needs have been met can one focus on locating family, providing social services, and disseminating information to the media.

110. Correct Answer: D

Sometimes, families do not have enough education to make proper decisions. In this case, the family needed to know that the patient was still quite capable of making decisions and his wishes would be honored.

111. Correct Answer: B

Even if this patient signed a consent form, either she is not certain about the procedure or she is not fully informed. The nurse must act as advocate and notify the physician.

112. Correct Answer: C

Sometimes the bed is needed emergently. Ideally, the military would arrange for compassionate leave for the military service member. Providers certainly should not simply go ahead and try to procure organs as soon as the family leaves.

113. Correct Answer: C

This is the best nursing response. All members of the healthcare team can join in the decision-making process. Visiting policies vary, but are primarily designed to protect children from disease and from being overwhelmed by equipment and the ICU milieu. Under the circumstances, most nurses would probably want to sneak the child in during the night shift, but many factors should weigh into the final decision. This situation could produce the child's last memory of his mother (intubated with tubes). Participants in the conference will weigh the child's maturity and coping ability; he and the father will probably lose the mother and the sibling. There is no simple answer.

114. **Correct Answer: B**
Ciprofloxacin, a fluoroquinolone antibiotic, is the drug of choice for inhalation anthrax. Doxycycline, a tetracycline derivative, may also be utilized but the dosage given in this question is incorrect. Penicillin G is not an option because the bacterium, *Bacillus anthracis,* becomes beta lactamase positive, making the penicillin ineffective. Augmentin would not be used for this situation and is only given orally.

115. **Correct Answer: C**
The incubation period for inhalation anthrax ranges from 7 days to as long as 60 days after exposure. Symptoms are initially vague and flu-like, such as malaise, low-grade fever, and nausea. These symptoms quickly progress to profound diaphoresis, chest discomfort, and rhonchi. The mild symptoms occur in the first 5 days of the illness and are followed by a brief rally. The patient then experiences an abrupt onset of high fever and severe respiratory distress. Death occurs as early as 24 to 36 hours after symptoms begin.

116. **Correct Answer: A**
Inhalation anthrax starts with mild, nonspecific symptoms such as malaise, low-grade fever, fatigue, and cough. If it is left untreated, death occurs within 24 to 36 hours from respiratory failure.

117. **Correct Answer: D**
Antibiotics for inhalation anthrax are continued for 60 days after exposure, even if the exposure is only suspected. Treatment is initially intravenous, but then changes to oral dosing for the remaining time. The 2 antibiotics most commonly given in this setting are ciprofloxacin and doxycycline.

118. **Correct Answer: C**
According to the CDC, contact precautions are all that is required for inhalation anthrax. Standard precautions may include the use of a face mask if the patient has a productive cough.

119. **Correct Answer: B**
Kathy has botulism from the old green beans she consumed. Because this patient ate the contaminated food a few days ago, it is too late to give her the antitoxin. She will be placed on a ventilator for an extended period until the *Clostridium botulinum* toxins clear her body. If she survives the acute phase, she may have lasting fatigue and dyspnea for years, requiring long-term therapy.

Many home-canned foods may contain botulism spores. These foods include beans, fermented fish, tomatoes, chili peppers, asparagus, corn, beets, improperly handled baked potatoes, and garlic or herbs in olive oil. All of these items have a low acid content, which encourages the survival of *Clostridium botulinum* spores. Proper sterilization of home-canning equipment and storage containers reduces the risk to those consuming these foods. Boiling the foods for at least 10 minutes will also kill the *Clostridium botulinum* spores.

120. **Correct Answer: B**

    Clostridium botulinum is a rod-shaped bacterium that is the causative organism of botulism. Only 25% of all U.S. cases of botulism are caused by food products, and most of these cases involve home-canned foods. The majority of botulism cases involve infant botulism, which accounts for more than 70% of all cases of botulism in the United States. Babies younger than 1 year old should not consume honey, especially raw or home-grown honey, because it may contain botulism spores. The third type of botulism is seen in wounds contaminated by soil containing the botulism spores.

121. **Correct Answer: C**

    Ricin is made from castor beans and is one of the most toxic substances known. It interferes with protein synthesis and causes cell death. Chewing castor beans may cause some symptoms, but the most lethal form is inhaled. Ricin is not spread by casual contact. The most likely victims of a terrorist attack involving ricin would be seen in enclosed areas such as subway trains, buses, or small rooms. It is usually aerosolized with a liquid, such as water or a weak acid.

122. **Correct Answer: D**

    Surveys can be used to anonymously identify staff perceptions and determine educational opportunities. Mental health issues impact every person at some point in their lives. Whether those problems arise from a catastrophic event or ongoing psychological issues, it is important that nurses understand their own biases regarding mental health disorders and be able to identify appropriate resources when caring for this population. If the nurses believe the survey results will be used punitively, then data may be skewed to reflect what the staff believe the surveyor is looking for, not the truth. Instead of changing assignments immediately, it is best to use the opportunity for education and professional growth.

123. **Correct Answer: B**

    A psychological crisis may precede an emergency, but not always. Although there is no specific definition for either term, accepted criteria for both are a crisis is a less immediate situation that has developed over time in the presence of a psychological situation. Coping mechanisms may be partially effective, but do not address the situation directly to lead to a satisfactory conclusion of the problem. A crisis may develop into an emergency if coping mechanisms fail or additional stressors appear. A psychological emergency has the following basic elements: a sense of urgency that, if the situation is not resolved, anxiety may be intolerable and may lead to feelings of being overwhelmed. In this situation, the person's coping skills have completely failed and the patient recognizes the need for help to alleviate the stressors. Suicide calls, notes, and messages meet these criteria.

124. **Correct Answer: D**

    The wife may need time to open up, so the nurse will need to ensure that his or her other patient is cared for while dealing with her. Even though the social worker and the spiritual advisor may need to be called, it is important not to overwhelm the person until the stressor and situation has been identified. It is not appropriate for the nurse to contact the wife's physician; although the wife may need prescriptions during this time, that decision should be made only by her physician upon direct assessment.

125. **Correct Answer: A**
    Although each of these situations can be classified as a crisis, the 80-year-old home-bound male without family resources is at greatest risk for an emergency. Because he is home-bound, it will be more challenging to get resources to him. Public assistance, friends, and seniors groups may be effective resources to ensure appropriate coping.

126. **Correct Answer: C**
    Anger, fear, and denial are normal emotions in this situation. Staff members who feel anxiety are at greater risk. Anxiety is a commonly encountered emotion in psychological emergencies. Anxiety involves uncertainty about the unknown and may limit the person's ability to identify resources or initiate appropriate coping mechanisms. Debriefings held after codes, successful and unsuccessful, are therapeutic and allow staff to verbalize their emotions in a safe and stable environment. As a team, the staff may identify ways to support families and each other during crises and emergency situations.

127. **Correct Answer: A**
    Rapid and pressured speech is a sign of tension and indicates that the patient needs support and assistance in coping with his diagnosis. Humor and social activities can be positive coping techniques, as long as they are not used to avoid the stressful situation. The patient will need assistance and education regarding his diagnosis so that he can effectively identify positive lifestyle changes.

128. **Correct Answer: D**
    The patient may feel as if he has failed the nurse by not remaining sober and that assistance may be withdrawn. This statement does not judge the patient and shows him that help is still available by initiating communication and encouraging the patient to talk about his struggles with maintaining sobriety. Answer A is judgmental and demeaning. Answer B limits support and indicates to the patient that he is unable to succeed. Answer C focuses on the nurse's feelings and not on the patient.

129. **Correct Answer: C**
    This response acknowledges the patient's situation without allowing the patient to manipulate the nurse and indicates that the nurse takes his suicidal talk seriously. This patient should be placed on suicide precautions and moved to a room where he is under direct supervision at all times. Both the physician and psychological services should be notified immediately. The patient will need continued physical and psychological support during his recovery. Careful monitoring for depression and suicidal thoughts and attempts must be done. At this point, the patient is unable to see options or acknowledge positive facts of being alive. Visitors may be seen as pitying him, rather than as being supportive of the patient. Medication may be necessary, but should not be implemented until the situation has been fully assessed.

130. **Correct Answer: A**
    Safety is your highest priority. By removing the daughter from the unit, hospital personnel can manage her behavior and anger more safely. It is important to address the daughter directly, acknowledge her anger, and avoid trapping her physically in any corner. Use quiet and even tones that will not escalate her emotions. Ignoring the behavior and making jokes will only further anger the daughter and may lead to physical acts of violence. Calling the police may elevate the situation if she has not directly made or acted on threats. If security is unable to assist in diffusing the situation, then police assistance may be needed.

131. **Correct Answer: C**

     The goal at this point is to regulate the patient's breathing and stabilize vital signs. Using a firm and quiet voice with simple sentences can help the severely anxious patient focus and diffuse the anxiety. Severely anxious individuals are less able to see options and cope at this stage. Goals should include decreasing any unnecessary stress and remaining available to the patient for communication. The other answers speak to facts not in the nurse's knowledge and may increase fear or lead to false hope.

132. **Correct Answer: A**

     The timing of the symptoms is consistent with alcohol withdrawal delirium tremens (DTs). DTs are typically seen 12 to 24 hours after last ingestion of alcohol as blood alcohol levels drop. Effects may peak as long as 15 days after DTs begin. Fluids, vitamins, nutrition, and short-term pharmacological treatments are appropriate. The severity of symptoms will be affected by the amount and duration of alcohol ingestion as well as his underlying physical health, the combination of other drugs he is taking, and his existing psychological status. There are no indications at this time that the patient is septic or has schizophrenia. There may be underlying drug withdrawal symptoms, but the patient history does not provide any indication in this regard.

BIBLIOGRAPHY

Ahmed, I., & Beckingham, I. G. (2007). Liver trauma. *Trauma, 9*(3), 171–180.

Ahrens, T. (2006). *Critical care nursing certification.* Columbus, OH: McGraw-Hill.

American Association of Critical-Care Nurses. (2006). *Core curriculum for critical care nursing* (6th ed.). Philadelphia: Saunders.

American Association of Critical-Care Nurses. (2007). *AACN certification and core review for high acuity and critical care* (6th ed.). Philadelphia: Saunders.

American Heart Association. (2007). *Guidelines 2005 for cardiopulmonary resuscitation and emergency cardiovascular care.* Retrieved July 24, 2008, from http://circ.ahajournals.org/content/vol112/24_suppl

Antunez, C., Martin, E., Cornejo-Garcia, J. A., et al. (2006). Immediate hypersensitivity reactions to penicillins and other betalactams. *Current Pharmaceutical Design, 12*(26), 3327–3333.

Atlas, R. M. (2002). Bioterrorism: From threat to reality. *Annual Review of Microbiology, 56,* 167–185. Retrieved March 1 , 2008, from Research Library database.

Audi, J., Belson, M., Patel, M., Schier, J., & Osterloh, J. (2005). Ricin poisoning: A comprehensive review. *Journal of the American Medical Association, 294*(18), 2342–2351.

Benson, A., Dickson, W. A., & Boyce, D. E. (2006). ABC of wound healing: Burns. *British Medical Journal, 332*(7542), 649–652.

Benson, L. S., Edwards, S. L., Schiff, A. P., Williams, C. S., & Visotsky, J. L. (2006). Dog and cat bites to the hand: Treatment and cost assessment. *Journal of Hand Surgery, 31*(3), 468–473.

Bergmann, J. F., & Kher, A. (2005). Venous thromboembolism in the medically ill patient: A call to action. *International Journal of Clinical Practice, 59*(5), 555.

Bistrian, B. (2007). Systemic response to inflammation. *Nutrition Reviews, 65*(12), S170–S172.

Borgel, D., Bornstain, C., Reitsma, P. H., Lerolle, N., Gandrille, S., Dali-Ali, F., et al. (2007). A comparative study of the protein C pathway in septic and nonseptic patients with organ failure. *American Journal of Respiratory and Critical Care Medicine, 176*(9), 878–885.

Bresolin, N. L., Carvalho, F. C., Goes, J. C., Fernandes, V., & Barotto, A. M. (2002). Acute renal failure following massive attack by Africanized bee stings. *Pediatric Nephrology, 17*(8), 625–627.

Bulger, E. M., Jurkovich, G. J., Nathens, A. V., Copass, M. K., Hanson, S., Cooper, C., et al. (2008). Hypertonic resuscitation of hypovolemic shock after blunt trauma. *Archives of Surgery, 143*(2), 139.

Burd, A., & Noronha, F. V. (2005). Theme symposium: What's new in burns trauma? *Surgical Practice, 9*(4), 126–136.

Burns, S. M. (Ed.). (2007). *American Association of Critical-Care Nurses (AACN): AACN protocols for practice: Healing environments* (2nd ed.). Sudbury, MA: Jones and Bartlett.

Cai, S., Singh, B. R., & Sharma, S. (2007). Botulism diagnostics: From clinical symptoms to in vitro assays. *Critical Reviews in Microbiology, 33*(2), 109–125. Retrieved March 1, 2008, from ProQuest Health and Medical Complete database.

Carter, C. (2005). Evaluation and treatment of brown recluse spider bites. *American Family Physician, 72*(7), 1372, 1376.

Cauwels, A. (2007). Nitric oxide in shock. *Kidney International, 72*(5), 557–565.

Centers for Disease Control and Prevention. (2006). Fast facts: Anthrax information for health care providers. Retrieved March 3, 2008, from http://emergency.cdc.gov/agent/anthrax/anthrax-hcp-factsheet.asp

Centers for Disease Control and Prevention. (2006). Ricin: Epidemiology overview for clinicians. Retrieved March 3, 2008, from http://emergency.cdc.gov.agent/ricin/clinicians/epidemiology.asp

Chauhan, D., Chari, P., Khuller, G., & Singh, D. (2004). Correlation of renal complications with extent and progression of tissue damage in electrical burns. *Indian Journal of Plastic Surgery, 37*(2), 99–104.

Co-Minh, H. B., Demoly, P., Guillot, B., & Raison-Peyron, N. (2007). Allergy Net: Anaphylactic shock after oral intake and contact urticaria due to polyethylene glycols. *Allergy, 62*(1), 92–93.

Conover, M. B. (2003). *Understanding electrocardiography* (8th ed.). St. Louis, MO: Mosby/Elsevier.

Copstead, L., & Banasik, J. L. (2000). *Pathophysiology: Biological and behavioral perspectives* (2nd ed.). Philadelphia: Saunders/Elsevier.

Cosgrove, S. E., Perl, T. M., Song, S., & Sisson, S. D. (2005). Ability of physicians to diagnose and manage illness due to Category A bioterrorism agents. *Archives of Internal Medicine, 165*(17), 2002–2006. Retrieved March 3, 2008, from Research Library database.

Curley, M. A. Q. (1998). Patient–nurse synergy: Optimizing patients' outcomes. *American Journal of Critical Care, 7*, 64–72.

De Waele, J. J. (2008). Abdominal compartment syndrome in severe acute pancreatitis: When to decompress? *European Journal of Trauma and Emergency Surgery, 34*(1), 11–16.

Diaz, J. H., & Leblanc, K. E. (2007). Common spider bites. *American Family Physician, 75*(6), 869–873.

Dossey, B. M., Keegan, L., & Guzzetta, C. (2003). *Holistic nursing: A handbook for practice* (3rd ed.). Sudbury, MA: Jones and Bartlett.

Edwards, D. F. (1999). The Synergy Model: Linking patient needs to nurse competencies. *Critical Care Nurse, 19*(1), 88–98.

Emergency Nurses Association, & Newberry, L. (2003). *Sheehy's emergency nursing: Principles and practice* (5th ed.). St. Louis, MO: Mosby/Elsevier.

Finkelmeier, B. A. (2000). *Cardiothoracic surgical nursing* (2nd ed.). Philadelphia: Lippincott, Williams & Wilkins.

Garretson, S., & Malberti, S. (2007). Understanding hypovolaemic, cardiogenic and septic shock. *Nursing Standard, 21*(50), 46–55; quiz, 58.

Gaspardone, A., & Versaci, F. (2005). Coronary stenting and inflammation. *American Journal of Cardiology, 96*(12A), L65–L70.

Gasparis Vonfrolio, L., & Noone, J. (1999). *Critical care examination review* (3rd ed. revised). Staten Island, NY: Power Publications.

Glapa, M., Kourie, J. F., Doll, D., & Degiannis, E. (2007). Early management of gunshot injuries to the face in civilian practice. *World Journal of Surgery, 31*(11), 2104–2110.

Gonzalez, N. C., Allen, J., Blanco, V. G., Schmidt, E. J., van Rooijen, N., & Wood, J. G. (2007). Alveolar macrophages are necessary for the systemic inflammation of acute alveolar hypoxia. *Journal of Applied Physiology, 103*(4), 1386.

Gueant, J. L., Gueant-Rodriguez, R. M., Viola, M., Valluzzi, R. L., & Romano, A. (2006). IgE-mediated hypersensitivity to cephalosporins. *Current Pharmaceutical Design, 12*(26), 3335–3345.

Hardin, S. R., & Kaplow, R. (Eds.). (2004). *Synergy for clinical excellence: The AACN Synergy Model for Patient Care*. Sudbury, MA: Jones and Bartlett.

Harman, K. R., & Herndon, T. M. (2006). Cold-water immersion in a 22-year-old service member. *Military Medicine, 171*(5), 459–462.

Harries, M. (2003). ABC of resuscitation: Near drowning. *British Medical Journal, 327*(7427), 1336–1338.

Hickey, J. V. (2002). *The clinical practice of neurological and neurosurgical nursing* (5th ed.). Philadelphia: Lippincott, Williams & Wilkins.

Holgate, S. T., & Polosa, R. (2008). Treatment strategies for allergy and asthma. *Nature Reviews. Immunology, 8*(3), 218–230.

Howell, J. M., Mayer, T. A., Hanfling, D., & Morrison, A. (2004). Screening for inhalational anthrax due to bioterrorism: Evaluating proposed screening protocols. *Clinical Infectious Diseases, 39*(12), 1842–1847. Retrieved March 1, 2008, from Research Library database.

Hurst, J. R., Perera, W. R., Wilkinson, T. M. A, Donaldson, G. C., & Wedzicha, J. A. (2006). Systemic and upper and lower airway inflammation at exacerbation of chronic obstructive pulmonary disease. *American Journal of Respiratory and Critical Care Medicine, 173*(1), 71–78.

Index case of fatal inhalation anthrax due to bioterrorism in the United States. (2002). *Journal of Cutaneous Medicine and Surgery, 6*(4), 379. Retrieved March 3, 2008, from ProQuest Health and Medical Complete database.

Inhalation anthrax. (2001). *Morbidity and Mortality Weekly Report.* Retrieved March 3, 2008, from http://www.cdc.gov/mmwr/preview/mmwrhtml/mm5043al.htm

Joulin, O., Petillot, P., Labalette, M., Lancel, S., & Neviere, R. (2007). Cytokine profile of human septic shock serum inducing cardiomyocyte contractile dysfunction. *Physiological Research, 56*(3), 291–297.

Kandil, E., Burack, J., Sawas, A., Bibawy, H., Schwartzman, A., Zenilman, M. E., et al. (2008). B-type natriuretic peptide. *Archives of Surgery, 143*(3), 242.

Karmy-Jones, R., Carter, Y., & Stern, E. (2002). The impact of positive pressure ventilation on the diagnosis of traumatic diaphragmatic injury. *American Surgeon, 68*(2), 167–172.

Keel, M., Eid, K., Labler, L., Seifert, B., Trentz, O., & Ertel, W. (2006). Influence of injury pattern on incidence and severity of posttraumatic inflammatory complications in severely injured patients. *European Journal of Trauma, 32*(4), 387–395.

Kemerer, J. J., Reitz, M., & Diaz, J. H. (2007). Diagnosis of brown recluse spider bites is overused/ In reply. *American Family Physician, 76*(7), 943–944; author reply, 944, 947.

Kozieras, J., Thuemer, O., & Sakka, S. G. (2007). Influence of an acute increase in systemic vascular resistance on transpulmonary thermodilution-derived parameters in critically ill patients. *Intensive Care Medicine, 33*(9), 1619–1623.

Kury Hughs, S., Nilsson, D. E., Boyer, R. S., Bolte, R. G., Hoffman, R. O., Lewine, J. D., et al. (2002). Neurodevelopmental outcome for extended cold water drowning: A longitudinal case study. *Journal of the International Neuropsychological Society, 8*(4), 588–595.

Legeza, V. I., Galenko-Yaroshevskii, V. P., Zinov'ev, E. V., et al. (2004). Effects of new wound dressings on healing of thermal burns of the skin in acute radiation disease. *Bulletin of Experimental Biology and Medicine, 138*(3), 311–315.

Leibovici, L., Gafter-Gvili, A., Paul, M., Paramonov, B. A., Kreichman, G. S., Turkovskii, I. I., et al. (2007). Relative tachycardia in patients with sepsis: An independent risk factor for mortality. *QJM, 100*(10), 629–634.

Lipson, J. G., Dibble, S. L., & Minarik, P. A. (Eds.). (1996). *Culture and nursing care: A pocket guide.* San Francisco, CA: UCSF Nursing Press.

McNally, P. (2001). *GI/liver secrets* (2nd ed.). Philadelphia: Hanley & Belfus/Elsevier.

McQuillan, K. A., Von Rueden, K. T., Hartsock, R. L., Flynn, M. B., & Whalen, E. (Eds.). (2002). *Trauma nursing: From resuscitation through rehabilitation* (3rd ed.). Philadelphia: Saunders/ Elsevier.

Medina, J., & Puntillo, K. (2006). *AACN protocols for practice: Palliative care and end-of-life issues in critical care.* Sudbury, MA: Jones and Bartlett.

Merchant, R. C., Zabbo, C. P., Mayer, K. H., & Becker, B. M. (2007). Factors associated with delay to emergency department presentation, antibiotic usage and admission for human bite injuries. *CJEM: Journal of the Canadian Association of Emergency Physicians, 9*(6), 441–448.

Mitchell, J. W., & Danska, J. (2007). Escharotic lesion after a "brown recluse spider bite." *American Family Physician, 75*(12), 1841–1842.

Modell, J. H., Idris, A. H., Pineda, J. A., & Silverstein, J. H. (2004). Survival after prolonged submersion in freshwater in Florida. *Chest, 125*(5), 1948–1951.

Monneuse, O., Al-Ahmadi, K., & Ahmed, N. (2006). The case of a migrating bullet. *Lancet, 368*(9544), 1392.

Moore, E. E., Cheng, A. M., Moore, H. B., Masuno, T., & Johnson, J. L. (2006). Hemoglobin-based oxygen carriers in trauma care: Scientific rationale for the US multicenter prehospital trial. *World Journal of Surgery, 30*(7), 1247–1257.

Norris, R. L., Wilkerson, J. A., & Feldman, J. (2007). Syncope, massive aspiration, and sudden death following rattlesnake bite. *Wilderness & Environmental Medicine, 18*(3), 206–208. Retrieved March 29, 2008, from Research Library database (Document ID: 1363946451).

O'Brien, J. M., Ali, N. A., Aberegg, S. K., & Abraham, E. (2007). Sepsis. *American Journal of Medicine, 120*(12), 1012.

O'Brien, K. K., Higdon, M. L., & Halverson, J. J. (2003). Recognition and management of bioterrorism infections. *American Family Physician, 67*(9), 1927–1934.

Pagana, K. D., & Pagana, J. (2005). *Mosby's manual of diagnostic and laboratory tests* (3rd ed.). St. Louis, MO: Mosby/Elsevier.

Petroianu, A. (2007). Arterial embolization for hemorrhage caused by hepatic arterial injury. *Digestive Diseases and Sciences, 52*(10), 2478–2481.

Prodan Lange, S., & Shank, S. L. (2008). *Managing the psychiatric crisis homestudy* (Catalog 50 JDE). Lakeway, TX: National Center for Continuing Education.

Ranasinghe, A. M., Hyde, J. A. J., & Graham, T. R. (2002). Management of flail chest: Trauma 3. *Trauma, 4*(3), 146.

Regueira, T., Hasbun, P., Rebolledo, R., Galindo, J., Aguirre, M., Romero, C., et al. (2007). Intra-abdominal hypertension in patients with septic shock. *American Surgeon, 73*(9), 865–870.

Rhoads, J. (2007). Epidemiology of the brown recluse spider bite. *Journal of the American Academy of Nurse Practitioners, 19*(2), 79–85.

Richardson, J. D., Franklin, G. A., Heffley, S., & Seligson, D. (2007). Operative fixation of chest wall fractures: An underused procedure? *American Surgeon, 73*(6), 591–596; discussion, 596–597.

Robin-Lersundi, A., Trancho, F. H., Gastardi, J. C., Martinez, A. G., García, A. T., & Balibrea Cantero, J. L. (2003). Penetrating chest gunshot wounds: Conservative treatment. *Surgical Endoscopy, 17*(10), 1677.

Rubin, A. E., Wang, K., & Liu, M. L. (2003). Tracheobronchial stenosis from acid aspiration presenting as asthma. *Chest, 123*(2), 643–646.

Seamon, M. J., Fisher, C. A., Gaughan, J. P., Kulp, H., Dempsey, D. T., & Goldberg, A. J. (2008). Emergency department thoracotomy: Survival of the least expected. *World Journal of Surgery, 32*(4), 604–612.

Seiler, J. G., & Shaw, B. A. (2003). Rattlesnake bite with associated compartment syndrome: What is the best treatment? *Journal of Bone and Joint Surgery, 85*(6), 1163.

Seth, R., Chester, D., & Moiemen, N. (2007). A review of chemical burns. *Trauma, 9*(2), 81–94.

Sharma, O. P., Oswanski, M. F., Singer, D., Raj, S. S., & Daoud, Y. A. H. (2005). Assessment of nonoperative management of blunt spleen and liver trauma. *American Surgeon, 71*(5), 379–386.

Shaw, B. A., & Hosalkar, H. S. (2002). Rattlesnake bites in children: Antivenin treatment and surgical indications. *Journal of Bone and Joint Surgery, 84*(9), 1624–1629.

Skidmore-Roth, L. (2004). *Mosby's 2004 nursing drug reference*. St. Louis, MO: Mosby/Elsevier.

Smeltzer, S., & Bare, B. G. (2003). *Brunner and Suddarth's textbook of medical–surgical nursing* (10th ed.). Philadelphia: Lippincott, Williams & Wilkins.

Sole, M. L., Hartshorn, J., & Lamborne, M. L. (2001). *Introduction to critical care nursing* (3rd ed.). Philadelphia: Saunders/Elsevier.

Spaniolas, K., Velmahos, G. C., Wicky, S., Nussbaumer, K., Petrovick, L., Gervasini, L., et al. (2008). Is upper extremity deep venous thrombosis underdiagnosed in trauma patients? *American Surgeon, 74*(2), 124–128.

Spencer, R. C. (2003). *Bacillus anthracis. Journal of Clinical Pathology, 56*(3), 182–187. Retrieved March 3, 2008, from ProQuest Health and Medical Complete database.

Spies, C., & Trohman, R. G. (2006). Narrative review: Electrocution and life-threatening electrical injuries. *Annals of Internal Medicine, 145*(7), 531–537.

Swanson, D. L., & Vetter, R. S. (2005). Medical progress: Bites of brown recluse spiders and suspected necrotic arachnidism. *New England Journal of Medicine, 352*(7), 700–707.

Taplitz, R. A. (2004). Managing bite wounds. *Postgraduate Medicine, 116*(2), 49.

Turk, T., Vural, H., Ata, Y., Eris, C., & Yavuz, C. (2007). Acute aortic insufficiency after blunt chest trauma: A case report. *Journal of Cardiovascular Surgery, 48*(3), 359–361.

Tzortzaki, E. G., Lambiri, I., Vlachaki, E., & Siafakas, N. M. (2007). Biomarkers in COPD. *Current Medicinal Chemistry, 14*(9), 1037–1048.

Urden, L. D., Stacy, K. M., & Lough, M. E. (2007). *Thelan's critical care nursing: Diagnosis and management* (5th ed.). St. Louis, MO: Mosby.

van Haren, F. M. P., Sleigh, J. W., Pickkers, P., & van der Hoeven, J. G. (2007). Gastrointestinal perfusion in septic shock. *Anaesthesia and Intensive Care, 35*(5), 679–694.

Vassilakopoulos, T., & Hussain, S. N. A. (2007). Ventilatory muscle activation and inflammation: Cytokines, reactive oxygen species, and nitric oxide. *Journal of Applied Physiology, 102*(4), 1687.

Vécsei, V., Arbes, S., Aldrian, S., & Nau, T. (2005). Chest injuries in polytrauma. *European Journal of Trauma, 31*(3), 239–243.

Warwick, A. M., Goonewardene, K., Burton, P. R., Usatoff, V., & Evans, P. M. (2007). HP38P Management of the traumatic pancreatic injury. *ANZ Journal of Surgery, 77*(s1), A48.

Weber-Carstens, S., Deja, M., Bercker, S., Dimroth, A., Ahlers, O., Kaisers, U., et al. (2007). Impact of bolus application of low-dose hydrocortisone on glycemic control in septic shock patients. *Intensive Care Medicine, 33*(4), 730–733.

Wiegand, D. J. L., & Carlson, K. K. (Eds.). (2005). *AACN procedure manual for critical care* (5th ed.). Philadelphia: Elsevier.

Woltmann, A., Beisse, R., Eckardt, H., Potulski, M., & Bühren, V. (2007). Combined abdominal and spine injuries after high energy flexion–distraction trauma. *European Journal of Trauma and Emergency Surgery, 33*(5), 482–488.

Woods, S., Sivarajan Froelicher, E. S., & Motzer, S. U. (2000). *Cardiac Nursing* (4th ed.). Philadelphia: Lippincott, Williams & Wilkins.

Zeller, J. L. (2007). Evaluation of white blood cell count, neutrophil percentage, and elevated temperature as predictors of bloodstream infection in burn patients. *Journal of the American Medical Association, 298*(9), 968.

Practice CCRN Examination

This practice test contains the same information that is found on the enclosed CD. The questions on the CD are in random order. Allow yourself 2½ hours to complete this practice test. The answers and rationale appear at the end of the exam.

Keep practicing until you can score at least 80%.

ADULT CCRN PRACTICE EXAMINATION

1. Michael is a 19-year-old college student. Last week he suffered an MI. He was pledging to a fraternity and, as part of the hazing ritual, he was required to consume large amounts of alcohol. He passed out and the other members left him on the lawn outside to, "sleep it off." Michael became hypoxic and had a left anterior wall MI. He was unresponsive when found. Michael was in a third-degree heart block when he was admitted to your unit and his 12-lead EKG showed primary lead changes in V_2–V_4. Michael regained consciousness and was extubated on the fifth day post admit day and suffered no neurological deficits. Today, he complains of precordial pain that radiates to the shoulder and neck and is worse when he coughs or takes a deep breath. Michael probably is symptomatic of
    A. An extending MI.
    B. A dissecting aortic aneurysm.
    C. Dressler's syndrome.
    D. Pneumonitis.

2. Diana had influenza 2 weeks ago. She was admitted to your MICU because she had an exacerbation of her COPD. Today she started having difficulty with repeated headaches. When you return to her room after notifying the physician about the headaches, you note that she is exhibiting a facial droop, yet her speech is clear. Because of her recent history, you suspect Guillain-Barré syndrome. What are the 4 types of Guillain-Barré syndrome?
    A. Ascending, progressive, relapsing-remitting, pure motor
    B. Ascending, descending, Miller–Fischer variant, pure motor
    C. Ascending, descending, relapsing, pure sensory
    D. Ascending, relapsing–remitting, pure motor, pure sensory

3. Doris is a 30-year-old admitted to your ICU with status asthmaticus. She has been taking Accolate, Allegra, and using a Proventil inhaler. Prior to her admission, Doris was coughing paroxysmally and her bronchospasms worsened so she was transported to the ED. In the ED, she received albuterol, oxygen, and epinephrine without significant improvement. On auscultation, inspiratory and expiratory wheezing with a prolonged expiratory phase is heard throughout the lung fields. She is using

accessory muscles for respiration and is tachycardic and tachypneic. She is placed on 2 L/min via NC and ABGs are drawn. Blood gas results show: pH 7.50, pO_2 96 mm Hg, pCO_2 28 mm Hg, and HCO_3 23 mEq/L. These blood gas results showed respiratory alkalosis and Doris was placed on a mask at 5 L/min. Her wheezing became less audible and her work of breathing increased. This probably indicates

A. Improvement.

B. A need to lower the O_2.

C. A need for epinephrine.

D. A worsening condition.

4. People who have emphysema develop chronic hypoxia. Which potential imbalance would be expected with this condition?

A. Hypokalemia

B. Hypochloremia

C. Decreased bicarbonate levels

D. Hyponatremia

5. Gerry was involved in an automobile accident and suffered multiple fractures and lacerations. He has been on TPN for nutritional needs. This morning he is confused and disoriented to place and time. He also exhibits orthostatic hypotension. The physician believes Gerry has HHNS. Which labs would you anticipate for a patient with HHNS?

A. Glucose 1,258, negative ketones, serum osmolality 375 mOsm/L

B. Glucose 550, positive ketones, serum osmolality 280 mOsm/L

C. Glucose 700, negative ketones, serum osmolality 270 mOsm/L

D. Glucose 600, positive ketones, serum osmolality 240 mOsm/L

6. You have just assisted with the insertion of an esophageal and gastric balloon. Tamponade therapy duration should be carefully documented because

A. Prolonged inflation may lead to necrosis or ulceration.

B. Patient comfort increases 24 hours after balloon placement.

C. Hgb and Hct should drop after balloon placement.

D. Enteral feeding may be given via the tube after 36 hours.

7. Marco was preparing his family's Sunday meal when he bumped a pan of boiling water and spilled it on his left arm. The burn on his left arm is pink and blistered. When it is touched, Marco screams with pain. This classification of burn is

A. First degree.

B. Second degree partial thickness.

C. Third degree full thickness.

D. Fourth degree full thickness.

8. Your patient was in full arrest following a root canal procedure. After a successful resuscitation, the patient has developed Ludwig's angina. This type of angina can be defined as

A. A type of painful bradycardia in which the Q-T interval is lengthened.

B. Cardiac ischemic post-code syndrome.

C. Dysrhythmia with severe pain secondary to inhalation of noxious gases.

D. An infectious process.

9. Acute post-hemorrhagic anemia develops after
   A. Rapid loss of erythrocytes.
   B. The spleen is damaged.
   C. Iron levels decrease by more than 15%.
   D. Bone marrow is damaged.

10. High blood viscosity and low oxygen tension are the cause of which of the following types of anemia?
   A. Pernicious
   B. Aplastic
   C. Sickle cell
   D. Hemolytic

11. You notice your patient's hand spasming when the automatic blood pressure cuff inflates. When you attempt a manual blood pressure measurement, the same thing happens when you inflate the cuff to just past the systolic pressure. This carpopedal spasm is indicative of
   A. Hypokalemia.
   B. Hyperphosphatemia.
   C. Hypocalcemia.
   D. Hypernatremia.

12. What is the mean arterial pressure (MAP) for a patient with a blood pressure of 95/50, and a heart rate of 85, PAP 29/14, and PAOP of 13?
   A. 65
   B. 1.9
   C. 72
   D. 3.5

13. Harold suffered a cardiac arrest at a picnic. The family did not perform CPR, and the paramedics arrived 6 minutes after the arrest occurred. The patient was found in pulseless V-tach. Defibrillation was performed and CPR was continuous during transport to the ED. The patient was transferred to the ICU because of a bed shortage in the ED. The physician initiated hypothermic measures and administered vecuronium. This medication was used to
   A. Control ventricular dysrhythmias.
   B. Prevent shivering.
   C. Stop bleeding.
   D. Prevent metabolic acidosis.

14. Normal values for pulmonary artery pressures would be:
   A. PAS 30–40 mm Hg, PAD 20–25 mm Hg, PAM 25–30 mm Hg
   B. PAS 20–30 mm Hg, PAD 4–10 mm Hg, PAM 10–15 mm Hg
   C. PAS 10–20 mm Hg, PAD 6–12 mm Hg, PAM 8–10 mm Hg
   D. PAS 5–10 mm Hg, PAD 4–8 mm Hg, PAM 6–9 mm Hg

15. You are discussing herbal remedies at work when you are approached by a family member of your patient with Alzheimer's disease who has been admitted with pneumonia. She asks if her mother would benefit from drinking Ginkgo Biloba at home once discharged because she had heard that it would decrease symptoms in early-stage Alzheimer's. You tell her:

A. "There is a lot of research, but nothing really supports its use."

B. "Sure, there are no interactions with other drugs, so she should be fine."

C. "Her doctor doesn't approve of any natural remedies, so don't tell him if you are using it."

D. "There could be very dangerous side effects if this herb is taken without consulting her physician. I will have him speak with you when he comes in."

16. Jonathan was admitted in hypertensive crisis. He has been receiving nitroprusside. As a critical care nurse, you know that when giving this medication, it is necessary to monitor for

A. Tachycardia.

B. Cyanide toxicity.

C. Retinal changes.

D. Ataxia.

17. Paula works in the fashion industry and is a cutter in the wool sweater section of her company. This morning, a fire broke out in her section. Paula did not suffer any burns, but she did inhale large quantities of smoke. What would be the most potent toxin she might have inhaled?

A. Carbon monoxide

B. Smoke

C. Inhaled nitrates

D. Cyanide

18. Your patient was stabbed during a gang fight in the right anterior chest and left shoulder area. He lost approximately 1,500 to 1,600 mL of blood. Which of the following signs and symptoms would be expected with this volume of blood loss?

A. BP decreased, pulse pressure normal, RR 20–30/min

B. BP normal, RR increased, capillary refill normal

C. RR increased, BP normal, pulse pressure normal

D. BP decreased, RR increased, CO decreased

19. Which of the following conditions would be contraindicated when scheduling a patient for a transesophageal echocardiogram (TEE)?

A. Cardiac tumors

B. Dysphagia

C. Vegetative endocarditis

D. Mitral valve regurgitation

20. What must be present for calcium to be utilized by the body?

A. Increased oral calcium

B. Increased phosphorus

C. Euthyroid state

D. Adequate vitamin D levels

21. **Which of the following statements is true about a pulmonary embolism?**
    A. Respiratory acidosis will occur.
    B. Heparin is used to dissolve clots.
    C. Normal D-dimer results can rule out a pulmonary embolism.
    D. Metabolic alkalosis will develop.

22. **Martha is now 45 years old and states she had, "some sort of reaction when she had her tonsils out at age 6." To determine whether Martha has a genetic predisposition for malignant hyperthermia, which of the following drugs might be used?**
    A. Halothane
    B. Caffeine
    C. Accolate
    D. Singulair

23. **When assessing a patient with a chest tube drainage system, which of the following statements would be correct?**
    A. Check for subcutaneous emphysema around the insertion site by auscultation.
    B. If using a Pleur-Evac with an auto-transfusion connection, make certain all clamps are open.
    C. The average chest tube size for an adult is 20 Fr.
    D. If using a chest tube drainage system with a one-way value and suction, water is required to maintain a seal.

24. **Your intubated patient has required frequent suctioning for tenacious secretion during the night. You are hesitant to irrigate with normal saline. Research has shown that use of normal saline does not thin secretions and may cause which of the following adverse effects?**
    A. Anxiety
    B. Depression
    C. Decreased mean arterial pressure
    D. Bronchodilation

25. **During a cardiac arrest, an end-tidal CO_2 device is placed on the patient's endotracheal tube. Which of the following statements is true regarding the use of capnography to verify endotracheal tube placement?**
    A. $ETCO_2$ is a moderately reliable indicator of correct tube placement.
    B. It is not necessary to auscultate lung sounds when an $ETCO_2$ device is used.
    C. Capnography is a substitute for pulse oximetry.
    D. Placement of an $ETCO_2$ device can be difficult to learn initially.

26. **Your patient with a Minnesota tube has a sudden drop in oral secretions and esophageal balloon pressures. You should**
    A. Provide oral care and check again in 2 hours.
    B. Document pressures and check again in 2 hours.
    C. Check for bleeding and notify the physician.
    D. Attempt to re-inflate the balloon to 70 mm Hg.

27. The daughters of your patient with severe biliary obstruction notice that their father has multiple scratches and excoriations all over his skin. They are concerned that their father is being abused. You explain:

    A. "Do not panic, we are not abusing him."

    B. "I understand you are concerned. Because of the high bilirubin levels, he scratches unconsciously."

    C. "He must have gotten out of the restraints."

    D. "He did it to himself as a result of ICU psychosis."

28. Susan, a 35-year-old executive, just had surgery for peritonitis related to diverticulitis. During drug reconciliation, which of the following medications should Joan continue?

    A. Advil for headaches

    B. Prednisone for bronchitis

    C. Morphine for surgical pain

    D. Verapamil for atrial fibrillation

29. Mannitol would be classified as which type of diuretic?

    A. Loop

    B. Thiazide

    C. Osmotic

    D. Potassium sparing

30. Which of the following types of cell would be considered a nongranular leukocyte?

    A. Eosinophil

    B. Neutrophil

    C. Basophil

    D. Monocyte

31. Blood component replacement therapy for DIC may include all but which of the following components?

    A. FFP

    B. Cryoprecipitate

    C. Amicar

    D. Platelets

32. Walter is a 76-year-old gentleman who was admitted for end-stage mesothelioma. Which of the following occupations would lend itself to a diagnosis of mesothelioma?

    A. Bricklayer

    B. Gardener

    C. Office manager

    D. Shipbuilder

33. Pernicious anemia results from a lack of

    A. Vitamin B_6.

    B. Vitamin A.

    C. Vitamin B_{12}.

    D. Vitamin E.

34. Ralph is an 87-year-old man who was found unconscious in his board and care. His blood sugar is 1,520, he has negative serum ketones, and his serum osmolality is 342. What do you anticipate for medical treatment of this condition?
    A. D_5 ½NS intravenous fluids 300 mL/h and an insulin drip with sliding-scale coverage
    B. Normal saline at 200 mL/h, subcutaneous insulin with sliding-scale coverage every 4 hours, and monitor potassium
    C. Intravenous fluids with normal saline in high volumes, insulin drip with sliding-scale coverage, and monitor electrolyte levels
    D. Normal saline intravenously, bicarbonate drip, and monitor electrolytes

35. Fred had a thyroidectomy yesterday for thyroid cancer. Today he is delirious, vomiting, hyperthermic, and tachycardic. It is imperative to notify the physician stat because
    A. Fred has a postoperative infection.
    B. Fred may have had a cerebrovascular accident.
    C. Fred may have thyrotoxic crisis.
    D. Fred is hypoxic and needs a tracheostomy.

36. Why are hyperglycemia and hyperlipidemia seen concurrently in diabetes mellitus?
    A. Very-low-density lipoprotein (VLDL) production increases in response to increased insulin production.
    B. Insulin resistance promotes VLDL production.
    C. Lipid breakdown is hindered by hyperinsulinemia.
    D. Increases in glucose levels cause the liver to increase lipid production.

37. What can trigger the renin–angiotensin mechanism?
    A. Aldosterone and diuretics
    B. Diuretics and decreased renal blood flow
    C. Diuretics and adrenergic blockers
    D. Increased renal blood flow and diuretics

38. Carl was admitted for diabetic ketoacidosis. His HCO_3 is 10 mEq/L. In addition to the insulin drip, you should anticipate which of the following therapies?
    A. Sodium bicarbonate drip with frequent HCO_3 levels
    B. Sodium bicarbonate bolus and repeat every 4–6 hours
    C. Increase the insulin drip to hasten the resolution of the metabolic acidosis
    D. Decrease the insulin drip as the acidosis is resolving

39. The most accurate method of measuring intracranial pressure is
    A. A subarachnoid bolt.
    B. Intraventriculosotomy.
    C. An epidural catheter.
    D. A subdural catheter.

40. Which of the cranial nerves (CN) are affected by a basilar skull fracture?
    A. I, VII, VIII
    B. I, II, III
    C. I, V, VIII
    D. II, III, VIII

41. **What are the most common causes of syndrome of inappropriate antidiuretic hormone (SIADH)?**
    A. Bronchogenic (oat cell) carcinoma, pneumonia, head injury
    B. Pneumonia, COPD, tuberculosis
    C. Brain tumors, pneumonia, polycystic kidney disease
    D. Polycystic kidney disease, cerebrovascular accident, oat-cell carcinomas

42. **Felix is an SICU patient who suffered a gunshot wound to his T11–T12 spine. Upon assessment, you find motor paralysis on the same side as the gunshot wound but loss of pain and temperature sensation on the opposite side. This is called**
    A. Grey–Turner syndrome.
    B. Cushing syndrome.
    C. Syndrome X.
    D. Brown–Sequard syndrome.

43. **Why is prednisone contraindicated in tuberculosis?**
    A. It masks the infection.
    B. It increases edema, leading to dyspnea.
    C. It decreases the effectiveness of isoniazid.
    D. It increases the effectiveness of isoniazid.

44. **In ARDS, pulmonary capillaries leak blood into the pulmonary interstitium. This phenomenon is due to:**
    A. Alveolar-oxygen gradient
    B. Colloid osmotic pressure
    C. A-a gradient
    D. Diffusion

45. **Bob is a 25-year-old construction worker who suffered a flail chest, fractured clavicle, and severely bruised hip after a fall from a roof. At first, he was ventilated using a high-frequency jet ventilator and is now on SIMV mode. Today, he is being weaned from the ventilator. About 45 minutes after the start of weaning, which change would indicate Bob might fail weaning at this time?**
    A. The minute ventilation is 7 L/min.
    B. His heart rate has increased from 86 to 108.
    C. His SpO_2 is 96.
    D. His respiratory rate has increased by 10 breaths per minute.

46. **Bob was attempting to wean from ventilator support, but failed. He was placed back on the ventilator, but was mistakenly placed on IMV instead of SIMV. He immediately started to override the ventilator and became quite anxious. ABGs were drawn before he was placed back on the correct mode. You would expect the results to show**
    A. Respiratory acidosis.
    B. Metabolic alkalosis.
    C. Respiratory alkalosis.
    D. Metabolic acidosis.

47. Connie, like many patients with flail chest, was initially placed on a high-frequency jet ventilator because
   A. It improves removal of CO_2.
   B. It increases tidal volume.
   C. It helps stabilize the chest wall.
   D. It reduces the need for humidification.

48. After 3 doses of Neupogen, your patient complains of bone pain and muscle aches. What do you tell him?
   A. These reactions are common side effects of the medication.
   B. His bone cancer has metastasized.
   C. His arthritis has flared up.
   D. He has gout.

49. Auto-PEEP
   A. Is the same as plateau pressure.
   B. Is the same as static pressure.
   C. Is a result of inadequate exhalation time.
   D. Decreases the work of breathing.

50. Which of the following would be considered a relative complication for performing a thoracentesis?
   A. Splenomegaly
   B. Coagulation disorder
   C. A previous pneumonectomy
   D. Pleural fluid protein to serum protein ratio greater than 0.5 g/dL

51. Which of the following statements is true regarding chest tube drainage systems?
   A. Drainage of frank blood in amounts greater than 100 mL/h is not significant.
   B. Drainage tubing should be placed horizontally on the bed and down to the collection chamber.
   C. All drainage tubing should be dependent to the insertion site.
   D. Chest tube drainage from a mediastinal tube should not bubble in the water seal chamber.

52. Steven is a 36-year-old patient originally admitted for a fractured femur and to rule out a coronary contusion following a skiing accident. While you are giving Steven his discharge teaching, he suddenly complains of pain in his left chest. He immediately becomes tachypneic and tachycardic. When you lay Steven back down in the bed, you note asymmetrical chest wall excursion and neck vein distention. He has absent breath sounds on the left side and his heart sounds are muffled. Steven rapidly becomes dyspneic and cyanotic. Steven's condition is likely due to
   A. Tension pneumothorax.
   B. Cardiac tamponade.
   C. Pulmonary embolism.
   D. Esophageal rupture.

53. Nursing actions that should be performed prior to initiating pronation therapy would include
    A. Secure EKG leads on the anterior chest with tape.
    B. Note the amount of all drainage for colostomies and ileostomies.
    C. Utilize capnography monitoring.
    D. Document existing drainage on any wound dressings.

54. A SpO$_2$ value of 94% correlates with which of the following PaO$_2$ values?
    A. 95
    B. 70
    C. 94
    D. 80

55. Subcutaneous emphysema usually occurs in the area of the
    A. Head.
    B. Neck.
    C. Thorax.
    D. Abdomen.

56. Pulse oximetry has not been shown to be affected by
    A. Dark skin.
    B. Elevated bilirubin.
    C. Dark nail polish.
    D. Presence of hemoglobin.

57. Your patient had a pulmonary artery catheter placed to closely monitor fluid status. The physician ordered PAWP pressures q 8 hours. You obtain the initial readings on your shift. The next afternoon, when you attempt another wedge pressure, you notice decreased resistance to the syringe. Which of the following complications may have occurred?
    A. Syringe malfunction
    B. Embolization
    C. Balloon rupture
    D. This is an expected finding.

58. Gertrude, age 76, is admitted to your unit with tachycardia (146), RR 34, BP 90/60, T 96.4°F. Her white count is 16,000. Gertrude states she was treated for a "kidney infection" 2 weeks ago. She denies pain at this time. Gertrude probably has
    A. MODS.
    B. A kidney stone.
    C. SIRS.
    D. Appendicitis.

59. Mr. M. was participating in a tailgate party when a barbeque flared up as he was walking by. He received partial-thickness burns of his neck, upper chest, and left shoulder. He has soot around his mouth and nose. He is now becoming more restless, and his blood pressure is 94/60. Which treatment would be most appropriate for Mr. M. at this time?

A. Fluid resuscitation at a rate of 300 cc/h

B. Monitor pulse oximetry continuously

C. Intubation and place on FiO_2 100%

D. Antibiotic therapy

60. A 36-year-old male was pumping gas when a spark ignited the fumes. He suffered full-thickness burns of the right arm. During your initial assessment, you note that eschar is present and the right radial pulse is not palpable. A Doppler pulse is also not discernible. Which of the following actions would be appropriate at this time?

A. Move the patient's arm away from his torso and elevate it on a pillow.

B. Escharotomy

C. Morphine 4 mg IV

D. Ice packs to reduce swelling

61. Your patient has burns on the right lower leg that are circumferential (all the way around the leg). What is a potential risk with this type of burn?

A. Infection into the bone

B. Difficulty removing dead tissue

C. Compartment syndrome

D. Escharotomy

62. Initially, a burned area is estimated by the Rule of Nines, or using the palm to represent 1% of the body surface area. There are many ways to calculate the body surface area involved in a burn. If your patient was burned over 40% of his body and weighs 75 kg, calculate his total fluid requirements during the first 24 hours using the Parkland formula.

A. 12,000 mL

B. 6,300 mL

C. 14,500 mL

D. 8,400 mL

63. When using the Parkland formula, the preferred fluid for burn resuscitation is

A. Normal saline.

B. D_5/Isolyte M.

C. Lactated Ringer's.

D. D_5W.

64. Parker is preparing to go home after treatment with antivenin for a black widow spider bite. Which of the following discharge instructions is correct?

A. You may experience muscle spasms for only a few days.

B. You may experience tingling and weakness for 5 years or more.

C. It is normal to have a rash or fever in the next 3 days.

D. Contact your physician immediately if you experience joint or abdominal pain or begin to have trouble breathing.

65. Harold is a 62-year-old male who has become septic following a TURP 1 week ago. During his course of treatment, he is prescribed naloxone. The purpose of the naloxone is
    A. To block prostaglandins.
    B. To stabilize the cell membrane.
    C. To block endorphins.
    D. To block histamine.

66. A nursing consideration with administration of norepinephrine (Levophed) would be
    A. To not administer it with alkaline solutions.
    B. To not administer it for low coronary artery perfusion states.
    C. It is not indicated for vasogenic shock.
    D. To not use it for hypotensive states.

67. Your patient was admitted for malaise, severe dyspnea, and he had a syncopal episode at work. The patient states he has a midline burning sensation in his chest that worsens when he is supine. You suspect
    A. A pleural effusion.
    B. Pericardial tamponade.
    C. GERD.
    D. Myocarditis.

68. Which of the following hemodynamic changes will occur with a cardiac tamponade?
    A. Increased cardiac output
    B. Decreased stroke volume
    C. Increased contractility
    D. Decreased heart rate

69. With regard to stable angina, which of the following statements is true?
    A. A positive treadmill test will indicate CAD.
    B. A thallium test will not diagnose LV dysfunction.
    C. The treadmill test may miss up to 20% of cases of single-vessel disease.
    D. CK-MB isoenzymes and troponins will not increase.

70. If the inferior wall of the heart is infarcted, the leads that will most directly reflect the injury are
    A. II, III, and aVF.
    B. I and aVL.
    C. V_1–V_2.
    D. V_5–V_6.

71. Stimulation of the vasomotor center in the medulla occurs when the partial pressure of oxygen changes. This is initiated by
    A. Baroreceptors.
    B. Chemoreceptors.
    C. The Purkinge system.
    D. Bainbridge reflex.

72. **Potential complications with use of an intra-aortic balloon pump (IABP) include**
    A. Decreased cardiac output.
    B. Gangrene of the lower extremity.
    C. A ruptured papillary muscle.
    D. Preoperative use prior to CABG.

73. **The drug of choice to treat AV nodal and atrioventricular re-entrant arrhythmias is**
    A. Amiodarone.
    B. Clonidine.
    C. Quinidine.
    D. Adenosine.

74. **An example of a systolic murmur would be**
    A. Tricuspid stenosis.
    B. Tricuspid insufficiency.
    C. Mitral stenosis.
    D. Pulmonic insufficiency.

75. **Francis was admitted for increased exercise intolerance, severe edema, and dyspnea at rest. A pulmonary artery catheter was placed and the following pressures were obtained: RAP = 18, PA = 62/30, RV = 66/26, PAOP = 14. You would suspect**
    A. Cardiac tamponade.
    B. Congestive heart failure.
    C. Pulmonary embolus.
    D. Pulmonary hypertension.

76. **Postrenal AKI may be caused by**
    A. Malignant hypertension.
    B. Transplant rejection.
    C. Neurogenic bladder.
    D. DIC, preeclampsia.

77. **A renal transplant that results from humoral rejection or acute cellular rejection may be definitively diagnosed only via**
    A. Ultrasound.
    B. Nuclear scan.
    C. Doppler scan.
    D. Renal biopsy.

78. **Nephrotoxity may be caused by**
    A. Furosemide.
    B. Aspirin.
    C. Irbesartan.
    D. Acyclovir.

79. **Medications that can decrease BUN levels include**
    A. Neomycin and rifampin.
    B. Chloral hydrate and furosemide.
    C. Bacitracin and gentamycin.
    D. Chloramphenicol and streptomycin.

80. Peter, a 63-year-old store clerk, is admitted to the intensive care unit for cocaine intoxication. He begins to complain of severe epigastric pain. His lab results are as follows:

    WBC 18.2 with 77% neutrophils

    Hematocrit 38%

    LDH 341

    Platelets 226

    BUN 7

    Creatinine 1.0

    Urine analysis shows traces of proteins, few RBCs, and positive urine toxicology for cocaine. What could cause Peter's pain?
    A. Peptic ulcer disease
    B. Renal infarction
    C. Gastroenteritis
    D. Infarcted mesenteric artery

81. Beatrice is a 60-year-old diabetic with congestive heart failure. After 4 days of no contact, her daughter went to her home, where she found Beatrice in bed, unresponsive. Beatrice has a red, dry swollen tongue, a temperature of 102°F, and flushed dry skin. She is tachycardic, hypotensive, with decreased reflexes. Her urine specific gravity is 1.050. You suspect
    A. Hypernatremia.
    B. Hypocalcemia.
    C. Hypermagnemesia.
    D. Hypokalemia.

82. Hypokalemia may cause
    A. Respiratory alkalosis only.
    B. Metabolic alkalosis only.
    C. Both respiratory and metabolic alkalosis.
    D. Metabolic acidosis only.

83. In Addison's disease, what influences the potassium level?
    A. Hyperkalemia related to the decrease in aldosterone secretion
    B. Hyperkalemia related to the increase in aldosterone secretion
    C. Hypokalemia related to the decrease in aldosterone secretion
    D. Hypocalcemia related to the increase in aldosterone secretion

84. Your patient was admitted and treated for polymorphic ventricular tachycardia. This rhythm was presumed to have been caused by a low magnesium level. The patient was found to have an underlying rhythm of atrial fibrillation, which required placement of an internal pacemaker. The patient asks about the types of food he could prepare that are rich in magnesium. Which of the following foods is low in (a poor source of) magnesium?
    A. Honey
    B. Broccoli
    C. Almonds
    D. Chocolate

85. **Your patient has a history of transphenoidal hypophysectomy. Which procedure is absolutely contraindicated?**
    A. Nasal placement of a gastric tube
    B. Oral placement of a gastric tube
    C. Oral intubation with an endotracheal tube
    D. Tracheal intubation

86. **The family members of your 48-year-old patient with chronic liver failure ask what they can do to make him more comfortable. You tell them that they can**
    A. Provide deep tissue massage every 2 hours.
    B. Apply a moisturizing lotion when visiting.
    C. Assist with rapid range-of-motion exercises every 4 hours.
    D. Limit visitation to once a day.

87. **Your 19-year-old patient is post MVA with blunt abdominal trauma related to the seat belt placement. He begins complaining of severe abdominal pain around the epigastric area, stating that the pain is knife-like and twisting. You also note a low-grade fever with diaphoresis, abdominal distention, decreased bowel tones, and rebound tenderness. You suspect**
    A. Pancreatitis.
    B. Acute liver failure.
    C. Gastrointestinal bleeding.
    D. Abdominal bruising.

88. **Bill, a 58-year-old construction worker with cirrhosis, was admitted yesterday after attending a weekend party with alcohol, drugs, and smoking. His A.M. labs were as follows:**
    ALT 250 U/L
    AST 150 U/L
    Bilirubin 10 mg/dL
    PT 23 sec
    PLT 76 × 10³/mm³
    Hgb 8.2 g/dL
    Hct 32%

    These findings would indicate a high risk for
    A. Peptic ulcer disease.
    B. Variceal bleeding.
    C. Gastritis.
    D. Boerhaave's syndrome.

89. **Mr. H. had abdominal surgery for perforation yesterday. Today's abdominal X rays show a double-bubble appearance. Mr. H. is complaining of nausea and has bile-stained emesis, abdominal distention, pain, and fever. You should**
    A. Contact the surgeon and prepare for immediate surgery.
    B. Administer morphine and Tylenol, then call the physician if there is no improvement.
    C. Position the patient flat and give him Tylenol.
    D. This is normal. The physician should be notified only if the abdomen becomes discolored.

90. Your patient just returned from abdominal surgery. Two hours later, you note decreased urine output, increased CVP, increased PAP, increased SVR, and decreased cardiac output. In addition, the ventilator continuously alarms low volume despite intact circuits. Based on these findings, you would expect which intra-abdominal pressure value?

    A. 5 mm Hg
    B. 15 mm Hg
    C. 25 mm Hg
    D. 50 mm Hg

91. Helen, a 26-year-old mother of 6, is 7 months pregnant and admitted to your unit for severe HELLP syndrome. She is also at risk for

    A. Intra-abdominal hypertension (IAH) and abdominal compartment syndrome (ACS).
    B. Decreased intracranial pressure (ICP).
    C. Hypocarbia.
    D. Increased platelets.

92. Joab, a 40-year-old Orthodox Jew, presents with an unintentional weight loss of 20 pounds, fatigue, anorexia, and chronic, watery diarrhea with bloody mucus. He is tachycardic, tachypneic, and hyperthermic. His Hgb is 7 g/dL and his Hct is 21%. You suspect

    A. Colonic diverticulitis.
    B. Ulcerative colitis.
    C. Pancreatitis.
    D. Cholecystitis.

93. Sam, a 60-year-old computer programmer, was hospitalized for a myocardial infarction with emergency cardiopulmonary artery bypass graft surgery yesterday. He has been having recurrent uncontrolled atrial fibrillation intermittently for the last 10 hours. This evening he complains of abdominal pain with distention, intolerance for soft diet with nausea and vomiting, and fever. The physician orders a plain film of the abdomen. Which of the following results would you expect to see?

    A. Air in the biliary tree with signs of small bowel obstruction and calculus in pelvis
    B. Dilated small bowel loops and air–fluid levels
    C. Dilation of the entire bowel including the stomach, "thumb printing," and pneumatosis intestinalis
    D. Air under the diaphragm on the right upper chest or over the right lobe of the liver

94. Management of pain may be challenging in the bariatric patient. Management with opioids via a patient-controlled analgesia (PCA) pump is necessary to do all of the following *except*

    A. Prevent pulmonary emboli.
    B. Early mobility.
    C. Prevent atelectasis.
    D. Early transition to oral pain medications.

95. **An indication for the use of PEEP would be**
    A. To reduce mediastinal bleeding post CABG.
    B. To help assess mean arterial pressure.
    C. To increase surfactant.
    D. To help reduce FiO_2.

96. **Multiple organ dysfunction syndrome (MODS) may be directly caused by**
    A. Venous thrombosis.
    B. Shunting.
    C. Oral estrogen therapy.
    D. Pulmonary embolism.

97. **Your patient has a confirmed flail chest. Which alteration in acid–base balance would you expect?**
    A. Metabolic alkalosis
    B. Metabolic acidosis
    C. Respiratory acidosis
    D. Respiratory alkalosis

98. **Seymour is a 64-year-old male with a significant history of COPD. He started smoking when he was 5 years old and up until this admission he continued to smoke as many as 5 packs of cigarettes per day. In addition, he has uncontrolled diabetes and peripheral vascular disease. Three days ago, Seymour had a major stroke when he was walking down the stairs. He suffered a broken pelvis, fractured right ulna, and fractured right patella. He has been comatose since his admission, with a flat-line EEG study. His wife has agreed that do not resuscitate (DNR) orders are appropriate; she has also agreed to ventilatory support. His physician recommends that Seymour receive morphine as a comfort measure during this process. Seymour's wife has been informed that the morphine will make him more comfortable, but may decrease his ability to ventilate and, in fact, may hasten his demise. This type of ethical dilemma is known as**
    A. A null ethical principle.
    B. Double effect.
    C. Slippery slope.
    D. Palliative principle.

99. **Sinusitis and ventilator-acquired pneumonia (VAP) pose many challenges for the critical care nurse. Which statement is true regarding these conditions?**
    A. Good hand washing technique is an effective way to reduce the incidence of VAP.
    B. Sinusitis can be prevented by using a smaller-diameter endotracheal tube.
    C. Nasogastric tubes are preferred to orogastric tubes.
    D. Oral tubes are associated with a higher incidence of sinusitis.

100. Analyze the following arterial blood gas results. Use the provided space to the right side to assist in interpretation by writing acidosis, alkalosis, compensated, or uncompensated. You may also use scrap paper.

pH 7.30

CO_2 61

HCO_3 25

  A. Uncompensated metabolic alkalosis
  B. Compensated respiratory acidosis
  C. Compensated metabolic acidosis
  D. Uncompensated respiratory acidosis

101. Your patient has the following parameters:

HR 95

BP 110/70

SV 50

BSA 1.9 m^2

Use the space provided to calculate the cardiac index (CI) for this patient:

  A. 4.95 L/min/m^2
  B. 55 L/min/m^2
  C. 2.5 L/min/m^2
  D. 30 L/min/m^2

102. Normal cerebral blood flow (CBF) averages

  A. 25 to 50 mmHg.
  B. 50 ml/100 g of brain tissue per minute.
  C. About 10 mmHg higher than metabolic demand.
  D. Less than 10 ml/50 g/min.

103. If your patient had a cardiac tamponade, which of the following findings would you expect on a chest X ray?

  A. A dilated superior vena cava
  B. Increased JVD
  C. Narrowed mediastinum
  D. Delineation of the pericardium and epicardium

104. An anterior wall infarction may be seen in leads

  A. V_4 R.
  B. V_5–V_6.
  C. V_7–V_9.
  D. V_2–V_4.

105. Alpha-adrenergic effects of norepinephrine include

  A. Increased force of myocardial contraction.
  B. Increased SA node firing.
  C. Increased AV conduction time.
  D. Peripheral arteriolar vasoconstriction.

106. **NSAIDs are contraindicated in the treatment of patients with heart failure because they**
    A. Decrease myocardial contractility.
    B. Cause atrial fibrillation in patients with heart failure.
    C. Promote fluid retention.
    D. May cause hypocalcemia.

107. **Contraindications for use of an intra-aortic balloon pump (IABP) would include**
    A. Cardiogenic shock.
    B. Aortic valve regurgitation.
    C. Left ventricular failure.
    D. Unstable angina.

108. **Calcium-channel blockers act primarily on**
    A. Reduction of cardiac output.
    B. Arteries to arterioles.
    C. Lung receptors only.
    D. Venules to veins.

109. **An example of a pansystolic murmur is**
    A. Pulmonic insufficiency.
    B. Tricuspid insufficiency.
    C. Atrial stenosis.
    D. Mitral stenosis.

110. **Norman is a 45-year-old steel worker who was admitted for acute dyspnea and chest pain. A pulmonary artery catheter was placed and the following readings were obtained: RAP = 16, RV = 68/26, PA = 68/34, PAOP = 24. The most probable diagnosis is**
    A. Congestive heart failure.
    B. Restrictive pericarditis.
    C. Pulmonary embolus.
    D. Pulmonary hypertension.

111. **If the international normalized ratio (INR) is above 5.0, the patient is at significant risk of bleeding. A drug that can cause a significant rise in the INR is**
    A. Ethacrinic acid.
    B. Penicillin.
    C. Amiodarone.
    D. A statin.

112. **Darlene was admitted 3 days ago for management of deep vein thrombosis. During your initial assessment this morning, you found her sitting on the side of the bed leaning forward. Darlene states that this position relieved her newly developed chest pain. She also states that the pain is worse on inspiration. You notify the physician, who orders a CXR and lab work. The sed rate and WBCs are elevated. Darlene most likely has**
    A. Pericarditis.
    B. A thoracic aneurysm.
    C. A pulmonary embolus.
    D. Pulmonary edema.

113. **Wellen's syndrome**
    A. Is the same as Prinzmetal's angina.
    B. Occurs with proximal stenosis of the LAD.
    C. Is called crescendo angina.
    D. Is variant angina.

114. **Leon is experiencing delirium tremens. Nursing interventions include keeping the room well lit and minimizing stimulation. Staff members continuously reorient Leon to time, place, and person. Haldol has been given as ordered, and the patient is in four-point restraints. Which of these interventions should be discontinued?**
    A. Reorientation
    B. Medication administration
    C. Restraints
    D. Controlling stimulation

115. **Brody is a 46-year-old male who was admitted to the ICU following a bar-room brawl during which he suffered multiple stab wounds. He is angry and verbally assaultive with the staff. The goal of anger management for this patient is to do all of the following *except***
    A. Confront him directly with whatever made him angry.
    B. Discuss what in the situation made him angry.
    C. Discuss with Brody alternative and positive ways to express his feelings.
    D. Decide on positive ways for Brody to express his feelings when confronted with frustrating situations in the future.

116. **Martha is the lone survivor of a car crash that killed her parents and 2 siblings. She is recovering from a pneumothorax, hemothorax, and bilateral broken legs. Martha has been extremely depressed and withdrawn. You are discussing medications, psychiatric therapy, and the increased risk of suicide and suicidal behavior with Martha's distant relatives. The family makes each of the following statements. Which of them is false?**
    A. "If Martha is considering suicide, she will make statements or give warnings of suicide."
    B. "We should trust our instincts if we feel Martha is in danger."
    C. "As she recovers from her depression, Martha is at greater risk of suicide."
    D. "If she talks about suicide or asks about pills, then Martha is just voicing the thought and will not attempt suicide."

117. **Amy is the sole survivor of a crash that killed her immediate family. While recovering from massive injuries, her behavior and moods change rapidly. Which of the following behaviors is most concerning and indicates suicidal behavior?**
    A. Drug seeking with multiple requests for pain medications and sedatives
    B. Withdrawal from conversation and other types of interaction
    C. Crying and statements of helplessness
    D. Screaming at her distant relatives

118. Timothy, a 56-year-old father of 6, has suffered a heart attack and requires an immediate coronary artery bypass graft. His children and wife are present as well as other family and church members. You overhear his wife and children speaking about complete insurance coverage; they state that Timothy's employer has approved significant sick level time for his recovery and has offered the ability to work from home if additional recuperation time is required. You are determining the level of psychiatric distress in this family. Your first priority is to
    A. Administer psychotropic medications.
    B. Examine the range and effectiveness of their coping mechanisms.
    C. Work with any available family members, friends, or religious support systems.
    D. Determine if there is a crisis.

119. Factors that may affect results of urine morphine levels include all the following *except*
    A. Poppy seed ingestion may produce false-positive results.
    B. 10 mg MS IV may remain detectable in urine for as long as 84 hours.
    C. Use of a stealth adulterant will cause negative results in a positive sample.
    D. High levels of lymphocytes will mask morphine in urine.

120. Your patient was admitted for severe flank pain and hematuria. He is scheduled for a kidney biopsy. Your patient and family teaching should include
    A. Report any pain in the flank or abdomen post-procedure.
    B. A small kidney stone may be passed after the procedure.
    C. The patient will be on bed rest for 24 hours.
    D. No teaching is necessary.

121. Acetaminophen overdose may take as long as 2 weeks to resolve. From 72 to 96 hours from ingestion, symptoms will include
    A. Pallor, lethargy, metabolic acidosis.
    B. Increased renal function.
    C. Right upper quadrant pain, increased serum hepatic enzymes.
    D. Jaundice, confusion, coagulation disorders.

122. If your patient was in the early stage of septic shock, you would expect which of the following hemodynamic parameters?
    A. SVR elevated, PAOP elevated, CO decreased
    B. CO decreased, RAP elevated, PAOP elevated
    C. RAP elevated, SVR decreased, PAOP increased
    D. CO increased, PAOP decreased, SVR decreased

123. Your patient is being evaluated for multiple organ dysfunction syndrome. Which of the following is an acronym for an outcome predictor score for MODS?
    A. SOFA
    B. TEARDROP
    C. CRIPE
    D. COOK

124. Calculate the fluid requirements (first 24 hours) for a patient who weighs 65 kg and is burned over 45% of his body using the Parkland formula:
    A. 29,250 mL
    B. 11,700 mL
    C. 26,000 mL
    D. 10,300 mL

125. You are treating Sid, a patient with long QT syndrome. Which of the following herbs should he avoid?
    A. Ginseng
    B. Ginkgo Biloba
    C. Marijuana
    D. Oregano

126. Jose is an alcoholic admitted to your unit with cirrhosis. Why is thiamine added to his IV fluids?
    A. Thiamine is a sedative and will ease agitation.
    B. Thiamine decreases the symptoms of DTs.
    C. Thiamine is used to prevent the damage to the brain as a result of Wernicke's syndrome.
    D. Thiamine is used to prevent complications of substance abuse.

127. Floyd was a spectator at a tennis tournament when he was struck by lightning. He was thrown about 10 feet into another set of seats. Floyd suffered a fractured left tibia, a concussion, and burns on his left arm, chest, and right leg. He has been somewhat confused since the accident. Which of the following statements about lightning injuries is true?
    A. Internal burns are common.
    B. Barotrauma is rare.
    C. Myoglobinuria is rarely seen.
    D. DC current will most likely cause ventricular fibrillation.

128. You are helping to evaluate victims of a bus accident. Your patient is a 20-year-old female who was trapped in her car for almost 2 hours by the steering column. She complains of left shoulder pain, left upper quadrant rebound tenderness, and she presents with an obviously fractured lower leg that was splinted by paramedics. The paramedics had listed her as stable and stated that she had no rebound tenderness or guarding at the accident scene. She is tachycardic at 116 and has fractures of ribs 9 and 10. You suspect
    A. A ruptured pancreas.
    B. Diaphragm rupture.
    C. A spleen injury.
    D. A lacerated liver.

129. Fred, an 18-year-old college student, was injured while skateboarding and has a T 8 spinal cord injury. He has been diagnosed with spinal shock. The critical care nurse knows the symptoms of spinal shock include

A. Areflexia, autonomic dysfunction, loss of sensation, and eliminatory dysfunction.

B. Areflexia, peripheral vasodilatation, decreased SVR, and loss of sensation.

C. Areflexia, heightened sensation, and cardiovascular shock.

D. Areflexia, bowel and bladder dysfunction, and bradycardia.

130. **Nursing management of a patient with a cerebral aneurysm includes**

A. Ambulation and monitoring of vital and neurologic signs.

B. Glasgow Coma Scale assessments and monitoring for cerebral vascular spasm.

C. Maintaining normal intracranial pressure.

D. Maintaining systolic blood pressure less than 120 mm Hg.

131. **The most accurate method of measuring intracranial pressure is**

A. A subarachnoid bolt.

B. Intraventriculosotomy.

C. An epidural catheter.

D. A subdural catheter.

132. **In the critical care setting, patients with DIC are at a high risk of developing**

A. Deficiencies in vitamin K and folate.

B. Increased fibrinogen levels.

C. A decreased D-dimer (less than 300).

D. Dependency on heparin to maintain hemostasis.

133. **Possible causes of thrombocytopenia in critical care could include**

A. Portal hypertension.

B. MI.

C. Latex.

D. Low-protein diet.

134. **Quincy had a renal transplant about 1 year ago. He was admitted to your unit for severe flu-like symptoms. Which sign or symptom would lead you to suspect that Quincy is having an acute rejection episode?**

A. Pelvic pain

B. Hypotension

C. Increased urine output

D. Decreased urine osmolality

135. **Following heart–lung transplants, prostaglandin (PGE$_1$) is used to**

A. Provide inotropic support.

B. Augment the heart rate.

C. Promote pulmonary vasodilation.

D. Promote wound healing.

136. **Jon, a 41-year-old Type 2 diabetic, is admitted to the intensive care unit for acute coronary syndrome (ACS). He is NPO for angiography. Jon calls you, stating that he feels funny. You find him pale, diaphoretic, anxious, and restless. What is your next step?**

A. Check vital signs and temperature.

B. Check vital signs, repeat cardiac enzymes, and stat EKG.

C. Check vital signs and blood sugar.

D. Check vital signs and pulse oximetry reading.

137. Frank has arterial blood gases drawn. Which of the following results would you expect to see with diabetic ketoacidosis?
    A. pH 7.55; CO_2 22 mm Hg; HCO_3 26 mEq/L
    B. pH 7.36; CO_2 54 mm Hg; HCO_3 33 mEq/L
    C. pH 7.15; CO_2 24 mm Hg; HCO_3 12 mEq/l
    D. pH 7.40; CO_2 41 mm Hg; HCO_3 25 mEq/L

138. Mrs. R. is admitted to the intensive care unit with myxedema coma. She is receiving intravenous thyroid replacement therapy when she suddenly develops hypotension, hypoglycemia, nausea, and vomiting. What has happened?
    A. Mrs. R. has had an allergic response to the thyroid medication.
    B. Mrs. R. needs an increased dose of thyroid medication.
    C. Mrs. R. needs a lower dose of thyroid medication.
    D. Mrs. R. is experiencing Addisonian crisis.

139. George is admitted to the intensive care unit in hypertensive crisis. You notice large fluctuations in his blood pressure even though you have not changed his nitroprusside drip. The physician orders a plasma catecholamine level. George's fractional epinephrine level is very high. What does this finding indicate?
    A. Cocaine use
    B. Pheochromocytoma
    C. Adrenal cortex tumor
    D. Hyperthyroidism

140. What is the most common presentation of a patient with syndrome of inappropriate antidiuretic hormone (SIADH)?
    A. Excessive, dilute urine output
    B. Hypotension
    C. Seizures
    D. Tetany

141. David is a 60-year-old male admitted to the intensive care unit for an acute myocardial infarction. He has a schizoaffective disorder for which he has taken lithium for 15 years. You note that David has a very high urine output—approximately 800 cc/h and a SpG of 1.001. What is wrong?
    A. David is experiencing the diuretic effect of a low-sodium diet.
    B. David has diabetes insipidus from long-term lithium use.
    C. David has excessive oral fluid intake.
    D. David has neurogenic diabetes insipidus.

142. Frank is admitted to the intensive care unit for diabetic ketoacidosis. As his nurse, you know his insulin drip will be titrated based on a sliding scale and the patient's anion gap. What does the anion gap measure?
    A. An estimate of cations and anions
    B. An estimate of unmeasured anions
    C. An estimate of anions in the blood
    D. An estimate of the correction of the acid–base balance

143. **Which of the following leads is best for monitoring for a RBBB?**
    A. Lead II
    B. Lead I
    C. Lead V_1
    D. Lead V_6

144. **A patient is at high risk for ventricular septal defect or rupture or even a ventricular aneurysm if an infarct occurs in the**
    A. Left anterior descending artery.
    B. Left main coronary artery.
    C. Left circumflex artery.
    D. Right coronary artery.

145. **Increased afterload would be seen with**
    A. Polycythemia.
    B. Aortic insufficiency.
    C. Hypovolemia.
    D. Sepsis.

146. **A sign of necrosis on an EKG would include**
    A. Acute ST elevation.
    B. A right BBB.
    C. A left BBB.
    D. A Q wave in Lead III.

147. **The physician has just informed your patient that she needs an LVAD. The patient is crying and says, "I just know I am going to die. What's the point? It must be my time." The patient is obviously quite stressed. The priority for the nurse at this time is to**
    A. Tell the patient she will not die.
    B. Explore possible suicidal ideation.
    C. Immediately place the patient in a single room.
    D. Notify the hospital's spiritual advisor.

148. **Your patient was admitted for pneumonia. He is 2 years post heart transplant. When you place the EKG monitoring leads, you note sinus tachycardia with PVCs and a 2-mm ST elevation. The patient denies pain. This finding is**
    A. Impossible.
    B. Normal.
    C. Indicative of a RBBB.
    D. Indicative of an inferior MI.

149. **Terrance had a pulmonary artery catheter placed. When a wedge pressure was initially obtained, large V waves were noted and the PAOP was 27. The probable cause of this reading is**
    A. A ventricular septal defect.
    B. Left heart failure.
    C. Papillary muscle rupture.
    D. Right heart failure.

150. The most common infection in patients with a ventricular assist device (VAD) is
   A. Septicemia.
   B. Pericarditis.
   C. Pneumonia.
   D. Pericardial effusion.

Congratulations! You have completed the practice examination. Keep reviewing the questions in the book and learn the rationale. Please contact us if you have any questions.

ADULT CCRN PRACTICE EXAMINATION ANSWERS

1. **Correct Answer: C**
Michael probably has Dressler's post infarction syndrome, a delayed form of acute pericarditis. The symptoms can appear from approximately a week to several months after an MI. The cause is suspected to be an immunologic response to necrotic myocardial tissue. Other symptoms may include a pericardial friction rub and a pleural effusion. The symptoms may be treated with steroids.

2. **Correct Answer: B**
Gloria is probably suffering from the descending form of this disease. The progression downward is rapid, so as the critical care nurse, you must be aware that the patient may need rapid-sequence intubation.
   Ascending, descending, Miller–Fischer variant, and pure motor are the 4 types of Guillain-Barré syndrome:
   - Ascending is the classic form; it is characterized by weakness and numbness that starts in the legs and moves up the trunk to involve the cranial nerves in some patients. The weakness is symmetrical.
   - The descending form of Guillain-Barré syndrome affects the cranial nerves first and the weakness progresses downward, toward the feet. Respiratory failure is a major problem for these patients.
   - Miller–Fisher variant is a very rare form of Guillain-Barré syndrome. It is characterized by a triad of symptoms that includes ophthalmoplegia, areflexia, and pronounced ataxia.
   - The pure motor form of Guillain-Barré syndrome is identical to the ascending form but there is limited sensory involvement and, therefore, no pain.

3. **Correct Answer: D**
Doris' condition is not improving. As air becomes trapped in the alveoli and excessive mucous is produced, the patient struggles to breathe and becomes exhausted. When the wheezing diminishes or stops altogether, it means air is not able to pass through an opening. This is a medical emergency, and the patient may need to be intubated. There is a lot of controversy about intubating patients with asthma, because it may cause barotrauma, hyperinflation and cardiac compromise.

4. **Correct Answer: B**
Chronic hypoxia leads to chronic respiratory acidosis. The kidneys retain bicarbonate in the form of sodium bicarbonate, which is then exchanged for sodium chloride. Ammonia is an acid, and excess amounts must be removed from the body. This is done by releasing ammonium chloride. In chronic hypoxia, there is an increase in bicarbonate levels and a decrease in chloride levels. Other causes of hypochloremia include NG suction, vomiting, and diarrhea.

5. **Correct Answer: A**
Blood sugars over 600 with negative serum ketones and a serum osmolality greater than 310 are typical of hyperglycemic, hyperosmolar, nonketotic syndrome (HHNS). The pH is usually greater than 7.3 and the blood urea nitrogen (BUN) may be elevated. Osmolality is the best predictor of survivability than the blood sugar levels.

6. **Correct Answer: A**

Maximum therapy time is 24 to 36 hours for esophageal balloons and 48 to 72 hours for gastric balloons related to increased risk for necrosis, ulceration, erosion of skin around the nares, airway obstruction, and aspiration of gastric or oropharyngeal contents. Patient comfort decreases over time and the risk of erosion to the mucosal lining increases. Hgb and Hct should increase or stabilize with cessation of bleeding and blood replacement. The patient's gastrointestinal lining may be inflamed related to blood in the system, and feedings should be held until bleeding is stopped.

7. **Correct Answer: B**

This type of burn may be superficial or a deep partial-thickness burn. The nerve endings are still intact, and this type of burn is very painful.

Sometimes burns can be deceptive. A reddened area may be diagnosed as a first-degree burn but then overlooked when requirements for fluid and nutrient resuscitation are calculated. After a few hours, these areas can develop blisters, and are only then recognized as dermal burns. A new way of assessing burn levels is by using a laser Doppler during the first week of treatment.

Assessing a burn depth can be tricky. The first thing to do is determine the factors that caused the burn (chemical, electrical, or thermal), the length of time for which the causative mechanism was in contact with the area, blood flow, and location of the burn. Another thing to consider is the thickness of the skin at the site. Elderly people and children have thinner skin, so burns in these populations tend to be more severe. Burns on the eyelids and genital area are about 1 mm thick, whereas burns on the palms and soles of the feet are on areas about 5 mm thick. Although the thicker skin offers a bit more thermal protection, the palms and soles of the feet become infected more easily.

8. **Correct Answer: B**

Ludwig's angina is a submaxillary infection. It is a cellulitis of the neck and floor of the mouth that usually occurs with, or after, dental disease.

9. **Correct Answer: A**

This type of anemia may be the result of hemorrhage, a cancerous lesion, an ulcerative lesion that erodes an arterial wall, trauma to a major vessel, or rupture of an aneurysm. After hemorrhage, plasma is lost and vasoconstriction takes place. The concentration of erythrocytes is increased because the volume is low. In other words, the amount of cells is not diluted in the usual amount of fluid, so the count is artificially high. It can take as long as 6 weeks for hemoglobin levels to return to normal.

10. **Correct Answer: C**

Sickle cell anemia occurs primarily in the African American population. Affected individuals are homozygous for HgS and have more HgS than HgA. This causes some of the cells to form a "sickle" shape—curved with rough edges. A crisis can occur when the low oxygen tension (postulated) causes a proliferation of these cells. The sharp edges of these cells travel through the microcirculation and damage capillaries. Even a simple thing like cold weather can precipitate massive sickling. Other identified risk factors include dehydration, vomiting, diarrhea, high altitude, excessive exercise, and stress. When the sickled cells break apart, they occlude the microcirculation and lower oxygen tension, which initiates more sickling. A crisis is a very painful time for the patient, and pain management and fluids are very important.

11. **Correct Answer: C**
This procedure elicits Trousseau's sign, an indication of hypocalcemia. You can also elicit this response by having the patient hyperventilate. When the patient becomes alkalotic, the serum calcium level decreases and a carpopedal spasm occurs.

12. **Correct Answer: A**
The MAP is a mean pressure that takes into account that the diastolic phase of the cardiac cycle comprises two-thirds of the cycle. The formula for the MAP is

$$MAP = 2(DBP) \times (SBP)/3$$

If you took the average of the 2 pressures, it would not account for the importance of the diastolic phase. The heart rate does not enter into this calculation. Patients should maintain a MAP of at least 60 to ensure adequate perfusion to the brain and kidneys.

13. **Correct Answer: B**
Vecuronium is a paralytic and will prevent shivering. If the patient shivers, the temperature will rise.

14. **Correct Answer: B**
Answer B represents the normal range of values.

15. **Correct Answer: D**
Although natural, herbal supplements and herbal use are not regulated, and they can have varying strengths and resultant side effects. Regardless of personal beliefs, it is vital that treating staff be aware of any herbal supplements taken separately or in drinks or foods. Although some research has favored Ginkgo's use in increasing cerebral blood flow, there have also been documented cases of severe bleeding, seizures, glucose instability, and allergic reactions with use of this herb. Extreme caution should be used with herbal supplements in patients on anticoagulation therapy, antiplatelet therapy, anti-inflammatories, diabetic regimen, MAO inhibitors, antipsychotic drugs, and anti-seizure medications.

16. **Correct Answer: B**
Sodium nitroprusside, when used in high doses (10 mcg/kg/min), or over a period of days, can raise blood concentrations of cyanide to toxic levels. Patients who are malnourished or who are stressed from surgery may have low thiosulfate reserves. These patients are at increased risk for developing symptoms, even with therapeutic dosing. These patients may become agitated and combative, and their symptoms may be mistaken for ICU psychosis. If patients are given hydroxocobalamin or sodium thiosulfate along with sodium nitroprusside, these symptoms may be prevented or at least mitigated.

17. **Correct Answer: D**
Wool and silk give off cyanide gas. Nitriles, like that found in the gloves we wear, will burn and give off cyanide. Household plastics such as melamine dishes, plastic cups, polyurethane foam in furniture cushions, and many other synthetic compounds may produce lethal concentrations of cyanide when burned under certain circumstances. Cyanide inhibits cellular respiration, even when the person has adequate oxygen stores. Cellular metabolism changes from aerobic to anaerobic, and produces lactic acid. The organs with the highest oxygen requirements are the most affected by cyanide inhalation.

18. **Correct Answer: D**
This patient is in hypovolemic shock. The normal blood volume in an adult is approximately 5,000 mL. A loss of 1,500 mL of blood would be equal to about one-third of the total blood volume. You would expect the patient to demonstrate an increased HR (120–150), increased BP, a narrowed pulse pressure, increased RR (25–40), and delayed capillary refill. The skin would be cool and clammy, and the patient might develop neurological issues such as restlessness, anxiety, and confusion.

19. **Correct Answer: B**
In a TEE, the patient is sedated and the gag reflex reduced by application of an oral numbing spray. A gastroscope is advanced and the patient swallows it. The tube is then positioned directly behind the heart and allows for sound waves to be reflected off the heart chambers and valves. The left mainstem bronchus can interfere with the view. Some types of scopes can generate a three-dimensional picture.

The TEE procedure carries a risk that the patient might experience reflex bradycardia, esophageal perforation, transient hypoxia, drug-initiated tachycardia, or oversedation. Additional contraindications to TEE would include stenosis and obstruction of the esophagus, penetrating chest injuries, central nervous system depression (no sedatives), and inability to lie flat.

20. **Correct Answer: D**
Calcium cannot be utilized by the body without adequate vitamin D levels. Fifteen minutes of daylight on the skin without use of sun block allows the body to create its own vitamin D. An increase in phosphorus would bind the calcium, making it unavailable.

21. **Correct Answer: C**
An elevated D-dimer level may be caused by other conditions. A normal D-dimer rules out a pulmonary embolism. Hyperventilation will occur subsequent to hypoxemia, resulting in respiratory alkalosis. Heparin does not dissolve existing clots.

22. **Correct Answer: B**
In malignant hyperthermia, use of anesthetic agents such as halothane causes muscles to contract and the patient to become hypothermic. Caffeine is used diagnostically because it can contract muscles at higher doses without the danger of depolarizing cell membranes. The antidote for malignant hyperthermia is dantrolene.

23. **Correct Answer: B**
When using an auto-transfusion drainage system, make sure to connect the system per manufacturer's recommendations. Most connections will be color coded for ease of connecting. Clamps must remain open to allow for blood collection and to prevent increased intrathoracic pressures. Subcutaneous air should be checked by palpation and borders marked for further monitoring. The average adult-size catheter is 28 or 36 Fr. If a one-way valve system and suction is used, water is not required to maintain a seal because the valve performs this function.

24. **Correct Answer: A**
Research utilizing various solutions has shown that normal saline use in tracheal suctioning causes anxiety, increases the risk for hospital-acquired pneumonia, and often leads to bronchoconstriction. Current recommendations focus on dry suctioning, frequent oral care, balanced hydration, and frequent position changes to prevent complications associated with intubation and mechanical ventilation.

25. **Correct Answer: C**

    The ETCO$_2$ is not a substitute for pulse oximetry. A pulse oximeter measures the availability of sites on the hemoglobin molecule for oxygen transport versus how many sites are occupied. ETCO$_2$ measures whether gas exchange is taking place at the cellular level. If CO$_2$ is being given off, it will react with chemically treated paper in the ETCO$_2$ detector. There is no excuse for not auscultating the patient's lungs to determine correct ET placement. If the esophagus has been intubated, the ETCO$_2$ device may give a false-positive reading if the patient has consumed a carbonated beverage within the past few hours.

26. **Correct Answer: C**

    A sudden drop in the balloon pressure and the patient's ability to swallow may indicate balloon or esophageal rupture as evidenced by bleeding. This problem should be reported to the physician immediately. The patient should not be able to swallow when the balloon is inflated properly, so these findings indicate a problem requiring investigation and reporting. A drop in balloon pressures may indicate a ruptured balloon or esophagus. An inflation pressure of 70 mm Hg is too high.

27. **Correct Answer: B**

    This response acknowledges the daughters' concerns and provides education. Elevated bilirubin levels deposited in the skin result in unconscious scratching and excoriations. With the presence of increased PT, PTT, and INR levels, hematomas may also be present. Answer A provides no explanation for the scratches and decreases communication with the family. Restraints are inappropriate for this patient. ICU psychosis can lead to abnormal behavior, but it is not the reason for this patient's behavior.

28. **Correct Answer: D**

    This patient may safely continue Verapamil for atrial fibrillation. Calcium-channel blockers have been found to provide some protection against complications of diverticulae. Nonsteroidal anti-inflammatory drugs (NSAIDs), corticosteroids, and opiate analgesics have been noted to increase the risk of perforation of diverticulae.

29. **Correct Answer: C**

    Mannitol and urea are osmotic diuretics. They act to increase osmotic pressure of the filtrate, which will in turn attract water and electrolytes and prevent reabsorption. The problem is that these agents can cause a rebound volume expansion, and hyponatremia. Mannitol may be used in lieu of sodium bicarbonate to manage hemoglobinuria and myoglobinuria secondary to rhabdomyolysis or severe crush injury. If large volumes of fluid are also used, this therapy may reduce or prevent renal tubular obstruction.

30. **Correct Answer: D**

    Monocytes and lymphocytes are classified as agranulocytes. The monocyte is the largest leukocyte, but comprises a small portion of the total cell count for WBCs. When the monocytes mature, they become a tissue macrophage and work as phagocytes. When a phagocyte lives in the liver, it is called a Kupffer cell. When a phagocyte is in the lungs, it is called an alveolar macrophage. When it is in the connective tissues, it is called a histiocyte.

    Macrophages contain lysosomal enzymes and chemicals that can destroy bacteria. If the macrophage is activated by an antigen, it will secrete monokines that control communication between all the cells involved in an immune response.

31. **Correct Answer: C**

Amicar is used to inhibit fibrinolysis. It is used in the treatment of DIC, but it may change a simple bleeding issue into DIC. For this reason, Amicar must be given in combination with heparin. DIC is usually treated with FFP, cryoprecipitate, and platelets. Cryoprecipitate contains 5 to 10 times more fibrinogen than FFP. A good rule of thumb is to give 10 units of cryoprecipitate for each 3 units of FFP. If the patient is actively bleeding, platelets are commonly used.

32. **Correct Answer: D**

Mesothelioma is a cancer of the mesothelium; it is a relatively rare cancer. Most cases of mesothelioma begin in the pleura or peritoneum. Symptoms include dyspnea, pleural effusions, weight loss, and abdominal pain and swelling due to an excess of fluid in the abdomen. Other symptoms of peritoneal mesothelioma may include bowel obstruction, clotting disorders, anemia, and fever. Symptoms with metastases may include pain, dysphagia, or swelling of the neck or face.

Approximately 2,000 new cases of mesothelioma are diagnosed in the United States each year. This cancer occurs more often in men than in women and risk increases with age. Symptoms of mesothelioma may not appear until 30 to 50 years after exposure to asbestos. An increased risk of developing mesothelioma was later found among shipyard workers, people who work in asbestos mines and mills, producers of asbestos products, workers in the heating and construction industries, and other tradespeople.

Asbestos has been widely used in many industrial products, including cement, duct linings, sound insulation, brake linings, roof shingles, flooring products, textiles, and thermal insulation. If tiny asbestos particles float in the air, especially during the manufacturing process, they may be inhaled or swallowed and can cause serious health problems. In addition to mesothelioma, exposure to asbestos increases the risk of lung cancer, asbestosis, and cancers of the trachea, larynx, and kidney. Smoking does not appear to increase the risk of mesothelioma, but the combination of smoking and exposure to asbestos increases a person's risk of developing bronchial cancer.

33. **Correct Answer: C**

Pernicious anemia results from lack of protein intrinsic factor in the stomach that helps the body absorb vitamin B_{12}. The stress on the heart from the resultant hypoxia can cause heart murmurs, tachycardias, arrhythmias, hypertrophy, and heart failure. A lack of vitamin B_{12} raises the homocysteine level. High levels of homocysteine add to the buildup of fatty deposits. A lack of vitamin B_{12} can damage nerve cells and cause problems such as paresthesias in the hands and feet and problems with ambulation and balance. Memory loss, visual disturbances, and confusion may develop. This condition was termed "pernicious" because it often proved fatal before the cause was discovered to be vitamin B_{12} deficiency.

34. **Correct Answer: C**

Large volumes of normal saline are given until depletion is corrected, and then D_5NS is administered once blood glucose is in the 250–300 mg/dL range. You can also use an insulin drip at about 15 units per hour with hourly glucose monitoring. Frequent electrolyte monitoring would also be performed. If the patient was given D_5 ½NS too early in the treatment, it could lead to cerebral edema.

35. **Correct Answer: C**

Thyrotoxic crisis is a rare but serious problem in post-thyroidectomy patients, patients with undertreated hyperthyroidism, patients with cardiopulmonary disease, and patients undergoing hemodialysis.

36. **Correct Answer: B**

Insulin resistance predisposes the patient to elevated blood glucose levels and increased insulin production. Very-low-density lipoprotein (VLDL) production increases with hyperinsulinemia.

37. **Correct Answer: B**

Anything that causes a perceived drop in renal blood flow may trigger the renin–angiotensin mechanism. Renin release can also be triggered by sodium and volume depletion, like that seen with diuretic use.

38. **Correct Answer: A**

A sodium bicarbonate drip should be anticipated to replace the HCO_3. This treatment will help resolve the metabolic acidosis. Boluses would be given only if the pH was very low. The insulin drip will not directly correct the HCO_3.

39. **Correct Answer: A**

A sodium bicarbonate drip should be anticipated to replace the HCO_3. This will help resolve the metabolic acidosis. Boluses would be given only if the pH was very low. The insulin drip will not directly correct the HCO_3.

40. **Correct Answer: A**

CN I is the frequently affected cranial nerve in a basilar skull fracture and leads to loss of the sense of smell. CN VII and CN VIII are less likely to be affected unless it is a severe head injury. CN VII (Facial nerve) injury causes ipsilateral (same side) paralysis. CN VIII (Acoustic nerve) injury can interrupt balance and hearing.

41. **Correct Answer: A**

The most common causes of SIADH include bronchogenic (oat cell) cancer, pneumonia, and head injury. Less common causes include stroke, tuberculosis, Guillain-Barré syndrome, meningitis, encephalitis, multiple sclerosis, subarachnoid hemorrhage, pancreatic cancer, and lymphoma.

42. **Correct Answer: D**

Brown–Sequard syndrome is ipsilateral (same side) motor paralysis and contralateral (opposite side) loss of pain and temperature sensation. This syndrome occurs because of the way the pyramidal tracts cross in the spinal column.

43. **Correct Answer: C**

Prednisone decreases the effectiveness of isoniazid.

44. **Correct Answer: B**

Normally the colloid osmotic pressure is 10 to 25 mm Hg higher than the pulmonary capillary wedge pressure (PAOP). Colloid osmotic pressure from proteins and albumin keep fluid in the intravascular space. If this pressure decreases, fluid leaks from the pulmonary capillaries. Fluid may also leak if the wedge pressure increases.

45. **Correct Answer: B**
An increase in heart rate is an early sign of failure to wean. If PaO_2 levels drop or the minute ventilation is increased to more than 10 L/min, the patient is considered as having failed the attempt at weaning.

46. **Correct Answer: C**
Bob's anxiety probably resulted in hyperventilation, causing him to override the ventilator. Carbon dioxide would be blown off and the pH would fall and he would become alkalotic. Flail chest is very painful, and this pain could have contributed to the failure. If Bob was medicated, it might also hinder his chance of successful weaning from the ventilator.

47. **Correct Answer: C**
Small tidal volumes are used and delivered at a high rate. The chest wall does not move as much which could cause pain and displace the fractures. Humidification is more critical with this type of ventilator because of the fast rate. Secretions may be thicker and suctioning may have to be performed more often.

48. **Correct Answer: A**
Neupogen stimulates the bone marrow to increase production of macrophages and granulocytes. Bone pain and muscle aches are common side effects.

49. **Correct Answer: C**
Physiologic PEEP is the amount of positive pressure that remains in the alveoli after exhalation and keeps the alveoli from totally collapsing. Auto-PEEP occurs when the patient is mechanically ventilated and an amount of PEEP remains in the alveoli. The Auto-PEEP occurs in addition to the physiologic PEEP. Causes of Auto-PEEP include use of small-diameter endotracheal tubes, bronchospasm, water in the ventilator tubing, high minute ventilation, and high respiratory rates. Patients actually have increased work of breathing in this situation because to initiate a breath on the ventilator, they have to overcome the set sensitivity and the amount of Auto-PEEP. Corrective measures include use of large-diameter endotracheal tubes, slower respiratory rates, emptying the water from the ventilatory tubing, use of sedatives and/or narcotics, and adjustment of the ventilator to shorten inspiratory time to allow more time for exhalation.

50. **Correct Answer: D**
A high ratio of pleural fluid to serum protein will cause a fluid shift and result in an effusion. This is a reason for performing a thoracentesis. Contraindications for performing a thoracentesis include coagulation disorders or patients receiving anticoagulants, abnormal anatomy—normal landmarks cannot be clearly identified—PEEP/CPAP, and splenomegaly. In patients who have undergone a pneumonectomy, thoracentesis may damage the remaining lung or drastically change intraplural pressure and possibly collapse the lung.

51. **Correct Answer: D**
If a mediastinal chest tube is in place, bubbling in the water seal chamber may indicate a communication between the mediastinal space and the pleural space. The physician should be notified immediately. Some sporadic bubbling typically occurs when suction is first turned on, because fluid must displace air in the collection chamber. Chest tube tubing that is dependent or coiled will allow for the accumulation of drainage. This obstruction may increase pressure in the lung.

52. **Correct Answer: A**

These are the classic symptoms for a tension pneumothorax. Air has leaked into the pleural space and, because the thorax is closed, the increasing pressure has caused the lung to collapse. This is a medical emergency.

53. **Correct Answer: C**

Adding a capnography device will help assure appropriate positioning of the endotracheal tube while turning the patient and while the patient is in a prone position. All EKG leads should be removed from the anterior chest wall. All wound dressings should be changed prior to placing the patient prone. All colostomy and ileostomy bags should be emptied because the patient's weight may cause the bags to rupture.

54. **Correct Answer: B**

Pulse oximetry values do not directly correlate with PaO_2. Instead, you must use ABGs to determine PaO_2, the amount of oxygen available to the tissues. SpO_2 measures the number of hemoglobin-binding sites that are occupied compared to the number of hemoglobin-binding sites that are available. The following data show this correlation.

Pulse Oximetry Values	Probable PaO_2
97	100
95	80
94	70
90	60
85	50
75	40
57	30
32	20
10	10

55. **Correct Answer: C**

Subcutaneous emphysema usually occurs in the thorax as a result of a pulmonary air leak. This air leak may occur secondary to the patient receiving positive-pressure ventilation or from alveolar rupture caused by a pneumothorax. The air travels along under the skin and may be easily palpated and may feel like a crackling sensation. Patients who have chest tubes often have at least a small amount of subcutaneous emphysema at the tube insertion site. Sometimes the patient will feel pain when palpation is performed because the air tears the tissue. The free air must be reabsorbed and this may take several days.

56. **Correct Answer: A**

Bilirubin is not within the color spectrum that will interfere with pulse oximetry results. Dark nail polish, especially black, brown, blue, and green, will interfere with light transmission and cause an artificially lowered SpO_2. Patients who have bruising under the nails may also have SpO_2 values that are artificially decreased.

57. **Correct Answer: C**

Sometimes balloons are old and weakened and rupture easily. The balloons are made of rubber and will disintegrate in the presence of circulating lipoproteins. If the balloon does rupture, it will not wedge, so you can attempt to aspirate blood through the inflation port. If you cannot aspirate blood, the balloon is probably ruptured. Immediately place a piece of tape with a notation that the balloon is ruptured so that the next person will not attempt to use the port and inject air into the pulmonary circulation. Sometimes the balloon shatters into small parts, which become rubber emboli. Another precaution is to determine if the patient has a preexisting rubber allergy.

58. **Correct Answer: C**
MODS is usually the result of a direct injury to an organ. A kidney stone or appendicitis should present with pain and tenderness. SIRS is a systemic infection that can present in an elderly person with hypothermia and even with a WBC of less than 4,000 or more than 12,000.

59. **Correct Answer: C**
Because of the immediate danger of airway closure, intubation should be done as soon as possible on a prophylactic basis. Once the airway begins to close, intubation may be impossible. At times, even a tracheostomy is extremely difficult to perform.

60. **Correct Answer: B**
This is an emergency. The pressure must be relieved via an escharotomy, an incision through multiple layers of tissue. Any circumferential burn of the body may lead to impaired function and require escharotomy.

61. **Correct Answer: C**
Escharotomy is a procedure, not a direct risk. The highest risk at this time is compartment syndrome. As a nurse, you must constantly assess the patient for quality of pulses. Edema may be so great as to completely cut off circulation in a limb and cause a myoglobin-related renal failure. Elevating the limb may help drain fluid and mitigate further edema. If the pulse is lost, compartment syndrome is not necessarily the cause. The problem could be due to failure to replace the lost volume secondary to the burn.

62. **Correct Answer: D**
The Parkland formula was developed by Dr. Charles Baxter at Parkland Hospital in Dallas, Texas, in the 1960s. It is still used nationwide as a standard for fluid resuscitation. Many other formulas are in use, but this one is widely known and will probably be on the CCRN examination. The Parkland formula is:

4 mL fluid × patient's weight (in kg) × body surface area burned (%)

In this case:

4 × 70 × 30 = 8,400 mL fluid requirement for the first 24 hours

Half of the calculated volume is given in the first 8 hours, and the remaining volume is given over the next 16 hours.

63. **Correct Answer: C**
Lactated Ringer's (LR) is used with many of the formulas for burn resuscitation. It is preferred for large-volume resuscitation because LR contains 130 mEq/L of sodium compared to normal saline that has 154 mEq/L of sodium. LR has a higher pH (6.5) compared to normal saline (5.0). The pH of the LR is close to a normal pH. The patient

will be in metabolic acidosis, so the metabolized lactate will buffer the acidosis. LR is also an isotonic crystalloid.

64. **Correct Answer: D**

    Joint and abdominal pain (pain related to splenomegaly) as well as dyspnea may be signs of anaphylaxis or serum sickness, which can occur as long as 2 to 4 weeks after antivenin administration. Patients should be taught to contact their physicians immediately if they experience these symptoms so that early treatment can be initiated to prevent complications. Administration of corticosteroids and antihistamines will aid in combating the inflammatory response to the animal proteins in the antivenin. The neurotoxin may cause residual muscle spasms, tingling, weakness, and nervousness for weeks to months after the exposure to the venom. Patients may need to slowly increase activity during their recovery.

65. **Correct Answer: C**

    Excess endorphins need to be mediated. Prostaglandin is blocked by ibuprofen. Corticosteroids are used to stabilize the cell membrane by modifying mediators.

66. **Correct Answer: A**

    Alkaline solutions may cause norepinephrine to precipitate. Also, do not use it if the solution is discolored. Answers B, C, and D are indications for use.

67. **Correct Answer: D**

    Myocarditis can also present with inspiratory pain. Pain that occurs when an individual is supine is a cardinal sign of myocarditis. Other findings can include symptoms that are consistent with a respiratory infection, and an S_3, S_4, and a pericardial friction rub may be present.

68. **Correct Answer: B**

    Because the heart cannot adequately fill or eject its contents adequately, stroke volume decreases, which in turn leads to decreased cardiac output. Contractility decreases because the muscle cannot adequately stretch and, therefore, cannot contract effectively.

69. **Correct Answer: D**

    Treadmill stress testing may miss as many as 40% of cases of single-vessel disease. LV dysfunction may be diagnosed via a thallium test (myocardial scintigraphy). A positive treadmill test may not be positive for CAD.

70. **Correct Answer: A**

    Leads I and aVL will show damage to the higher areas of the lateral wall. Leads V_1 and V_2 show septal wall damage. Leads V_5 and V_6 show damage to the apical area.

71. **Correct Answer: B**

    Minute changes in the partial pressure of oxygen, pH, and the partial pressure of carbon dioxide result in changes in the heart rate and respiratory rate. These changes are initiated by the chemoreceptors located in the carotid and aortic bodies.

72. **Correct Answer: B**

    The size of the femoral sheath may occlude or diminish circulation to the lower extremities. A thrombus could also form. Rarely, tearing or rupture of the aorta will occur. Other potential complications include infection, emboli, equipment malfunction, balloon leaks, and aortic dissection.

73. **Correct Answer: D**

    Amiodarone and quinidine are antiarrhythmic agents, whereas clonidine is an anti-hypertensive. Adenosine occurs naturally in the body and has a very short half-life (only a few seconds). Adenosine slows AV nodal conduction or can interrupt it altogether, potentially causing a transient AV block (seen as asystole). The patient may experience mild to moderate chest discomfort, slight hypotension, bradycardia, and possibly flushing.

74. **Correct Answer: B**

    A heart murmur is a sound produced from turbulent blood flow. By definition, a systolic murmur would be heard during systole when the ventricles are contracting. The mitral and tricuspid valves should be closed. If these valves are incompetent (insufficiency), blood will flow back through the valve (regurgitation). Thus, pulmonic and aortic stenosis, as well as mitral and tricuspid insufficiency, are systolic murmurs.

75. **Correct Answer: D**

    The elevated right ventricular pressure and the elevated right atrial pressure indicate pulmonary hypertension. The wedge pressure is normal. The wedge pressure reflects the status of the left side of the heart. Fluid cannot clear the lungs, so pressure builds and the right-side pressures rise due to the increased workload. Edema results from the fluid backup. The dyspnea and exercise intolerance are attributable to excess fluid in the lungs.

76. **Correct Answer: C**

    Other causes include tumors, tricyclic antidepressants, fibrosis, BPH, prostate cancer, urethral obstruction, stone disease, and ligation during surgery. Answers A, B, and D are causes of intrinsic failure/injury.

77. **Correct Answer: D**

    Ultrasound readings may be difficult to obtain or interpret due to ascites, obesity, or fluid in the retroperitoneal area. Doppler scans measure blood flow; this flow is diminished due to prerenal and intrinsic AKI. Nuclear scans are of limited value because the excretion rates may be slowed by disease. The renal biopsy is the gold standard for diagnosing rejection.

78. **Correct Answer: D**

    Acyclovir can crystallize in the kidney and cause AKI. It is important for the nurse to carefully monitor the infusion time and the amount of fluid used to dilute intravenous drugs. Additional drugs that can crystallize in the kidney include sulfonamides, idinivir, and triamterine.

79. **Correct Answer: D**

    Answers A, B, and C are medications that increase BUN levels.

80. **Correct Answer: B**

    Renal infarction can occur with cocaine intoxication. Cocaine abuse can lead to an MI. The proteinuria and RBCs in the urine are indicative of renal infarction.

81. **Correct Answer: A**

    Due to her medical condition, Beatrice was unable to drink, which led to dehydration and hemoconcentration. Because of her diabetes, she may have additional renal injury. Coupled with the decreased blood flow through the kidneys from the CHF, the kidneys were unable to filter the excess sodium from her body.

82. **Correct Answer: C**

Potassium and hydrogen move in opposite directions to each other. With hypokalemia, hydrogen moves into the extracellular fluid, leading to both respiratory and metabolic alkalosis.

83. **Correct Answer: A**

Addison's disease results in a decrease in aldosterone secretion. This leads to hyperkalemia and hyponatremia, because sodium cannot be retained and potassium cannot be removed from the body.

84. **Correct Answer: A**

Honey has the lowest amount of magnesium. It is better to recommend foods such as leafy vegetables that have a deep, green color, whole grains, nuts, legumes, seafood, cocoa, and chocolate.

85. **Correct Answer: A**

This surgical procedure predisposes the gastric tube's placement into the cranial vault. Oral gastric tube placement, by contrast, is safe. Oral intubation is not associated with any increase in complications. Similarly, tracheal intubations carry no increase in complications related to this history.

86. **Correct Answer: B**

The patient's skin may become very dry and gentle application of a moisturizer may relieve discomfort. Deep tissue massage is contraindicated due to the patient's decreased platelet count and increased risk of bruising. Development of orthostatic hypotension prohibits any rapid movement due to dizziness and risks of falls. Patients and family members are at risk for depression and visits may decrease the risk and will provide staff the opportunity to assess for and intervene if depression is observed.

87. **Correct Answer: A**

Acute pancreatitis may occur as a result of seat-belt trauma to the pancreatic duct or abdominal ischemia. Acute liver failure is characterized by flu-like symptoms, jaundice, confusion, and enlarged liver. Gastrointestinal bleeding may be associated with a history of ulcers and/or esophageal varices with hemodynamic changes, narrowing pulse pressures, hematemesis, and hyperactive bowel tones. Abdominal trauma does not produce the knife-like and twisting pain, and tenderness and a marbled appearance would be noted.

88. **Correct Answer: B**

Approximately 50% of deaths of patients with cirrhosis are from variceal bleeding. These lab tests are used to differentiate the causes of bleeding. History and lab values lean toward a diagnosis of varices. Although Hgb and Hct would be decreased in patients with peptic ulcer disease and gastritis, the other lab changes would not be diagnostic. Boerhaave's syndrome is a full-thickness rupture or perforation of the esophageal wall caused by prolonged and frequent vomiting related to eating disorders.

89. **Correct Answer: A**

The patient is exhibiting signs and symptoms of malrotation and duodenal obstruction related to a volvulus. The nurse should contact the physician immediately and prepare for surgery before necrosis of the bowel occurs. Tylenol and morphine will mask these serious symptoms. Pain is related to ischemia experienced by the intestines as blood supply is impaired by the malrotation. The fever may indicate perforation or necrosis of the intestines impacted by the volvulus. The patient will need to sit upright to prevent aspiration post vomiting. These symptoms are not normal, and discoloration of the abdomen indicates greater ischemia and a higher risk of perforation.

90. **Correct Answer: A**
Due to her pregnancy and resulting HELLP syndrome, there is an increased risk of fluid collecting in the abdominal cavity and tissue edema. Signs and symptoms of IAH and ACS include increased ICP, hypercarbia and decreased platelet values, decreased cardiac output, poor or absent urinary output, and abdominal wall rigidity.

91. **Correct Answer: C**
Intra-abdominal pressures of 5 to 15 mm Hg indicate a low to moderate pressure problem. When respiratory function is impaired, these values may increase to 25 to 40 mm Hg. You would expect to see increased respiratory distress and compromise. Severe compromise is seen with intra-abdominal pressures exceeding 40 mm Hg. Thoracic pressures increase as intra-abdominal pressures increase, inhibiting lung expansion and diaphragm movement, resulting in hypoventilation and hypoxia.

92. **Correct Answer: B**
Based on his presenting symptoms and ethnicity, Joab has ulcerative colitis. He may also present with leukocytosis and cachexia. Colonic diverticulitis presents with left upper quadrant pain, hyperthermia, vomiting, chills, diarrhea, and tenderness over the descending colon. Pancreatitis presents with left upper quadrant pain that radiates to the back or chest, hyperthermia, rigidity, rebound abdominal tenderness, nausea and vomiting, jaundice, Cullen's sign, Grey–Turner's sign, abdominal distention, and diminished bowel sounds. Cholecystitis presents with right upper quadrant or epigastric pain, pain that persists as long as 6 hours after a fatty meal, vomiting, and increased white blood cell counts.

93. **Correct Answer: B**
This patient is exhibiting signs of early ischemic bowel. At this time there will be some dilation of the bowel, with loops behind the ischemic bowel, because the ischemic bowel is not performing peristaltic actions. Late signs, if the condition is not diagnosed and treated early, include dilation of the entire bowel including the stomach. "Thumb printing" is when edema of the bowel wall shows the convex indentations of the lumen. Pneumatosis intestinalis is a mottled gas pattern in the bowel wall. Air in the biliary tree is indicative of a gallbladder emergency, and air under the diaphragm is a sign of pneumoperitoneum.

94. **Correct Answer: D**
Pain management via a PCA pump should be used only to facilitate the transition to oral pain medications after anastamoses have healed. Effective pain management allows for early ambulation to improve lung expansion and blood circulation to prevent atelectasis, pneumonia, and pulmonary embolism. Due to the high fat ratio, pain medications may need to be adjusted to ensure their greatest effectiveness.

95. **Correct Answer: D**
PEEP helps keep alveoli open, thereby raising PaO_2 and will decrease need for FiO_2.

96. **Correct Answer: D**

    If a pulmonary embolism decreases oxygen availability, the work of breathing increases, as does the respiratory rate. The thoracic respiratory muscles and the diaphragm will both increase their demands for oxygen, and respiratory muscle fatigue may result. Oxygen may be diverted to these muscles, depleting the oxygen and nutrient supplies available to other vital organs. These organs may become ischemic and develop multiple organ dysfunction. Answers A, B, and C may contribute to the formation of a pulmonary embolus.

97. **Correct Answer: C**

    Flail chest is a very painful condition that limits respiratory effort because of the pain; analgesia and sedation may be required. CO_2 will increase, PO_2 will decrease, and the pH will be below 7.35. The patient will develop respiratory acidosis.

98. **Correct Answer: B**

    Double effect is a common ethical dilemma. Here an action is justified as long as there is no intent to do further harm. Neither the physician nor the wife desire to hasten the patient's death, but they do want to make him more comfortable. It is the intent of the use of the narcotic—rather than the use itself—that defines double effect. At least some good is done as a result of the outcome of the discussion and resolution of the dilemma.

99. **Correct Answer: A**

    Sinusitis cannot be prevented simply by using a smaller-diameter ETT. If anything, it will make the patient's work of breathing more difficult, though it will not necessarily contribute to an infectious process. Orogastric tubes are preferable to nasogastric tubes whenever possible. Good hand washing technique has been shown to be effective in reducing all types of hospital-acquired infections.

100. **Correct Answer: D**

    This is uncompensated respiratory acidosis. The pH is less than 7.35—the value is uncompensated. To determine whether the acidosis is respiratory or metabolic, find the value that represents acidosis, the $CO_2 > 45$ mm Hg.

101. **Correct Answer: C**

    The CI is a more specific indicator of hemodynamic status. The CO has a broad range of 4–8 L/min. To make the numbers specific to an individual, their body surface area is entered in the equation; the normal range then becomes 2.5–4.5 $L/min/m^2$.

    First, you must calculate the cardiac output. Then, use the following equation:

    $$CI = CO/BSA$$

102. **Correct Answer: B**

    Cerebral blood flow must be maintained at 50 ml/100 g of brain tissue per minute. If the pressure becomes too low, ischemia and death result.

103. **Correct Answer: A**

    The vena cava is dilated because blood cannot empty into the right atrium. JVD would not be visible on a CXR. The mediastinum would be widened. A CXR will not show delineation of the pericardium or epicardium.

104. **Correct Answer: D**

    Leads V_4 and R indicate right ventricular damage. Leads V_5 and V_6 indicate apical injury. Leads V_7–V_9 are specific to the posterior wall.

105. **Correct Answer: D**
Answers A, B, and C are the effects of beta-adrenergic sympathetic stimulation.

106. **Correct Answer: C**
NSAIDs cause fluid retention and can contribute to renal insufficiency.

107. **Correct Answer: B**
Other contraindications include coagulopathy, aortic aneurysm, aortic dissection, and irreversible brain damage. Absolute contraindications include history of hemorrhagic stroke, acute pericarditis, pregnancy, bleeding disorders, and current abdominal bleeding.

108. **Correct Answer: B**
Large-lumen vessels in the arterial system are affected. The advantage of this action is that both systolic and diastolic pressures are reduced and the patient will not experience a drop in blood pressure. The blood pressure may be lowered slightly, which may cause a reflex baroreceptor response to speed up the heart rate to maintain cardiac output.

109. **Correct Answer: B**
By definition, "pansystolic" means the murmur is heard throughout systole. The only systolic murmur listed as an option here is tricuspid insufficiency. All of the other answers are diastolic murmurs.

110. **Correct Answer: B**
All the pressures are above normal. In restrictive pericarditis, the entire heart is affected and compressed, so the pressures are above normal.

111. **Correct Answer: C**
Answers A, B, and D cause only a moderate rise in the INR. Other drugs that significantly raise the INR include aspirin, sulfonamides, cimetidine, fluoroquinolones, and macrolide antibiotics.

112. **Correct Answer: A**
The CXR will probably show a pericardial effusion. The elevated sed rate and WBC indicate infection. In pericarditis, leaning forward often relieves the chest pain and lying supine makes it worse. If the pain worsens on inspiration, it is because the lungs expand and come in contact with the pericardium. The patient will probably also have a fever. The patient should be monitored for any signs of cardiac tamponade, and anticoagulants must be discontinued.

113. **Correct Answer: B**
Wellen's syndrome is a type of angina that occurs when the LAD is stenosed proximally. The ST segment is not elevated more than 1 mm in leads V_1–V_3, there is mild T wave inversion in leads V_2–V_3, and Q waves are not pathologic (greater than 25% of the total length). Because of the location of the stenosis, surgery is required emergently.

Variant angina is the same as Prinzmetal's angina. In this type of angina, the pain occurs at rest and is associated with vasospasm. Crescendo angina means that over time it takes less to initiate the pain; the pain also lasts longer.

114. **Correct Answer: C**
Restraints should be used only if alternative methods for behavioral correction prove ineffective. There is no indication that this patient is violent or poses any threat to staff

or self. Restraints should be used only as a last resort to prevent injury to self and staff. Reorientation, medications, and controlling external stimulation are all effective methods for controlling behavior.

115. **Correct Answer: A**

Direct confrontation with the object of anger may further exacerbate the situation and limit the person's ability to deal positively with the situation. Instead, engage the person in a conversation regarding the stressor and assist him in identifying his feelings and options.

116. **Correct Answer: D**

Careful consideration and observation should be given to any person voicing any thought or plan regarding suicide. Many individuals will provide warning about their suicidal thoughts, providing those in the family or in proximity with an opportunity to intervene. Warnings are often cries for help and intervention. Family members should pay close attention to any impression or instinct that the person is considering suicide. As individuals enter and exit depression, they are at greatest risk for suicide as they have sufficient mental focus to form a plan and energy or motivation to carry it out.

117. **Correct Answer: C**

Feelings of helplessness or hopelessness indicate psychotic emergencies. Extreme anxiety or inability to recognize options should alert staff and family that the person is at greater risk of suicide—the patient may see suicide as the only option. The other answers indicate depression and/or levels of grief and emotional expression.

118. **Correct Answer: D**

When assessing any potential psychiatric emergency or crisis, it is important to first determine if one actually exists. In this scenario, the patient has an extensive and involved support system, financial stability, and effective coping mechanisms; thus a psychiatric crisis is not likely to develop. It is important to carefully monitor the patient and family members for any change in status.

119. **Correct Answer: D**

The stealth adulterant will mask morphine in the urine. When heroin is taken, it breaks down into morphine. Ten milligrams of morphine remains detectable in urine for as long as 84 hours and can be measured in corpses for about a week.

120. **Correct Answer: A**

The biopsy may cause bleeding from highly vascular tissue. Flank pain may be the first sign.

121. **Correct Answer: D**

Renal function may be decreased and the patient may have increased ALT and AST levels. At about 4 days to 2 weeks after the overdose, the symptoms abate.

122. **Correct Answer: D**

The patient may have a mild fever and will be in a hyperdynamic state. The endotoxins that are circulating in the body will have vasodilatory effects, so RAP, PAOP, and SVR are decreased. The increase in CO is compensatory.

123. **Correct Answer: A**

SOFA is an acronym for sequential organ failure assessment. SOFA is therapy-related and is a reliable predictor for organ failure.

124. **Correct Answer: B**
The formula is

$$4 \times 65 \times 45 = 11{,}700 \text{ mL}.$$

125. **Correct Answer: A**
Ginseng has been known to increase the QT interval, thus putting this patient at greater risk for cardiac rhythm complications. Advise patients to carefully read the label before consuming any sports or high-energy drink, as some products contain various herbs and high levels of caffeine. Ginseng, which has effects similar to those seen with estrogen, may also cause breast tissue enlargement in men and erectile dysfunction. In women, there may be increased menstrual bleeding and hormone imbalances in conjunction with breast cancer, uterine cancer, or endometriosis. In addition, ginseng may cause complications or have interactions with anticoagulation therapy, calcium-channel blockers, and diabetes management, and will increase the potency of some sedatives.

126. **Correct Answer: C**
Wernicke's syndrome is a result of thiamine deficiency. It will result in brain damage if not treated immediately.

127. **Correct Answer: C**
AC current usually causes ventricular fibrillation and DC current usually causes asystole. In some cases, arrhythmias may be delayed for up to 12 hours.
  The mechanism of lightning strikes is quite complex. Lightening can injure a person in 5 ways:
  - A side splash from another object, which is probably the cause of this patient's injuries
  - Lightning hitting something like a post, and then bouncing off
  - A direct strike
  - A person touches an object that is struck
  - Ground current effect, which occurs when energy spreads out across the surface of the earth

  Lightning has 2 strokes, upward and downward. If these strokes do not meet, energy can be directed outward. Internal burns are rare, and myoglobinuria rarely occurs. Generally, lightning will cause cardiac and respiratory arrest, burns from metals touching the victim (watches, necklaces), and neurological damage.

128. **Correct Answer: C**
Splenic injury should be suspected when the 9–10th ribs on the left side are fractured, or when left upper quadrant tenderness and tachycardia are present. This patient has not complained of pain in the left shoulder, but it is a common complaint. Peritoneal signs such as rebound sensitivity and guarding will be delayed until the blood has had enough time to cause local irritation of the peritoneum. This patient was trapped in her car for almost 2 hours. Hypotension is a sign of an active bleed.

129. **Correct Answer: A**
Spinal shock occurs hours to weeks after a cord injury causing autonomic loss. The severity of a spinal cord injury cannot be fully assessed until the shock has resolved.

130. **Correct Answer: B**
Glasgow Coma Scale assessment is imperative in monitoring for vascular spasm, a potentially life-threatening problem for a patient with a cerebral aneurysm. Vascular spasm occurs secondary to meningeal irritation from the blood in the subarachnoid space.

131. **Correct Answer: B**
Because the catheter is inserted directly into one of the lateral ventricles, it is the most direct and accurate method of measuring intracranial pressure. The drain is inserted on the right side of the head. Ventriculostomy allows for not only drainage of excess CSF, but also sampling of CSF to monitor for infection.

132. **Correct Answer: A**
DIC often leads to malnutrition and nutritional deficits.

133. **Correct Answer: A**
Other potential causes include sepsis, viral infection, burns, and radiation therapy. Medications such as thiazides, furosemide, penicillins, sulfonamides, ranitidine, and heparin may cause thrombocytopenia. Chemotherapy is another cause.

134. **Correct Answer: A**
The transplanted kidney is placed in the pelvic area, so pelvic pain is an ominous sign. Patients who have undergone kidney transplants should be educated to notify their physicians immediately if they experience pelvic pain, as it is a symptom of rejection.

135. **Correct Answer: C**
Prostaglandin relaxes the smooth muscles within the pulmonary airways and produces vasodilation within arteries. Inotropic support is usually accomplished with epinephrine. The heart rate is usually augmented with isoproterenol. Wound healing is promoted with a single small dose of methylprednisolone.

136. **Correct Answer: C**
Jon is most likely experiencing a hypoglycemic event due to his NPO status. The other options are not wrong, but the question asks about a person with diabetes who is NPO.

137. **Correct Answer: C**
This blood gas results show uncompensated metabolic acidosis. The body has depleted its HCO_3 level in trying to correct the acidosis. The ABG is uncompensated because the pH is low and the CO_2 is elevated. Answer A is acute respiratory alkalosis; answer B is respiratory acidosis with metabolic alkalosis; and answer D is a normal ABG. Normal values for ABGs are pH 7.35–7.45, CO_2 35–45 mm Hg, and HCO_3 22–27 mEq/L.

138. **Correct Answer: D**
Subclinical adrenal insufficiency may co-exist with myxedema. The treatment of choice is intravenous hydrocortisone therapy.

139. **Correct Answer: B**
Pheochromocytoma is a tumor of the adrenal medulla. These tumors are rarely malignant. They cause the release of large amounts of catecholamines such as dopamine, epinephrine, and norepinephrine. Hypertension with pheochromocytoma can be triggered by foods such as cheese, alcohol, yogurt, and caffeine.

140. **Correct Answer: C**

Seizures are one of the most common presenting symptoms of syndrome of inappropriate antidiuretic hormone (SIADH). SIADH causes hemodilution and a relative decrease in serum sodium levels. Once the sodium level falls below 120, the patient is at great risk for seizures. Excessive urine output and hypotension are both symptoms of diabetes insipidus.

141. **Correct Answer: B**

This patient has nephrogenic diabetes related to his lithium use. Lithium causes insensitivity to vasopressin in the renal tubules, making the tubules incapable of absorbing water. Treatment involves administration of hydrochlorothiazide or indomethicin.

142. **Correct Answer: B**

The anion gap measures anions not generally quantified in routine lab tests. The result estimates the degree of lactic acidosis. The formula for calculating the anion gap is $Na - (HCO_3 + Cl)$, where the normal level is in the range of 10–20 mEq/L. With diabetic ketoacidosis, the anion gap is greater than 30 mEq/L.

143. **Correct Answer: C**

Lead V_1 is the best choice to monitor for RBBB. This lead should definitely be used when inserting a pulmonary artery catheter.

144. **Correct Answer: B**

An infarct in the left main coronary artery is ominous. Sudden death may occur, along with heart blocks and atrial and ventricular dysrhythmias.

145. **Correct Answer: A**

Hypovolemia and sepsis decrease afterload. Aortic insufficiency also decreases afterload. Aortic stenosis increases afterload, as does peripheral vasoconstriction and hypertension.

146. **Correct Answer: A**

Along with the acute ST elevation, an abnormal Q wave is an indicator of necrosis. If the Q wave appears within approximately 6 hours of a transmural MI, it is an ominous sign. If the Q wave is more than 0.04 seconds long, it is a sign of necrosis. In an inferior MI, the Q wave should not exceed 0.03 seconds or it is indicative of necrosis.

147. **Correct Answer: B**

The patient is approaching crisis and may feel hopeless. The nurse should take the time to fully explore and validate the patient's feelings, then decide the appropriate course of action.

148. **Correct Answer: B**

Patients with heart transplants do not feel cardiac pain because the heart has been denervated.

149. **Correct Answer: C**

The large V wave may be mistaken for the right ventricular tracing or even a pulmonary artery tracing. Large V waves usually occur with a papillary muscle rupture (sometimes ischemia) secondary to mitral regurgitation or an acute lateral wall MI.

150. **Correct Answer: C**

Pneumonia secondary to immobility is the primary reason for infection with VADs. The patient may also need some type of ventilatory support. The mere fact that tubes are placed into the body is a potential source of infection, but this risk is usually minimized by good hand washing and aseptic technique.

PRACTICE TEST ANSWER SHEETS

Use this sheet to test yourself with the Practice Exam.

1. A B C D	26. A B C D	51. A B C D
2. A B C D	27. A B C D	52. A B C D
3. A B C D	28. A B C D	53. A B C D
4. A B C D	29. A B C D	54. A B C D
5. A B C D	30. A B C D	55. A B C D
6. A B C D	31. A B C D	56. A B C D
7. A B C D	32. A B C D	57. A B C D
8. A B C D	33. A B C D	58. A B C D
9. A B C D	34. A B C D	59. A B C D
10. A B C D	35. A B C D	60. A B C D
11. A B C D	36. A B C D	61. A B C D
12. A B C D	37. A B C D	62. A B C D
13. A B C D	38. A B C D	63. A B C D
14. A B C D	39. A B C D	64. A B C D
15. A B C D	40. A B C D	65. A B C D
16. A B C D	41. A B C D	66. A B C D
17. A B C D	42. A B C D	67. A B C D
18. A B C D	43. A B C D	68. A B C D
19. A B C D	44. A B C D	69. A B C D
20. A B C D	45. A B C D	70. A B C D
21. A B C D	46. A B C D	71. A B C D
22. A B C D	47. A B C D	72. A B C D
23. A B C D	48. A B C D	73. A B C D
24. A B C D	49. A B C D	74. A B C D
25. A B C D	50. A B C D	75. A B C D

(Over for questions 76–150)

76. A B C D	101. A B C D	126. A B C D
77. A B C D	102. A B C D	127. A B C D
78. A B C D	103. A B C D	128. A B C D
79. A B C D	104. A B C D	129. A B C D
80. A B C D	105. A B C D	130. A B C D
81. A B C D	106. A B C D	131. A B C D
82. A B C D	107. A B C D	132. A B C D
83. A B C D	108. A B C D	133. A B C D
84. A B C D	109. A B C D	134. A B C D
85. A B C D	110. A B C D	135. A B C D
86. A B C D	111. A B C D	136. A B C D
87. A B C D	112. A B C D	137. A B C D
88. A B C D	113. A B C D	138. A B C D
89. A B C D	114. A B C D	139. A B C D
90. A B C D	115. A B C D	140. A B C D
91. A B C D	116. A B C D	141. A B C D
92. A B C D	117. A B C D	142. A B C D
93. A B C D	118. A B C D	143. A B C D
94. A B C D	119. A B C D	144. A B C D
95. A B C D	120. A B C D	145. A B C D
96. A B C D	121. A B C D	146. A B C D
97. A B C D	122. A B C D	147. A B C D
98. A B C D	123. A B C D	148. A B C D
99. A B C D	124. A B C D	149. A B C D
100. A B C D	125. A B C D	150. A B C D

PRACTICE TEST ANSWER SHEETS

Use this sheet to test yourself with the Practice Exam.

1. A B C D	26. A B C D	51. A B C D
2. A B C D	27. A B C D	52. A B C D
3. A B C D	28. A B C D	53. A B C D
4. A B C D	29. A B C D	54. A B C D
5. A B C D	30. A B C D	55. A B C D
6. A B C D	31. A B C D	56. A B C D
7. A B C D	32. A B C D	57. A B C D
8. A B C D	33. A B C D	58. A B C D
9. A B C D	34. A B C D	59. A B C D
10. A B C D	35. A B C D	60. A B C D
11. A B C D	36. A B C D	61. A B C D
12. A B C D	37. A B C D	62. A B C D
13. A B C D	38. A B C D	63. A B C D
14. A B C D	39. A B C D	64. A B C D
15. A B C D	40. A B C D	65. A B C D
16. A B C D	41. A B C D	66. A B C D
17. A B C D	42. A B C D	67. A B C D
18. A B C D	43. A B C D	68. A B C D
19. A B C D	44. A B C D	69. A B C D
20. A B C D	45. A B C D	70. A B C D
21. A B C D	46. A B C D	71. A B C D
22. A B C D	47. A B C D	72. A B C D
23. A B C D	48. A B C D	73. A B C D
24. A B C D	49. A B C D	74. A B C D
25. A B C D	50. A B C D	75. A B C D

(Over for questions 76–150)

76. A B C D	101. A B C D	126. A B C D
77. A B C D	102. A B C D	127. A B C D
78. A B C D	103. A B C D	128. A B C D
79. A B C D	104. A B C D	129. A B C D
80. A B C D	105. A B C D	130. A B C D
81. A B C D	106. A B C D	131. A B C D
82. A B C D	107. A B C D	132. A B C D
83. A B C D	108. A B C D	133. A B C D
84. A B C D	109. A B C D	134. A B C D
85. A B C D	110. A B C D	135. A B C D
86. A B C D	111. A B C D	136. A B C D
87. A B C D	112. A B C D	137. A B C D
88. A B C D	113. A B C D	138. A B C D
89. A B C D	114. A B C D	139. A B C D
90. A B C D	115. A B C D	140. A B C D
91. A B C D	116. A B C D	141. A B C D
92. A B C D	117. A B C D	142. A B C D
93. A B C D	118. A B C D	143. A B C D
94. A B C D	119. A B C D	144. A B C D
95. A B C D	120. A B C D	145. A B C D
96. A B C D	121. A B C D	146. A B C D
97. A B C D	122. A B C D	147. A B C D
98. A B C D	123. A B C D	148. A B C D
99. A B C D	124. A B C D	149. A B C D
100. A B C D	125. A B C D	150. A B C D

PRACTICE TEST ANSWER SHEETS

Use this sheet to test yourself with the Practice Exam.

1. A B C D	26. A B C D	51. A B C D
2. A B C D	27. A B C D	52. A B C D
3. A B C D	28. A B C D	53. A B C D
4. A B C D	29. A B C D	54. A B C D
5. A B C D	30. A B C D	55. A B C D
6. A B C D	31. A B C D	56. A B C D
7. A B C D	32. A B C D	57. A B C D
8. A B C D	33. A B C D	58. A B C D
9. A B C D	34. A B C D	59. A B C D
10. A B C D	35. A B C D	60. A B C D
11. A B C D	36. A B C D	61. A B C D
12. A B C D	37. A B C D	62. A B C D
13. A B C D	38. A B C D	63. A B C D
14. A B C D	39. A B C D	64. A B C D
15. A B C D	40. A B C D	65. A B C D
16. A B C D	41. A B C D	66. A B C D
17. A B C D	42. A B C D	67. A B C D
18. A B C D	43. A B C D	68. A B C D
19. A B C D	44. A B C D	69. A B C D
20. A B C D	45. A B C D	70. A B C D
21. A B C D	46. A B C D	71. A B C D
22. A B C D	47. A B C D	72. A B C D
23. A B C D	48. A B C D	73. A B C D
24. A B C D	49. A B C D	74. A B C D
25. A B C D	50. A B C D	75. A B C D

(Over for questions 76–150)

76.	A B C D	101.	A B C D	126.	A B C D
77.	A B C D	102.	A B C D	127.	A B C D
78.	A B C D	103.	A B C D	128.	A B C D
79.	A B C D	104.	A B C D	129.	A B C D
80.	A B C D	105.	A B C D	130.	A B C D
81.	A B C D	106.	A B C D	131.	A B C D
82.	A B C D	107.	A B C D	132.	A B C D
83.	A B C D	108.	A B C D	133.	A B C D
84.	A B C D	109.	A B C D	134.	A B C D
85.	A B C D	110.	A B C D	135.	A B C D
86.	A B C D	111.	A B C D	136.	A B C D
87.	A B C D	112.	A B C D	137.	A B C D
88.	A B C D	113.	A B C D	138.	A B C D
89.	A B C D	114.	A B C D	139.	A B C D
90.	A B C D	115.	A B C D	140.	A B C D
91.	A B C D	116.	A B C D	141.	A B C D
92.	A B C D	117.	A B C D	142.	A B C D
93.	A B C D	118.	A B C D	143.	A B C D
94.	A B C D	119.	A B C D	144.	A B C D
95.	A B C D	120.	A B C D	145.	A B C D
96.	A B C D	121.	A B C D	146.	A B C D
97.	A B C D	122.	A B C D	147.	A B C D
98.	A B C D	123.	A B C D	148.	A B C D
99.	A B C D	124.	A B C D	149.	A B C D
100.	A B C D	125.	A B C D	150.	A B C D